Bedside Proce

Heidi L. Frankel · Bennett P. deBoisblanc
Editors

Bedside Procedures
for the Intensivist

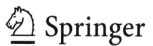 Springer

Editors

Heidi L. Frankel, MD, FACS, FCCM
Chief
Division of Trauma Acute Care and
Critical Care Surgery and Director
Shock Trauma Center
Penn State Milton S. Hershey
Medical Center
Hershey, Pennsylvania
hfrankel@hmc.psu.edu

Bennett P. deBoisblanc, MD
Professor of Medicine
and Physiology
Section of Pulmonary/
Critical Care Medicine
Louisiana State University Health
Sciences Center
New Orleans, Louisiana
bdeboi@lsuhsc.edu

ISBN 978-0-387-79829-5   e-ISBN 978-0-387-79830-1
DOI 10.1007/978-0-387-79830-1
Springer New York Dordrecht Heidelberg London

Library of Congress Control Number: 2010930507

Printed on acid-free paper

Springer is part of Springer Science+Business Media (www.springer.com)

*On December 25, 2008 while
serving his second tour of duty,
an a combat surgeon for the
U.S. Army, Dr. John Pryor,
"JP," was felled by enemy
fire. We are extraordinarily
grateful to him for his many
contributions in the field of
trauma and critical care surgery
and his accomplishments and
spirit that lives on in all of us
whose lives he touched.
This book is but one of those
accomplishments. We dedicate it
this book to his wife, Carmella,
and three children and to all of
those who serve their country
and profession so selflessly.*

Preface

Since the establishment of the first intensive care unit (ICU) in 1953 by Danish anesthesiologist Bjorn Ibsen at Copenhagen's university hospital, critical care medicine has evolved from a specialty focused primarily on mechanical ventilation of polio patients into a complex multidisciplinary specialty that provides care for a broad range of life-threatening medical and surgical problems. Dramatic technological advances in monitoring equipment and treatment modalities have improved the clinical outcomes for such patients. The miniaturization of microprocessors and the refinement of minimally invasive techniques have allowed many critical care procedures that were once performed in the operating room (OR) to now be performed at a patient's bedside in the ICU.

This evolution towards performing procedures at the bedside instead of in the OR has had distinct advantages for both patients and hospitals. First, it avoids the potential hazards and manpower costs of having to transport a critically ill patient out of the ICU. Second, procedures do not have to be worked into a busy OR schedule; they can be performed when they are needed – immediately, if necessary. This saves OR time and expense. Finally, by their nature, bedside procedures are less invasive than the parent procedures that they replace and therefore are usually associated with less risk to the patient, e.g., transbronchial lung biopsy versus open lung biopsy.

All procedures undergo refinement as more and more operators gain experience with them. The idea for *Bedside Critical Care Procedures* was born out of the idea that there should be a "how-to" reference that consolidates the cumulative experience of expert proceduralists into a single pocket manual that students, residents, fellows, and staff intensivists of diverse training can reference. Within these pages, practitioners will find easy-to-read descriptions of all aspects of the performance of safe, efficient, and comfortable procedures in the ICU. Each chapter includes bulleted lists of needed supplies and equipment, patient preparation and positioning, and the step-by-step technique. Included are procedures performed with and without ultrasound guidance.

Heidi Frankel, MD, FACS, FCCM
Ben deBoisblanc, MD, FACP, FCCP, FCCM

Contents

Contributors

Murtuza J. Ali, MD
Assistant Professor, Department of Internal Medicine,
Section of Cardiology, Louisiana State University School
of Medicine, New Orleans LA, USA

Gabriel T. Bosslet, MD
Fellow, Departments of Pulmonary and Critical Care Medicine,
Indiana University, Indianapolis IN, USA

Christian H. Butcher, MD
Staff Pulmonary and Critical Care Physician and Assistant Program
Director, Department of Medicine, Carilion Clinic and Virginia Tech
Carilion School of Medicine, Roanoke VA, USA

Chirag Choudhary, MD
Clinical Associate, Respiratory Institute, Cleveland Clinic,
Cleveland OH, USA

A. Britton Christmas, MD, FACS
Attending Surgeon Trauma, Critical Care, and Acute Care Surgery,
Department of General Surgery, Carolinas Medical Center,
Charlotte NC, USA

Steven A. Conrad, MD, PhD, FCCM
Professor, Department of Medicine, Emergency Medicine,
Pediatrics and Anesthesiology, Louisiana State University
Health Sciences Center, Shreveport LA, USA

Bennett P. deBoisblanc, MD
Professor of Medicine and Physiology, Section of Pulmonary/Critical
Care Medicine, Louisiana State University Health Sciences Center,
New Orleans LA, USA

Matthew J. Diamond, DO, MS
Assistant Professor, Department of Hypertension and Transplant
Medicine, Section of Nephrology, Medical College of Georgia,
Augusta GA, USA

Mary Ferguson, RDCS
Supervisor of Adult Echocardiography, Departments of Medicine
and Surgery, University of Maryland Medical Center,
Baltimore MD, USA

Erik E. Folch, MD, MSc
Fellow, Interventional Pulmonary Medicine, Respiratory Institute,
Cleveland Clinic, Cleveland OH, USA

Heidi L. Frankel, MD, FACS, FCCM
Chief, Division of Trauma Acute Care and Critical Care Surgery
and Director, Shock Trauma Center, Penn State Milton S. Hershey
Medical Center, Hershey PA, USA

Mark E. Hamill, MD
Assistant Professor of Surgery, Department of Surgery,
State University of New York Upstate Medical University,
Syracuse NY, USA

Jennifer Lang, MD
Resident, Department of Surgery, UT
Southwestern Medical Center, Dallas TX, USA

Albert Lee, MD, MSECE
Department of Neurosurgery, UT
Southwestern, Dallas TX, USA

Alexander B. Levitov, MD
ICU Director, Departments of Pulmonary and Critical Care
Medicine, Carilion Clinic, Virginia Tech Carilion School
of Medicine, Roanoke VA, USA

Christopher Madden, MD
Associate Professor, Department of Neurological Surgery,
The University of Texas Southwestern Medical Center,
Dallas TX, USA

Praveen N. Mathur, MBBS
Professor of Medicine, Departments of Pulmonary and Critical Care
Medicine, Indiana University, Indianapolis IN, USA

Stephan A. Mayer, MD
Director, Neurological Intensive Care Unit, Department of Neurology,
Columbia New York Presbyterian Hospital, New York NY, USA

Atul C. Mehta, MBBS, FACP, FCCP
Chief Medical Officer, Sheikh Khalifa Medical City managed
by Cleveland Clinic, Abu Dhabi, United Arab Emirates

Mark M. Melendez, MD, MBA
Chief Resident, Department of Surgery, Stony Brook University
Medical Center, Stony Brook NY, USA

Russell R. Miller III, MD, MPH
Medical Director, Respiratory ICU, Department of Pulmonary
and Critical Care Medicine, Intermountain Medical Center,
Murray UT, USA
Department of Pulmonary and Critical Care Medicine,
University of Utah, Salt Lake City UT, USA

Sarah B. Murthi, MD, FACS
Surgical Critical Care Attending and Assistant Professor of Surgery,
Department of Surgery, University of Maryland Medical Center,
Baltimore MD, USA

Irene P. Osborn, MD
Director of Neuroanesthesia, Department of Anesthesiology,
Mount Sinai Medical Center, New York NY, USA

James Parker, MD
Fellow, Section of Cardiology, Department of Internal Medicine,
Louisiana State University School of Medicine,
New Orleans LA, USA

John P. Pryor, MD
Assistant Professor of Surgery and Trauma Program Directory,
Division of Traumatology and Surgical Critical Care,
Department of Surgery, University of Pennsylvania School
of Medicine and University of Pennsylvania Medical Center,
Philadelphia PA, USA

Patricia Reinhard, MD
Attending Anesthesiologist, Munich, Germany

Shahid Shafi, MBBS, MPH
Staff Surgeon, Department of Surgery, Baylor Health Care System,
Grapevine TX, USA

Marc J. Shapiro, BS, MS, MD
Professor of Surgery and Anesthesiology and Chief, General Surgery,
Trauma, Critical Care and Burns, Department of Surgery,
SUNY – Stony Brook University and Medical Center,
Stony Brook NY, USA

Adam M. Shiroff, MD
Fellow, Department of Trauma and Surgical Care,
University of Pennsylvania and Hospital of the University
of Pennsylvania, Philadelphia PA, USA

Ronald F. Sing, DO
Trauma Surgeon, Department of General Surgery,
Carolinas HealthCare System, Charlotte NC, USA

Amy C. Sisley, MD, MPH
Section Chief, Emergency General Surgery, Department of Trauma
and Critical Care, R. Adams Cowley Shock Trauma Center,
University of Maryland, Baltimore MD, USA

R. Morgan Stuart, MD
Neurosurgeon, Department of Neurosurgery, Columbia University
Medical Center, New York NY, USA

Harold M. Szerlip, MD, MS(Ed)
Vice-Chairman, Section of Nephrology, Department of Hypertension and Transplant Medicine, Medical College of Georgia, Augusta GA, USA

Kathryn M. Tchorz, MD, RDMS
Associate Professor, Department of Surgery, Wright State University – Boonshoft School of Medicine, Dayton OH, USA

Sonali Vadi, MD, FNB
Department of Internal Medicine, Maryland General Hospital, Baltimore MD, USA

General Considerations

Heidi L. Frankel and Mark E. Hamill

■ INTRODUCTION

As ICU patient volume and acuity increase, there has been a parallel growth in the use of technology to assist in management. Several issues must be considered when determining where and how to perform certain procedures in critically ill and injured patients. Much forethought and planning are required to establish a successful intensive care unit (ICU)-based procedural environment – from concerns regarding the availability and reliability of pertinent equipment to more complex issues of acquiring competency and pursuing credentialing. It is essential to pay adequate attention to these general considerations to ensure that ICU-based procedures are accomplished with equivalent safety and results as those performed in more traditional settings.

■ WHY PERFORM BEDSIDE PROCEDURES

Shifting the venue of procedure performance into the ICU from the operating room, interventional radiology, or gastroenterology suite may benefit the patient, the unit staff, and the hospital in general.

H.L. Frankel (✉)
Division of Trauma Acute Care and Critical Care Surgery, Shock Trauma Center, Penn State Milton S. Hershey Medical Center, Hershey, PA, USA
e-mail: hfrankel@hmc.psu.edu

H.L. Frankel and B.P. deBoisblanc (eds.), *Bedside Procedures for the Intensivist*, DOI 10.1007/978-0-387-79830-1_1,

In the ensuing chapters, we will demonstrate that procedures as diverse as open tracheostomy and image-guided inferior vena cava insertion can be performed in the ICU setting with equivalent safety and lower cost. For example, Grover and colleagues demonstrated that an open tracheostomy performed in the ICU resulted in a cost savings of over $2,000 compared to a similar procedure performed in the operating room.[1] Upadhay noted that elective tracheostomy can be performed as safely in the ICU as in an operating room (complication rates of 8.7% vs. 9.4%, p=NS).[2] In fact, with the increased availability of ultrasound guidance for procedures such as thoracentesis and central venous catheter placement, it is possible to both improve the success and decrease the complication rate of procedures.[3,4] Moreover, it is apparent that a well-trained intensivist can perform a variety of bedside procedures with minimal focused training that can be acquired at such venues as the Society of Critical Care Medicine's annual Congress.[5] Some skills, such as open tracheostomy and performance of focused bedside echocardiography may require additional training and experience.[6,7] Multiple groups have suggested training guidelines to ensure accurate and reproducible exams.[8–10] Nonetheless, it is apparent that ICU practitioners from diverse backgrounds – be they pulmonary critical care, anesthesiology, surgery, or pediatrics – are able to perform a host of bedside procedures safely and competently after adequate training.[11]

Bedside performance of procedures diminishes the need to transport complex patients and incur adverse events. Indeck stated that, on an average, three personnel were required to supervise each trip out of the ICU for diagnostic imaging with two-thirds of the patients suffering serious physiologic sequelae during the transport.[12] In another study, a significant number of patients experienced a ventilator-related problem during transport, leading to two episodes of cardiac arrest in 123 transports.[13]

The benefits of avoiding transport must be balanced with the additional requirements placed upon the bedside ICU nurse to assist in the performance of the procedure. At our institution, we have created an additional float/procedural nurse position during daytime hours to assist in this role. Moreover, even though we have eliminated many transports from the ICU by performing bedside procedures, there are still many instances of travel for our patients. Finally, to assist the intensivist to perform some of these "bedside" procedures, we often move the patient from his ICU bed onto a narrower gurney, making it easier for the intensivist to be properly positioned. Alternatively, the so-called "cardiac" chair used in many ICUs can be flattened out to accomplish this end.

Some facilities are expanding the availability of procedures undertaken at the bedside in the ICU in an effort to streamline their ability to take care of their patients in an expeditious and safe manner.[14] Simpson found that after the introduction of bedside percutaneous tracheostomy, the percentage of patients receiving tracheostomies doubled (8.5–16.8%, $p < 0.01$) and the amount of time from ICU admission to tracheostomy was cut in half (median of 8 to 4 days, $P=-0.016$).[15] Limitations in scheduled time slots in the operating room, endoscopy suite, or interventional radiology suite have also pushed some centers to expand the use of bedside procedures in an effort to expedite patient care.

■ EQUIPMENT

Ultrasound

Many of the procedures discussed later in this text use ultrasound guidance. Ultrasound technology has advanced dramatically over the past several years, with economical portable or hand-held units now providing many of the same capabilities formally found only on expensive, full-sized units. The availability of portable ultrasound has dramatically increased the placement success of peripherally inserted central venous catheters (PICC).[16] Portable and hand-held ultrasound units can also provide valuable clinical information regarding volume status and cardiac function in high acuity populations.[7,17] Ultrasound devices have proved useful in a variety of image-guided ICU procedures, ranging from thoracentesis to placement of central venous catheters and inferior vena cava filters, to drainage of abscesses in multiple locations.[18] The features available on different portable and hand-held units range from simple 2D imaging with single-frequency transducers to units with advanced cardiology packages and Doppler imaging with the availability of multiple, interchangeable transducers. The specific features of different units can vary dramatically. However, with the rapid advancement of technology, even portable "laptop" style units are now available with interchangeable transducers in both lower frequency probes (suitable for abdominal imaging and procedure guidance) as well as higher frequency models (with increased image resolution at the expense of tissue penetration). In our institution, we have two units available in the ICU: a small, extremely portable unit with a fixed transducer used solely for the guidance of vascular access, as well as a more robust "lap-top" style unit with interchangeable transducers that functions in a variety of roles including focused echocardiography. Both units are dedicated to our surgical ICU; however, in a lower volume center, it might be possible to share the units between different procedure areas to limit cost.

Procedure Kits

In order to ensure a successful ICU bedside procedure environment, it is vital to guarantee the immediate availability of required supplies and instruments. Many common procedures utilize all-inclusive commercially available kits (e.g., for central venous catheter placement and percutaneous tracheostomy insertion). These kits can be further customized

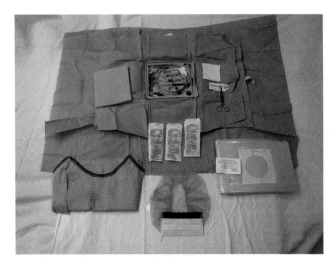

Figure 1-1. Customized central line kit components at Parkland Memorial Hospital.

to include drapes, gowns, caps, and masks, so that the only additional component necessary is the provider's gloves. This customization can dramatically improve compliance with maximal barrier precautions and can lower iatrogenic infection rates. Figure 1-1 demonstrates the contents of our customized central catheter insertion kit. We believe that this customized kit obviates the need for a dedicated "line cart" that is referenced in the literature.[19] However, kit contents can vary from one manufacturer to another; so, prior to use, the available components should be evaluated.

Generic Procedure Cart

At our institution, we have developed a self-contained cart to assist in the performance of a variety of procedures including open tracheostomy, open abdominal washout, and chest tube insertion. We have customized our instrument kits to ensure that all necessary components are present without redundancy. The cart is restocked by our team of nurse practitioners assisted by the bedside nurses. Mounted to the top of the cart are both a small headlight and an electrocautery. Table 1-1 lists the contents by drawer; Fig. 1-2 illustrates the cart. Although there are many medical manufacturers of such carts, it is also possible to utilize a commercially available tool chest at a substantial cost savings. The cart should be locked or stored in a secure location that can be readily accessed in case of emergency.

Table 1-1. Contents of the generic procedure cart of the surgical intensive care Unit at Parkland Memorial Hospital.

Drawer Number	Contents
1	Sterile surgical gloves: size 6–8½ (4 each)
2	Sutures/ties (1 box each)
	• 2-0 silk multipack on SH needle
	• 3-0 vicryl on SH needle
	• 2-0 silk tie multipack
	• 0 nylon (Ethilon) on CT needle
	• 2-0 Nylon (Ethilon) of FS needle
	• 5-0 Prolene on FS2 needle
	• 2-0 Prolene on SH needle
3	10 cc syringes (10)
	25 gage needles (10)
	21 gage needles (10)
	18 gage needles (10)
4	1% Lidocaine with epinephrine (2 bottles)
	1% Lidocaine without epinephrine (2 bottles)
	2% Chlorhexadine prep sticks (6)
	Betadine (2)
	Surgical lubricant (2 multiuse tubes)
5	Bovie pencils (2)
	Bovie grounding pads (2)
	JP drains (2)
	Sterile towel multipacks (4)
6	Sterile gowns (2)
	Sterile drapes (4)
7	8 Shiley tracheostomy tube (4)
	6 Shiley tracheostomy tube (2)
	Sterile suction tubing (2)
	Nasotracheal suction catheter (2)
	Trach accordion tubing (6)
	Endotracheal tube exchanger (2)
	Bougie (2)
	Yaunker suction catheter (2)
8	Blue Rhino Perc Trach Kit (1)
	4×4 multipacks (6)
	PEG kit (1)
	Minor procedure tray (1)
	Sterile gowns (2)
	Face shields (4)
	Bouffant surgical caps (4)
9	Surgical headlight
	Sterile saline irrigation 1,000 cc (2)
	Ioban surgical drape (2)
	Bowel bags (2)
	Burn dressings (2)
	Radio-opaque 4×4 multipacks (6)
	Laparotomy pad multipacks (2)

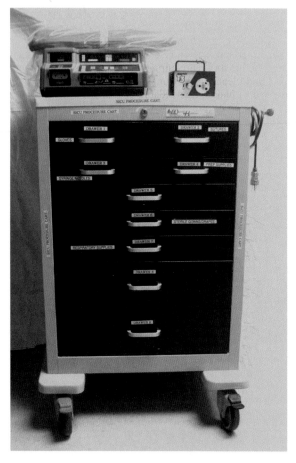

Figure 1-2. Procedure cart at Parkland Memorial Hospital with drawers labeled.

Endoscopy Cart

It must be determined who will own and service the equipment prior to embarking upon an ICU-based endoscopy program. Ideally, a central entity in the hospital would purchase, house, and service all endoscopes and would offer 24-h availability. In many institutions this is not the case. At our institution, although we have purchased our own bronchoscope, GI endoscope, and tower, we have partnered with both the operating room and the gastroenterology suite to take advantage of resources and expertise and to minimize costs to the ICU. Endoscopes are very expensive and finicky; improper handling and cleaning can result in the transmission of disease and the breaking of equipment. Regardless of where endoscopes are housed and cleaned, we would recommend that a service contract be maintained to handle unavoidable endoscope damage that occurs in the ICU setting. To ensure rapid availability of endoscopy equipment at the bedside, mobile endoscopy towers should be employed. These carts should be stocked with all necessary video imaging equipment as well as replacement endoscope valves, tubing, and bite blocks.

Fluoroscopy

Procedures that utilize fluoroscopy for imaging may require a separate procedure area to store bulky radiologic equipment and to shield or minimize the radiation exposure of those not involved.

Centralized Procedure Areas

Some hospitals have set aside specific procedure areas in their ICUs. While the use of these areas requires patient transport within the ICU, it does provide several advantages. First, a separate ICU procedure area allows for a more controlled environment, reduced traffic, and fewer breaches of sterile areas. In addition, centralized procedure areas may help minimize disruptions in the ICU routine for other patients and families while the procedures are in progress. Finally, use of such a strategy may allow for centralized storage of procedure-specific items.

If space constraints prevent the use of a separate procedure room, most ICU procedures may be performed at the bedside. A few specific details must be kept in mind before deciding to perform a procedure at the bedside: First, depending on the physical setup of the ICU, it might be necessary to limit visitors to either the immediately surrounding patients or possibly the entire unit while an ICU-based procedure is underway. This may be necessary both to ensure that a sterile field can be maintained as well as to provide some measure of privacy. Secondly, there must be adequate means to separate the procedure area from the rest of the ICU. This is necessary both to minimize distractions and disruptions while the procedure is being performed and maintain a sterile procedure field. While some units may provide adequate separation by virtue of physical barriers, others may use simple curtains or mobile partitions. Finally, several of the procedures discussed in later chapters involve some degree of radiation exposure. As long as adequate spacing is provided between the C-arm of an X-ray machine nearby patients and staff and as long as standard protective equipment is utilized, exposure risk from fluoroscopic-guided procedures is small.[20] Certainly, prior to embarking on a protocol of fluoroscopically guided procedures, the institution's radiation safety personnel should be involved to ensure that appropriate safety measures are being applied.

■ PERSONNEL AND CREDENTIALING

Credentialing for providers who perform ICU-based procedures should follow the same principles that the institution applies to practitioners who perform these procedures elsewhere. Application of guidelines established by the Society of Critical Care Medicine (SCCM) for Granting Privileges for the Performance of Procedures in Critically Ill Patients may be helpful.[5] In addition, once privileges have been granted, a mechanism must be easily available to verify privilege status at the areas where the procedures will be performed (i.e., electronically). Quality assurance and improvement mechanisms must also be put in place, along with an appeals process for any denials or revocations of privileges.

A variety of pathways should be made available for initial credentialing. In general, privileges should be granted based on a training pathway (i.e., competency by virtue of graduate medical education or continuing medical education), a practice pathway (i.e., competency inferred from credentials granted at other institutions or in other hospital areas outside the ICU), or an examination pathway (i.e., competency demonstrated by examination and demonstrated performance). Following initial privileging, maintenance of certification should be subjected to demonstration of continuing experience as well as participation in quality assurance and improvement mechanisms to ensure acceptable outcomes.

Various societies and boards are presently at work to further describe the components of successful maintenance of certification.[21] Several procedures associated with relatively steep learning curves, such as the insertion of intracranial pressure monitors and bedside ultrasonography, may require more specific guidelines to ensure competency. Training curricula for the use of ultrasound in critical care have been proposed, requiring a specific number of proctored exams to demonstrate competency.[22] Considering ventriculostomy placement, performance outside the realm of neurosurgical practice would require extensive training with monitored procedures until competency has been established. Percutaneous airway techniques, which can certainly be performed by nonsurgeons, require the ability to immediately convert to an open procedure in an urgent fashion. If these techniques are to be used outside the surgical realm, advance arrangements should be in place to ensure the immediate availability of surgical back up should it be required.

A recent review of privileging practices in community hospitals revealed that strict adherence to the SCCM guidelines is not always observed.[23]

Most small hospitals used an inclusive rather than an exclusive privileging process. Many do not distinguish ICU admission privileges from procedure privileges. Finally, most small community hospitals do not require documentation of previous or direct observation of current successful procedure performance before granting privileges. These less stringent requirements likely reflect the realities of the local or regional practice of medicine. However, due to the high acuity of patients involved, more stringent privileging practices may be recommended. The use of actual numbers as a benchmark for competency is very controversial, although many hospitals are actively pursuing credentialing language that incorporates this concept. On the other hand, Sloan and colleagues found no consistent relationship between more stringent credentialing practices and improved outcome.[24] Indeed, the successful acquisition of procedural skills in medicine is a complex issue. The adage of "see one, do one, teach one" with the assumption of competency is not valid today.[25] Even in areas such as endoscopy where a national society does make specific recommendations for procedure numbers for credentialing, Sharma and Eisen found that most centers do not follow the recommendations when considering the credentialing of individual providers.[26,27]

Nursing and support staff members also require education regarding proper conduct around and safety concerns regarding ICU bedside procedures. It is essential that all ICU staff members involved are familiar with the nuances of the procedure. While some aspects, such as the administration of adequate procedural sedation, should be commonplace for the ICU staff, in other areas these practices would be considered unusual. Prior to assisting in new procedures, adequate in-service training is essential. A period of observation in specialty areas is advisable if staff members do not have prior experience. For low-volume units, periodic retraining of support personnel is necessary to ensure staff familiarity with the details of each procedure. ICU bedside nurses should play an important role in development of local institutional policies governing bedside procedures. For example, due to the small size of ICU rooms at our institution, it is very difficult to access a patient's arms and torso during performance of certain bedside procedures. To overcome this obstacle, our nurses have developed practice guidelines for the administration of conscious sedation through intravenous lines placed in the foot.

■ CONSIDERATIONS FOR THE ACTUAL PROCEDURE

There are several general considerations applicable to all procedures. These include the use of sedation, adequacy of intravenous access, preprocedure preparation, and intraprocedure monitoring to maximize patient safety.

Conscious sedation is an important consideration for most bedside ICU procedures and will be discussed in detail in an upcoming chapter. Specific guidelines for sedation, analgesia, and monitoring have been established by a number of national societies including the American Society of Anesthesiologists (ASA), the American Academy of Pediatrics, and the Association of Operating Room Nurses.[28] While guidelines for the use of sedatives and analgesics for specific procedures are beyond the scope of this chapter, several general principles are important to note. Foremost, to ensure patient safety during the procedure, all procedures should have at least one care provider assigned specifically to administer sedatives and analgesics and to monitor the patient's physiologic response. For conscious sedation involving stable patients, this task is easily be accomplished by appropriately trained nursing staff; however, for either deeper levels of sedation or with hemodynamically unstable patients, this task may need to be delegated to an appropriately trained physician not otherwise involved with the procedure. When a patient does not already have an adequate artificial airway, advanced airway equipment must be immediately available both during and postprocedure.[29]

Another important area is the status of the patient's oral intake prior to the procedure. While tradition may dictate that all patients be made *nil per os* from midnight on the day of the procedure, this practice has been reexamined by a number of different groups over recent years. A recent Cochrane review demonstrated that, compared to usual fasting practices, a less restrictive fasting policy in adults was associated with similar risks of aspiration, regurgitation, and related morbidity.[30] A similar review in children demonstrated no benefit to withholding liquids more than 2 h prior to procedures compared to 6 h.[31] At our institution, patients undergoing either surgical or ICU procedures continue enteral nutrition throughout the procedure as long as the procedure does not involve the airway or GI tract and the airway is protected by tracheal intubation or tracheostomy.

It is important that intravenous access be adequate, redundant, and obtained prior to the start of the procedure. In choosing specific sites for intravenous access, attention must be given to the specific procedure being performed. At our institution, as noted previously, it is a common practice to obtain lower extremity access for procedures involving the chest and airway. This ensures that the site is easily accessible while the procedure is in process.

Except in emergency situations, adequate informed consent must be obtained from either the patient or a legally authorized representative prior to commencing any procedure. It is important to realize that many patients, either by virtue of illness or the administration of sedation, have some degree of altered sensorium.[32] Some institutions have adopted special procedures for ensuring a patient's competency for consent in the ICU setting.[33] At our institution, we utilize a universal ICU consent obtained shortly after unit admission that covers many commonly performed ICU procedures (Fig. 1-3). A separate consent is used for more

PARKLAND HEALTH & HOSPITAL SYSTEM
Dallas, Texas

INTENSIVE CARE UNIT
CONSENT FORM

INTRODUCTION:

Welcome to the Intensive Care Unit (ICU). As part of the regular care for you/your family member, the Intensive Care physicians at Parkland may need to perform a variety of procedures to help you/your family member recover from your/their illness. Any number of these procedures (from none to all) may be required during your/your family member's ICU stay; some may be performed more than once; some or all may be lifesaving.

These procedures may include any of the following:

- Breathing tube insertion (tube in airway to connect to a breathing machine)

- Central venous access catheter (tube in a large vein for fluids or medications)

- Pulmonary artery catheter (tube through a large vein that measures pressures in the heart)

- Chest tube (tube between the lung and chest wall to drain air or fluid) or sampling of chest or abdominal fluid

- Arterial catheter (tube in artery to measure blood pressure)

- Fiber optic bronchoscope (flexible lighted viewing device to look in the airway)

- Peritoneal lavage (fluid used to wash out the abdomen)

- Wound debridement (cutting away of dead tissue from a wound), incision and drainage or repair, escharotomy (cutting into the burned tissue that is harming circulation)

- Lumbar puncture (sampling of fluid around the spine to test for infection)

- Transfusion of blood or blood products

- Ventriculostomy (brain pressure monitor/drainage tube in or around the brain to measure and relieve pressure)

This protocol does not attempt to restrict the performance of emergent, immediately life-saving procedures in the judgement of the treating physician (patient will die or suffer harm if not performed at once).

RISK OF PROCEDURES:

Each of these procedures has unique risks. In general, the major risks for this group of procedures includes: pain, scar, bleeding, infection, failure of procedure, repeat procedure, and injury to adjacent structures. Given the nature of critical illness that requires ICU level care, death is possible as well.

Risks of blood transfusion: fever, transfusion reaction that may include kidney failure or anemia, heart failure, hepatitis, AIDS or other infections.

E10

6427 (Front) Revised 10/26/07 SRC

Figure 1-3. Universal consent form used in the intensive care units at Parkland Memorial Hospital.

invasive bedside procedures, such as tracheostomy. It is important that patients and families be familiar with the specific policies in place at the practice location.

The Joint Commission on Accreditation of Healthcare Organizations has developed a universal protocol for preventing wrong site, wrong procedure, and wrong person surgery.[34] Many institutions have expanded this process to include virtually all procedures. Our institution has a formal policy with the inclusion of a "time out" documentation form that is completed before the procedure begins (Fig. 1-4). It is important to note that protocols involving correct site/procedure/patient can vary widely among different institutions.[35] However, even strict adherence to verification protocols does not completely eliminate the incidence of wrong site events. In one recent review, wrong site events still occurred despite adherence to site identification procedures, although two-thirds less frequently.[36]

The unintentional retention of surgical instruments and sponges during invasive procedures is another area of concern. This may be less of an issue for some bedside procedures (e.g., tracheostomy with its limited surgical field), whereas a retained instrument or sponge becomes more of a possibility during others (e.g., bedside washout and dressing change for an open abdomen). In the operating theater, the practice of counting instruments and sponges has been a standard for many years. However, Egorova and colleagues recently examined the utility of this practice. They studied 1,062 incorrect counts over 153,263 operations and determined that an incorrect count identified only 77% of retained objects.[37] Some have described potential technologic solutions, including routine postoperative X-rays and electronic tagging of instruments and sponges.[38,39]

■ INFECTION CONTROL ISSUES

Several infection control issues should be considered in preparation for performing bedside ICU procedures. Proper hand hygiene, appropriate site selection, use of appropriate skin preparation agents, and an aseptic technique with a full body drape during device insertion have been shown to reduce the rate of nosocomial device-related infections.[40]

A recent Cochrane review of the effects of a variety of antiseptic skin preparation techniques for noncatheter procedures did not demonstrate any particular technique to be superior.[41] Different drape and gown materials have also been evaluated. The use of disposable gowns and paper drapes resulted in a significantly lower wound infection rates for all wound classes than did the use of cloth gowns and drapes.[42] Another recent Cochrane review found no evidence to show that adhesive plastic drapes reduced surgical wound infection rates.[43]

The use of antibiotic prophylaxis for ICU procedures is another area of controversy. Antibiotic prophylaxis for invasive surgical procedures should follow established guidelines for timing and duration as well as choice of specific antibiotic agents.[44,45] However, the need

PARKLAND HEALTH & HOSPITAL SYSTEM
Dallas, Texas

TIME OUT CHECKLIST

Date: Time:	Location:
A time out must be performed immediately before the start of any invasive procedure. **Time-out may be waived if:** • The provider states that the risk to life and limb exceeds the benefit of the time out	**Time out waived by** ____________ **ID #** _____ **Reason for waiver:**
Diagnostic Studies/Implants/Equipment • Available or transport confirmed	**Yes** **NA**
Continued Fertility: • **Patient states desire for permanent sterilization**	**Yes** **No** **NA**
All participants must agree • Correct name and medical record number* • Correct procedure, site, side, position • Consent verified if applicable • Correct surgical site marking if applicable • Review and circle **ONE** additional Admit diagnosis History/Physical Day Surgery Note Chief complaint Progress Note Pre-natal record • Desires permanent sterilization when applicable * Two identifiers must be verified. Name and date of birth may be used for outpatient settings * If the patient or family is capable of participation, ask them to state name, date of birth, procedure, site and side	**All staff members participating in the time out must verbalize joint agreement**** **Yes** **No** **Procedure** ____________ **Staff Member** ________ **ID #** _____ **Provider** ________ **ID #** _____ **Anesthesia** ________ **ID #** _____
Time Out Reconciliation** • If agreement has not been reached, notify the charge nurse or manager and activate Nursing Procedure, 21-04, "Procedure for Questioning Physician's Orders" or appropriate unit specific procedure	**Resolution Notes: Document Decision and Outcome** 409

PS 4753 Revised 07/23/04 SRC

Figure 1-4. "Time out" checklist employed for all procedures at Parkland Memorial Hospital.

for antibiotic prophylaxis for other procedures is not as clear. With respect to central venous catheter insertion, a literature review demonstrated no benefit from prophylactic antibiotics in adults and only a minor benefit in children that was offset by an increase in resistant organisms.[40] For other procedures such as percutaneous gastrostomy tube insertion, conflicting evidence exists regarding the usefulness of prophylactic antibiotics. It is our practice to utilize a first generation cephalosporin for prophylaxis prior to performance of a percutaneous gastrostomy, unless the patient is already receiving an antibiotic that will address Gram-positive skin organisms.

■ FAMILY PRESENCE DURING PROCEDURES

There is controversy regarding family presence during the performance of sterile bedside ICU procedures. While literature in the adult population is sparse, there have been several publications in the pediatric literature regarding this topic. Potential advantages of family presence during procedures include the ability to calm the patient and an increased awareness of the procedure.[46] This may be offset by more breaks in sterile technique, higher levels of anxiety and increased rates of failure among operators while performing the procedure.[47] Regarding endoscopy, Shapira found that the presence of a family member during the procedure led to increased patient satisfaction, improved patient perception regarding the severity of the procedure, and a general sense from the escorts that their presence was supportive to the patient.[48] MacLean and colleagues found that only 5% of units had specific written policies allowing family member to be present during procedures but 51% permitted the practice if requested. Furthermore, a survey of nursing personnel indicated that family members often asked to be present during procedures.[49] We suggest that units develop a written policy regarding family member presence, with appropriate exceptions to ensure patient safety and privacy. Importantly these policies should address the need for family members to rapidly escape if desired.

■ REFERENCES

1. Grover A, Robbins J, Bendick P, et al. Open versus percutaneous dilational tracheostomy: efficacy and cost analysis. *Am Surg*. 2001;67(4): 297–301.
2. Upadhyay A, Maurer J, Turner J, et al. Elective bedside tracheostomy in the intensive care unit. *J Am Coll Surg*. 1996;183(1):51–55.
3. Jones PW, Moyers J, Rogers J, et al. Ultrasound guided thoracentesis: is it a safer method? *Chest*. 2003;123(2):418–423.
4. Hind D, Calvert N, McWilliams R, et al. Ultrasonic devices for central venous cannulations: meta-analysis. *BMJ*. 2003;327(7411):361.
5. Society of Critical Care Medicine. Guidelines for granting privileges for the performance of procedures in critically ill patients. *Crit Care Med*. 1993;19(2):275–278.

6. Martin LD, Howell R, Ziegelstein R, et al. Hospitalist performance of cardiac hand-carried ultrasound after focused training. *Am J Med.* 2007;120(11):1000–1004.

7. Gunst M, Sperry J, Ghaemmaghami V, et al. Accuracy of cardiac function and volume status estimates using the bedside echocardiographic assessment in trauma / critical care: the BEAT exam. *J Trauma.* 2007;63(6):1432.

8. Mazareshahi RM, Farmer JC, Porembka D, et al. A suggested curriculum in echocardiography for critical care physicians. *Crit Care Med.* 2007;35(8 Supp):S431–S433.

9. Alexander JH, Peterson E, Chen A, et al. Feasibility of point-of-care echocardiography by internal medicine house staff. *Am Heart H.* 2004;147(3):476–481.

10. Langlois SLP, FRANZCR. Focused ultrasound training for clinicians. *Crit Care Med.* 2007;35(5 suppl):S138–S143.

11. Gardiner Q, White PS, Carson A, et al. Technique training: endoscopic percutaneous tracheostomy. *Br J Anaesth.* 1998;81(3):401–403.

12. Indeck M, Peterson S, Smith J, et al. Risk, cost and benefit of transporting ICU patients for special studies. *J Trauma.* 1988;28(7):1020–1025.

13. Damm C, Vandelet P, Petit J, et al. Complications [Complications during the intrahospital transport in critically ill patients. *Ann Fr Anesth Reanim.* 2005;24(1):24–30.

14. Jaramillo EJ, Trevino JM, Berghoff KR, et al. Bedside diagnostic laparoscopy in the intensive care unit: a 13-year experience. *J Soc Laparoendoscopic Surg.* 2006;10(2):155–159.

15. Simpson, Day, Jewkes, et al. The impact of percutaneous tracheostomy on intensive care unit practice and training. *Anaesthesia* 1999;54(2): 186–189.

16. Hunter M. Peripherally inserted central catheter placement at the speed of sound. *Nutr Clin Pract.* 2007;22(4):406–411.

17. Carr BG, Dean A, Everett W, et al. Intensivist bedside ultrasound (INBU) for volume assessment in the intensive care unit: a pilot study. *J Trauma.* 2007;63(3):495–500.

18. Nicolaou S, Talsky A, Khashoggi K, et al. Ultrasound-guided interventional radiology in critical care. *Crit Care Med.* 2007;35(5 Suppl): S186–S197.

19. Berenholtz SM, Pronovost P, Lipsett P, et al. Eliminating catheter-related bloodstream infections in the intensive care unit. *Crit Care Med.* 2004;32(10):2014–2020.

20. Sing RF, Smith C, Miles W, et al. Preliminary results of bedside inferior vena cava filter placement: safe and cost-effective. *Chest.* 1998;114(1):315–316.

21. Nussbaum MS. Invited lecture: American Board of Surgery Maintenance of Certification explained. *Am J Surg.* 2008;195:284–287.

22. Neri L, Storti E, Lichtensetein D, et al. Toward an ultrasound curriculum for critical care medicine. *Crit Care Med.* 2007;35(5 suppl):S290–S304.

23. Powner DJ. Credentialing for critical care in small hospitals. *Crit Care Med.* 2001;29(8):1630–1632.
24. Sloan FA, Conover C, Provenzale D, et al. Hospital credentialing and quality of care. *Soc Sci Med.* 2000;50(1):77–88.
25. Kovacs G. Procedural skills in medicine: Linking theory to practice. *J Emerg Med.* 1997;15(3):387–391.
26. Eisen DM, Baron T, Dominitz J, et al. Methods of granting hospital privileges to perform gastrointestinal endoscopy. *Gastrointest Endosc.* 2002;55(7):780–783.
27. Sharma VK, Coppola A, Raufman J, et al. A survey of credentialing practices of gastrointestinal endoscopy centers in the United States. *J Clin Gastroenterol.* 2005;39(6):501–507.
28. American Society of Anesthesiologists Task Force on Sedation and Analgesia by Non-Anesthesiologists. Practice guidelines for sedation and analgesia by non-anesthesiologists. *Anesthesiology.* 2002;96(4): 1004–1017.
29. Soifer BE. Procedural Anesthesia at the bedside. *Crit Care Clin.* 2000;16(1):7–28.
30. Brady M, Kinn S, O'Rourke K, Stuart P. Preoperative fasting for adults to prevent perioperative complications. Cochrane Database of Systematic Reviews 2003, Issue 4. Art. No.: CD004423. DOI: 10.1002/14651858. CD004423
31. Brady M, Kinn S, O'Rourke K, Randhawa N, Stuart P. Preoperative fasting for preventing perioperative complications in children. Cochrane Database of Systematic Reviews 2005, Issue 2. Art. No.: CD005285. DOI: 10.1002/14651858.CD005285
32. Davis N, Pohlman A, Gehlbach B, et al. Improving the process of informed consent in the critically ill. *JAMA.* 2003;289(15):1963-1968.
33. Fan E, Shahid S, Kondreddi V, et al. Informed consent in the critically ill: a two-step approach incorporation delirium screening. *Crit Care Med.* 2008;36(1):94–99.
34. Joint Commission on Accreditation of Healthcare Organizations. Universal Protocol for Preventing Wrong Site, Wrong Procedure, Wrong Person Surgery.http://www.jointcommission.org/PatientSafety/Universal Protocol as accessed on 4/23/08
35. Michaels RK, Makary M, Dahab Y, et al. Achieving the National Quality Forum's "Never Events": prevention of wrong site, wrong procedure, and wrong patient operations. *Ann Surg.* 2007;245(4):526–532.
36. Clarke JR, Johnston J, Finley E, et al. Getting surgery right. *Ann Surg.* 2007;246(3):395–403.
37. Egorova NN, Moskowitz A, Gelijns A, et al. Managing the prevention of retained surgical instruments – what is the value of counting? *Ann Surg.* 2008;247(1):13–18.
38. Ponrartana S, Coakley F, Yeh B, et al. Accuracy of plain abdominal radiographs in the detection of retained surgical needles in the peritoneal cavity. *Ann Surg.* 2008;247(1):8–12.

39. Greenberg CC, Diaz-Flores R, Lipsitz S, et al. Bar-coding surgical sponges to improve safety: a randomized controlled trial. *Ann Surg.* 2008;247(4):612–616.
40. O'Grady NP, Alexander M, Dellinger EP, et al. Guidelines for the prevention of intravascular catheter related infections. Centers for Disease Control and Prevention. *MMWR Recomm Rep.* 2002;51(RR-10):1–29
41. Edwards PS, Lipp A, Holmes A. Preoperative skin antiseptics for preventing surgical wound infections after clean surgery. *Cochrane Database Syst Rev.* 2004;3:CD003949
42. Moylan JA, Fitzpatrick KT, Davenport KE. Reducing wound infections. Improved gown and drape barrier performance. *Arch Surg.* 1987;122(2):152–157
43. Webster J, Alghamdi AA. Use of plastic adhesive drapes during surgery for preventing surgical site infection. *Cochrane Database Syst Rev.* 2007;4: CD006353.
44. Bratzler DW, Dale W, Houck PM, et al. Antimicrobial prophylaxis for surgery: an advisory statement from the National Surgical Infection Prevention Project. *Clin Infect Dis.* 2004;38(12):1706–1715.
45. Bratzler DW, Houck PM, Surgical Infection Prevention Guidelines Writers Workgroups. Antimicrobial prophylaxis for surgery: an advisory statement from the National Surgical Infection Prevention Project. *Am J Surg.* 2005;189(4):395–404
46. Fein JA, Ganesh J, Alpern ER. Medical staff attitudes toward family presence during pediatric procedures. *Pediatr Emerg Care.* 2004; 20(4):224–227.
47. Bradford KK, Kost S, Selbst S, et al. Family member presence for procedures: the resident's perspective. *Ambul Pediatr.* 2005;5(5):294–297.
48. Shapira M, Tamir AD. Presence of family member during endoscopy. What do patients and escorts think? *J Clin Gastroenterol.* 1996;22(4): 272–274.
49. MacLean SL, Guzzetta CE, White C, et al. Family presence during cardiopulmonary resuscitation and invasive procedures: practices of critical care and emergency nurses. *Am J Crit Care.* 2003;12(3):246–257.

2

Conscious Sedation and Deep Sedation, Including Neuromuscular Blockade

Russell R. Miller III

■ INTRODUCTION

Conscious sedation and deep sedation of intensive care unit (ICU) patients requiring procedures is both common and necessary. Guidelines exist for the sustained use of sedatives, analgesics, and paralytics[1,2] but not for their procedural use. Anecdotal experience serves as the basis for using analgesia when a critically ill patient undergoes bronchoscopy and to not do so when that same patient gets endotracheally suctioned. Few investigations have questioned the historically firm notion that some procedures require sedation and others do not.

R.R. Miller III (✉)
Respiratory ICU, Department of Medicine Pulmonary and Critical Care Division, Intermountain Medical Center, Murray, UT, USA
e-mail: russ.miller@imail.org

H.L. Frankel and B.P. deBoisblanc (eds.), *Bedside Procedures for the Intensivist*,
DOI 10.1007/978-0-387-79830-1_2,
© Springer Science+Business Media, LLC 2010

This chapter has three goals as they relate to bedside procedures for the intensivist:

- To review existing guidelines for sedation and analgesia, including those that address the appropriate depth and monitoring procedures both during and after the procedure
- To overview clinical factors that influence the selection of sedative, analgesic, and paralytic agents, for example, the duration and degree of pain, patient history, and the existing level of patient care
- To review commonly used sedatives, analgesics, and paralytics, including their pharmacologic properties and adverse effects that influence their selection.

■ EXISTING GUIDELINES

Depth of Sedation

As with hemodynamics and oxygenation, depth of sedation for bedside ICU procedures must be assessed routinely. The American Society of Anesthesiologists in 2002 characterized four levels of intended drug-induced sedation/analgesia: 1. Minimal sedation/anxiolysis 2. Conscious sedation 3. Deep sedation/analgesia 4. General anesthesia

Each level is defined by cognitive responsiveness, airway patency, spontaneous ventilation, and cardiovascular function (Table 2-1).[3]

Hemodynamic monitoring in sedated patients before, during, and after the institution of sedative, analgesic, and paralytic agents includes:

- Ventilatory function, using direct observation or auscultation
- Oxygenation, using a continuous, variable-pitch beep based upon the oxygen saturation reading
- Capnometry (end-tidal CO_2), particularly when deep sedation is planned or develops or in moderate sedation if the evaluation of ventilation is difficult
- Blood pressure, either every 5 min in patients wearing a cuff or continuously in those with an arterial catheter
- Electrocardiographic monitoring, both in all those undergoing deep sedation and in those receiving moderate sedation who have pre-existing cardiovascular disease or who are undergoing procedures expected to result in dysrhythmia (e.g., electrical cardioversion).

To make valid, reliable, subjective assessments of the level of consciousness in the ICU, tools such as the Richmond Agitation-Sedation Scale[4] (RASS) (Table 2-2) or Sedation Agitation Scale[5] (SAS) may be employed with the procedure to guide the need for initial as well as supplemental sedation and analgesia. Each tool provides standardized language for the assessment of a patient's level of consciousness, allowing

Table 2-1. Continuum of depth of sedation: definition of general anesthesia and levels of sedation/analgesia.

	Minimal Sedation (Anxiolysis)	Moderate Sedation/Analgesia (Conscious Sedation)	Deep Sedation/Analgesia	General Anesthesia
Responsiveness	Normal response to verbal stimulation	Purposeful[a] response to verbal or tactile stimulation	Purposeful[a] response after repeated or painful stimulation	Unarousable, even with painful stimulus
Airway	Unaffected	No intervention required	Intervention may be required	Intervention often required
Spontaneous ventilation	Unaffected	Adequate	May be inadequate	Frequently inadequate
Cardiovascular function	Unaffected	Usually maintained	Usually maintained	May be impaired

Minimal Sedation (Anxiolysis) = a drug-induced state during which patients respond normally to verbal commands. Although cognitive function and coordination may be impaired, ventilatory and cardiovascular functions are unaffected.

Moderate Sedation/Analgesia (Conscious Sedation) = a drug-induced depression of consciousness during which patients respond purposefully[a] to verbal commands, either alone or accompanied by light tactile stimulation. No interventions are required to maintain a patent airway, and spontaneous ventilation is adequate. Cardiovascular function is usually maintained.

Deep Sedation/Analgesia = a drug-induced depression of consciousness during which patients cannot be easily aroused but respond purposefully[a] following repeated or painful stimulation. The ability to independently maintain ventilatory function may be impaired. Patients may require assistance in maintaining a patent airway, and spontaneous ventilation may be inadequate. Cardiovascular function is usually maintained.

General Anesthesia = a drug-induced loss of consciousness during which patients are not arousable, even by painful stimulation. The ability to independently maintain ventilatory function is often impaired. Patients often require assistance in maintaining a patent airway, and positive pressure ventilation may be required because of depressed spontaneous ventilation or drug-induced depression of neuromuscular function. Cardiovascular function may be impaired.

Because sedation is a continuum, it is not always possible to predict how an individual patient will respond. Hence practitioners intending to produce a given level of sedation should be able to rescue patients whose level of sedation becomes deeper than initially intended. Individuals administering *Moderate Sedation/Analgesia (Conscious Sedation)* should be able to rescue patients who enter a state of *Deep Sedation/Analgesia*, while those administering *Deep Sedation/Analgesia* should be able to rescue patients who enter a state of general anesthesia.

Reproduced with permission from [3].

[a]Reflex withdrawal from a painful stimulus is not considered a purposeful response.

Table 2-2. Richmond agitation sedation scale.

Score	Term	Description
+4	Combative	Violent, immediate danger to staff
+3	Very agitated	Pulls at tube(s) or catheter(s); aggressive
+2	Agitated	Nonpurposeful movement, fights ventilator
+1	Restless	Anxious but movements are not aggressive
0	Alert and calm	Awake, alert
−1	Drowsy	Not fully alert, but sustained eye-opening and eye contact to *voice* > 10 s
−2	Light sedation	Briefly awakens with eye-opening and eye contact to *voice* < 10 s
−3	Moderate sedation	Movement or eye opening to *voice*, but no eye contact
−4	Heavy sedation/ stupor	No response to voice, but movement or eye opening to *physical* stimulation
−5	Unarousable/coma	No response to verbal or physical stimulation

Adapted from Sessler et al[4].

for a more objective assessment of the need to increase or decrease the amount or frequency of sedation.

Bispectral index (BIS) monitors are used in the operating room to provide an objective assessment of the level of sedation. These monitors could theoretically facilitate the titration of sedatives during neuromuscular blockade or bedside procedures in the ICU. The BIS[6] mathematically analyzes the electroencephalogram and provides the user with a numerical estimate of the level of consciousness. In the operating room, the BIS monitor cable is connected to the patient's forehead using an adhesive electrode. The bedside display is monitored to ensure adequate suppression of consciousness among those receiving general anesthesia. While monitors assign a numerical value to the BIS, their accuracy may not be good enough to reliably differentiate between inadequate and adequate sedation in the ICU, since critical illness encephalopathy and muscle activity may have confounding effects on the BIS. It is therefore unclear if the BIS can perform better than subjective sedation scales for guiding the bedside proceduralist.

One prescriptive approach would be to rely upon the sedation scale (e.g., RASS or SAS) for procedures requiring minimal, moderate, or deep sedation, and to consider more objective tools for cases of deep sedation or general anesthetic administration.

Patient Monitoring

There are three compelling reasons to carefully monitor patients receiving sedation and analgesia in the ICU. First, critically ill patients may be constantly under the influence of sympathetic drive, and sedatives, analgesics, and paralytics might blunt this drive, resulting in cardiovascular collapse. Second, these drugs may blunt the body's physiologic response to procedure-related complications and thereby delay the recognition of a complication.

And finally, hemodynamic monitoring helps determine whether the levels of sedation and analgesia are adequate to insure patient comfort.

The first step in the safe monitoring of critically ill patients undergoing conscious or deep sedation is to have physicians, nursing staff, and respiratory therapists focused on patient safety rather than simply on procedural technique. Anticipation of potential complications – for example, airway obstruction, apnea, hypoxia, or cardiovascular compromise – is the most important step in avoiding sedation related sequelae. Unfortunately, physicians commonly underestimate pain when compared to the self-reports of ICU patients.[7]

For communicative ICU patients undergoing invasive procedures requiring light or moderate sedation, a verbal pain scale has been successfully used.[8] For noncommunicative critically ill patients, such as those receiving deep sedation, there are numerous tools for assessing pain but none has good reliability.

In a review of instruments for use in noncommunicative patients, Sessler and colleagues stated that, "Current practice for adult ICU patients commonly includes a combination of [the numeric pain scale] or similar self-reported pain quantification tool, plus an instrument designed to identify pain using behavior and physiologic parameters in the noncommunicative patient."[9] The Critical Care Pain Observation Tool[10] may prove useful in monitoring procedural pain in a general ICU population. A comprehensive approach to monitoring the use of analgesics in the critically ill is advocated by the Society of Critical Care Medicine.[1]

Hemodynamic monitoring in patients before, during, and after the institution of sedative, analgesic, and paralytic agents includes:

- Ventilatory function, using direct observation or auscultation
- Oxygenation, using a continuous, variable-pitch beep based upon the oxygen saturation reading
- Capnometry (end-tidal CO_2), particularly when deep sedation is planned or develops or in moderate sedation if evaluation of ventilation is difficult
- Blood pressure, either every 5 min in patients wearing a cuff or continuously in those with an arterial catheter
- Electrocardiographic monitoring, both in all those undergoing deep sedation and in those receiving moderate sedation who have pre-existing cardiovascular disease or who are undergoing procedures expected to result in dysrhythmia (e.g., electrical cardioversion).

Clinical monitoring for procedural pain or discomfort is potentially fraught with problems,[11] particularly when moderate or deep sedation is employed. In deeply sedated or anesthetized patients, clinicians look for signs of sympathetic hyperactivity, such as tachycardia, hypertension, and diaphoresis as evidence of pain because behavioral signs of pain are often not apparent. During light or moderate sedation, behavioral markers may be more predictive of pain than physiologic observations when using self-report of patients as the standard.

Patients experiencing procedural pain are twice as likely to exhibit behavioral markers as those who do not report procedural pain.[8] In a descriptive study among nearly 6,000 patients from six countries, Puntillo et al noted the noxiousness of six common bedside ICU procedures: femoral sheath removal, central venous catheter placement, tracheal suctioning, wound care, wound drain removal, and turning [8,12]. Using a numeric rating scale (with range from 0 to 10, where 10 represents the worst pain), the authors reported that wincing, rigidity, forced eye closure, verbal complaints, and grimacing were behavioral markers consistent with discomfort. In the population studied, almost two-thirds received no analgesia, and only 10% received a combination of sedative and analgesic.

It is unclear if these findings apply to other, more noxious bedside ICU procedures where sedation and analgesia are routinely employed. Further study is important as we begin to learn more about the potential contribution of pain to psychiatric sequelae (e.g., posttraumatic stress disorder) following an ICU stay.

■ CLINICAL FACTORS INFLUENCING DRUG SELECTION

Type, Duration, and Noxiousness of the Bedside Procedure

Procedures in the ICU can be generally grouped according to type, duration, and noxiousness (Table 2-3).[8,12] For example, placement of peripheral or central intravenous catheters turning patients is of short duration and mildly painful in most circumstances. Endoscopy or bronchoscopy are usually of longer duration and are more unpleasant. Intubation, cardioversion, abscess drainage, and fracture reduction are often of fairly short duration but can be very noxious. Finally, placement of a chest tube, percutaneous tracheostomy, percutaneous gastrostomy, or ventriculostomy both require more time and are uniformly noxious. It is important to note, that the noxiousness of bedside procedures in the ICU often exceeds clinician expectations.

Patient History

Patient factors readily impact the selection of sedative or analgesic, the depth of sedation, and the risks involved with bedside procedures in the ICU. These factors include:

- Age
- Preprocedure level of consciousness, or awareness

Table 2-3. Interaction of duration and noxiousness of common bedside procedures in the ICU.

Procedure Duration	Procedure Noxiousness		
	Mild	Moderate	Severe
Short (<10 min)	Peripheral IV Central IV Arterial catheter Oral suctioning Nasogastric tube Foley catheter	Endoscopy Bronchoscopy Tracheal suctioning[a] Wound dressing change[a] Turning[a] Wound drain removal[a]	Intubation Cardioversion Ventriculostomy Chest tube
Long (>10 min)	± Central IV	Endoscopy Bronchoscopy	Percutaneous tracheostomy Percutaneous gastrostomy Burn debridement

[a]Clinicians uncommonly administer analgesia for tracheal suctioning, wound changes, turning, and drain removals even though patients undergo these procedures more frequently than endoscopy; correspondingly, patients remember the pain associated with them and rate the pain from them as severe.[8,12]

- Difficulty of the airway in nonintubated patients
- Prior cardiac, pulmonary, renal, or hepatic disease
- Recent use of sedatives or analgesics

While uncommonly the sole determinant of whether a bedside procedure in the ICU should be performed, age is especially important in considering the volume of distribution and clearance of sedatives, analgesics, and paralytic agents. At the extremes of age, pharmacokinetic and pharmacodynamic properties of drugs become less reliable.

A critically ill patient's level of consciousness is highly relevant in determining the type and amount of sedative or analgesic required. Patients with depressed consciousness generally require less sedation or analgesia and often require airway protection or ventilatory support for procedures. Patients who are more alert, however, can tolerate larger doses or combination doses with less fear of adverse effects.

A common and potentially life-threatening adverse effect of most sedatives and analgesics is depression of upper airway reflexes and respiratory drive.

A patient who has a difficult airway poses two potential problems. First, due to anatomical considerations, the upper airway may be more prone to occlude during sedation. If this is the case, the proceduralist may be required to use a lighter level of sedation that in turn may lead to patient discomfort and technical difficulty. And secondly, if airway management becomes necessary during the procedure, it is more likely to be problematic. During procedures that are noxious and/or long, it is sometimes best to electively intubate such patients to permit adequate pain and anxiety control.

Predictors of difficult airway include:

- Sleep apnea or morbid obesity
- Micrognathia or macroglossia
- Loose or carious teeth
- Large incisors or scleroderma (limited interincisor gap)
- Acute cervical/facial surgery or trauma
- Prior cervical spine surgery or advanced rheumatoid arthritis

Finally, a patient's medical history and comorbidities are relevant to drug selection. For example, a history of prior difficulty with sedation or anesthesia, hepatic or renal dysfunction, and/or chronic heart or lung disease will impact decisions regarding the optimum drug and dosage to be used. Special attention should be paid to the potential for additive or synergistic effects, both intended and adverse, of various medications. For example, patients who have been chronically receiving opiates or benzodiazepines may demonstrate tolerance to usual doses of the same drug given for a procedure. In contrast, a usual dose of an opiate or benzodiazepine given to a patient who has only recently been started on the same drug could have an additive effect on respiratory depression.

■ MEDICATION SELECTION

Sedatives

Sedatives and analgesics are often used in combination because they have complementary effects. For example, opiates give excellent pain relief while benzodiazepines provide anxiolysis and retrograde amnesia. However, it is important to remember that combinations of centrally acting drugs are often additive, not only in terms of efficacy but also in terms of adverse effects.

Sedative medications that can prolong the need for mechanical ventilation and ICU and hospital stay increase the risk of nosocomial pneumonia and deep venous thrombosis and sometimes cause death. How these adverse events come about is less clear, though over sedation can attend any sedative medication. Acutely, over sedation may be associated with hypotension, arrhythmia, gastrointestinal hypomotility, inhibition of cough, and excessive loss of spontaneous ventilation.

An ideal sedative for use during procedures in the ICU would have a rapid onset and a predictable duration of action, have minimal adverse cardiopulmonary effects, be easily reversible, not generate active metabolites, possess a high therapeutic index, and be inexpensive. Four categories of commonly used intravenous sedatives – benzodiazepines, propofol, etomidate, and central α_2-agonists – are compared in Table 2-4.

Table 2-4. Pharmacologic properties of sedatives commonly used for procedural sedation IN mechanically ventilated ICU patients.

Variable	Midazolam	Lorazepam	Etomidate	Propofol	Dexmedetomidine
Bolus dose (70 kg man)	1–5 mg	1–5 mg	0.1–0.3 mg/kg	2 mg/kg	0.2–1.0 µg/kg/h[a]
Intermittent dosing	Yes	Yes	No	No	No
Onset	2–5 min	2–20 min	1–3 min	1–2 min	1–2 min
Elimination half-life	1–5 h	10–40 h	75 min	30–60 min	2 h
Metabolism	Hepatic	Hepatic	Hepatic	Hepatic	Hepatic
Excretion	Renal	Renal	Renal	Renal	Renal
Lipophilic	High	Moderate	Minimal	High	Minimal
Complications	Respiratory suppression Long elimination Withdrawal	Respiratory suppression Longer elimination Withdrawal	Apnea (transient) Hypotension (delayed)	Respiratory suppression Hypotension ± Withdrawal	Hypotension Bradycardia
Active metabolites	Yes	No	No	No	No

[a]Dexmedetomidine may be initiated either without a bolus or with a small bolus (and careful hemodynamic monitoring). See text for further details.

Benzodiazepines

Among the forms of sedation used in critically ill patients, benzodiazepines have been studied most extensively and are nearly ubiquitously employed. Benzodiazepines bind to specific, high-affinity receptors in the brain that facilitate γ–aminobutyric acid (GABA) neurotransmitter activity. In addition to causing sedation-hypnosis and anxiolysis, benzodiazepines are anticonvulsant and amnestic, cause muscle relaxation, and potentiate analgesia. The benzodiazepines most commonly used in critically ill patients are midazolam and lorazepam.

Both midazolam and lorazepam are inexpensive benzodiazepines and are widely used for procedural sedation. Midazolam has rapid onset of action due in part to its high lipid solubility. It rapidly redistributes into fat stores giving it a short duration of action when given by intravenous bolus. Chronic infusions, however, allow the drug to depot in fat stores giving it a much longer pharmacodynamic effect than would be predicted based upon its terminal half-life after a single bolus. HIV protease inhibitors can further inhibit clearance, leading to severe respiratory depression and prolonged sedation. In contrast, lorazepam is intermediate-acting and requires several hours to reach maximal effect. Lorazepam does not share the interaction with protease inhibitors, but its clearance is generally slower than that of midazolam in other situations. It can also depot in fat tissues leading to prolonged sedation following repeated or continuous dosing. Liver failure reduces midazolam, but not lorazepam, metabolism because the glucuronidation process for lorazepam is commonly spared in liver failure. Propylene glycol toxicity with lorazepam is related to long-term, not short-term, procedural sedation.

Adverse effects of short-term benzodiazepine use include hemodynamic and respiratory suppression. Benzodiazepines can cause acute venodilation and impaired myocardial contractility that can lead to hypotension, especially in hypovolemic patients. Paradoxical excitation occurs in some patients that can mistakenly lead to additional benzodiazepine administration. In addition to neuroexcitation, benzodiazepines are known to be deliriogenic.

The effects of benzodiazepines are theoretically reversible with the administration of an antagonist. Flumazenil is approved for reversal of benzodiazepine-induced sedation in the ICU to enable neurologic evaluation, to hasten preparedness for extubation, or to treat overdose. However, use of the competitive GABA-receptor antagonist can increase myocardial oxygen consumption and/or induce withdrawal symptoms after administration of only 0.5 mg.[13] It is not indicated for routine use in ICU patients who have been on continuous benzodiazepine infusion.

Etomidate

Etomidate is a short-acting, GABA-like sedative-hypnotic with a rapid onset of action. It rarely has significant hemodynamic and respiratory effects and is a nearly ideal agent for use in rapid sequence endotracheal intubation.

Delayed effects include lowering of intracranial pressure. Since etomidate can inhibit the production of cortisol, hypotension in the 24–48 h following etomidate administration may be due to adrenal insufficiency, prompting some to suggest it should be avoided in septic patients. Extensive study has not yet resolved this controversy.

Propofol

A general anesthetic with sedative and hypnotic properties at lower doses, propofol causes GABA-mediated central nervous system depression. Propofol also has anxiolytic, anticonvulsant, antiemetic, amnestic, and intracranial pressure lowering effects. Its rapid onset and unimpaired elimination are particularly important qualities during endotracheal intubation and occasionally during other bedside procedures such as bronchoscopy. Like benzodiazepines, the length of recovery following discontinuation of infusions appears to be dose- and time-related, where higher or longer dosing predict longer recovery.

Propofol can be associated with myocardial suppression, tachyphylaxis, and paradoxical neurological excitation, such as myoclonus. The propofol infusion syndrome, nosocomial infection, and hypertriglyceridemia have not been reported with short-term use for procedural sedation.

Dexmedetomidine

Dexmedetomidine is a highly selective α_2-agonist that has sedative-analgesic properties. Sedation appears to be mediated by the α_2-adrenergic receptors located in the locus ceruleus of the brainstem that inhibit norepinephrine release. Concomitant analgesia may occur via spinal cord nociceptors. Dexmedetomidine has been most widely studied among postsurgical patients, where the goal is sedation and analgesia that does not interfere with respiration. It has been shown to enable easy arousability, a theoretically beneficial feature of sedation for ICU procedures. When given with a loading dose, dexmedetomidine can cause transient hypertension followed by bradycardia and hypotension. Bradycardia and hypotension usually resolve during the first few hours of infusion. As with benzodiazepines and propofol, dexmedetomidine may have exaggerated effects on heart rate or cardiac output in hypovolemic patients.

Analgesics

Analgesics are underutilized for ICU procedures. There appear to be several reasons for this. First, there may be concern that analgesics will obscure intraprocedural signs of a complication. Second, side-effects such as decreased bowel motility and cardiopulmonary instability have discouraged their use. And finally, ICU clinicians mistake signs of pain (e.g., hypertension and tachycardia) as signs of anxiety and thereby titrate sedatives instead of analgesics. Unfortunately, unrelieved pain results in psychological distress and may be related to development of delirium and agitation.

Ideal procedural analgesics in the ICU should have rapid onset, predictable duration of action, minimal adverse cardiopulmonary effects, easy administration, available reversing agents, no active metabolites, a favorable therapeutic index, and favorable cost. Three types of analgesics are commonly used in the ICU – opioid agonists, acetaminophen, and nonsteroidal anti-inflammatory drugs (NSAIDs).

Opioids

Acting centrally at stereospecific opioid receptors, opioid agonists block pain nociception while also causing dose-related sedation (Table 2-5). Titration to patient response is necessary; however, accurate assessment of the level of discomfort may be difficult in the ICU setting, since tachycardia and hypertension/hypotension may result from the underlying disease process. Monotherapy with opioid analgesics may allow for both adequate pain control and procedural sedation. Minimizing opioid complications requires using the lowest effective dose, using slow administration, and adequately repleting intravascular volume prior to administration. Adverse effects of short-term opioid use include suppression of spontaneous ventilation, hypotension, decreased gastrointestinal motility, and cognitive abnormalities (including delirium).

Morphine is a pure opioid receptor agonist that induces both sedation and euphoria that begins within minutes and lasts for 2–3 h. It may be administered via oral, intramuscular, subcutaneous, intrathecal, epidural, or intravenous route. Of these, the intravenous route is the most commonly employed in ventilated ICU patients. Dose-dependent respiratory depression occurs. When administered as a large (>10 mg) intravenous bolus, additional cardiopulmonary complications may occur, apparently as a result of histamine release. Constipation, urinary retention, nausea,

Table 2-5. Pharmacologic properties of selected opioids used for procedural analgesia in mechanically ventilated ICU patients.

Variable	Morphine	Fentanyl	Remifentanil
Intermittent dosing	Yes	Yes	No
Onset	1–3 min	<30 s	1–3 min
Elimination half-life	2–3 h	3–4 h	10–20 min
Metabolism	Hepatic	Hepatic	Plasma/tissue esterase
Excretion	Renal	Renal	Renal
Active metabolites	Yes	No	No
Reversible	Yes	Yes	Yes
Serious complications	Hypotension ± Bradycardia	Hypotension Muscle rigidity	Bradycardia Muscle rigidity Cost

vomiting, and bronchial constriction may complicate therapy. A reduction in dose or use of another agent is prudent in patients with renal, hepatic, or cardiac failure.

Fentanyl, a lipophilic synthetic opioid receptor agonist, is more potent than morphine. It has an extremely rapid onset of action when administered intravenously but this effect may be mitigated somewhat by initial redistribution to inactive tissues (muscle and fat). Transient profound chest wall rigidity has been noted anecdotally, particularly in elderly patients receiving large intravenous doses. Histamine release and hypotension are less common with fentanyl than with morphine. The drug accumulates with repeated administration. As with morphine, a reduction in dose and an increase in dosing interval are prudent in patients with liver or kidney disease.

A newer synthetic opioid, remifentanil, may prove useful for procedural sedation. It reportedly does not require adjustment in patients with liver and/or renal failure because it is metabolized in the plasma by nonspecific esterases. Remifentanil also avoids histamine release and only causes hypotension via bradycardia. The drug does not appear to accumulate over time, avoiding prolongation of mechanical ventilation. It lacks anxiolytic or amnestic properties and may enable neurologic assessment. Preliminary investigation suggests it may not cause as much delirium as other opioids. Because of these favorable properties, remifentanil may prove increasingly useful for procedural sedation in the ICU.

Reversal of opiates is achieved using the specific antagonist naloxone. In intravenous doses of 0.4–2.0 mg, naloxone reverses respiratory suppression. If administered in repeated low doses or by a slow infusion, it can do so without reversing analgesia. A single dose is likely to be insufficient in reversing respiratory suppression in patients who have accumulated drug in tissues during long-term narcotic infusions. Naloxone use in patients receiving remifentanil may be unnecessary given the rapidity of reversal of respiratory suppression with remifentanil.

Acetaminophen

Combining oral acetaminophen with opiates has been shown to produce better analgesia than the use of either drug alone. However, there is risk of hepatotoxicity with repetitive or high dose use, particularly in patients with preexisting hepatic dysfunction.

Nonsteroidal Anti-inflammatory Drugs (NSAIDs)

Combining NSAIDs with opiates for procedural sedation may allow lower opioid requirements. NSAIDs are commonly given orally although intravenous preparations are available. Short-term use of NSAIDs has not been shown to cause significant adverse effects. Renal dysfunction is frequently multifactorial, and its relationship to limited doses of NSAIDs is unclear and perhaps incorrect. However, concern over gastrointestinal bleeding, renal impairment, and platelet inhibition have led to the preferential use of opiates.

Neuromuscular Blocking Agents

Paralysis of patients in the ICU has come under increased scrutiny in the last decade due to a poor risk-to-benefit ratio, difficulty in monitoring the level of sedation and analgesia in paralyzed patients, and lack of demonstrable need for facilitating mechanical ventilation. Short-term paralysis for procedures likewise has become less common with the exception of rapid sequence intubation, where control of the airway is of utmost importance. Unlike sedatives and analgesics, the effects are not reversible with specific antagonists.

The pharmacological properties of three types of NMBA – succinylcholine, benzylisoquiliniums, and the aminosteroidals – are summarized in Table 2-6. The ideal paralytic for procedural use in the ICU would have rapid onset, minimal adverse effects on cardiovascular stability and respiratory function, easy administration, short duration of action and/or available reversing agents, no active metabolites, a favorable therapeutic index, and favorable cost.

When neural impulses reach the neuromuscular junction, they provoke the release of acetylcholine from presynaptic vesicles into the junction. The released acetylcholine binds to specific receptors on the motor endplate, causing sodium–potassium flux and depolarization. NMBAs work via one of two mechanisms: (1) persistent depolarization of the motor end-plate or (2) blockade of acetylcholine receptors without activation. Succinylcholine stereochemically resembles acetylcholine and binds and activates acetylcholine receptors. Because succinylcholine is not degraded by acetylcholinesterase, persistent depolarization occurs until the drug diffuses out of the synaptic cleft. Alternatively, the nondepolarizing NMBA, including the benzylisoquiliniums and the aminosteroidals, block acetylcholine receptors without activating them.

A combined approach of objective bedside assessment and peripheral nerve stimulation testing has been recommended to monitor paralysis during long-term use, but peripheral nerve stimulation is rarely necessary for short-term procedural paralysis. The diaphragm, larynx, and laryngeal adductor muscles require higher levels of receptor blockade to achieve relaxation than other skeletal muscles.[14] The diaphragm, in particular, is thought to require >90% receptor blockade to effect paralysis. Objective evaluation of respiratory effort, patient-ventilator dyssynchrony, tachypnea, diaphoresis, lacrimation, hypertension, tachycardia, and occasionally overt agitation with facial or eye movements can indicate incomplete or awake paralysis in most patients.

Nondepolarizing NMBA are preferred over succinylcholine for paralysis lasting more than a few minutes. The adverse effects of long-term use of nondepolarizing NMBA use are primarily myopathy, neuropathy,

Table 2-6. Selected neuromuscular blocking agents used for procedural paralysis of mechanically ventilated patients in the ICU.

Variable	Succinylcholine	Cisatracurium	Atracurium	Doxacurium	Pancuronium	Vecuronium	Rocuronium
Initial dose (mg/kg)	0.3–1.5[a]	0.1–0.2	0.4–0.5	0.025–0.05	0.06–0.1	0.08–0.1	0.6–1.0
ED_{95}[b] dose (mg/kg)	0.3	0.05	0.25	0.025–0.030	0.05	0.05	0.3
Onset of action (min)	0.25–1	2–3	2–3	5–11	2–3	2–5	1–4
Duration (min)	3–5	45–60	25–35	120–150	90–100	35–45	30
Recovery (min)	5–10	90	40–60	120–180	120–180	45–60	20–30
Duration in renal failure	No change	No change	No change	Increased	Increased	Increased	Minimal
Duration in hepatic failure	No change	Minimal/none	Minimal/none	N/A	Mild increase	Mild, variable	Moderate increase
Active metabolites	No	No	No	N/A	Yes	Yes	No
Vagolysis	No	No	No	No	Yes	No	Yes (high doses)

[a] For rapid sequence intubation, the standard dose is 1.5 mg/kg; otherwise, 0.3–1.1 mg/kg is generally recommended.
[b] ED_{95} = effective dose for 95% of patients

and the acute quadriplegic myopathy syndrome. Short-term effects of NMBAs are discussed in further detail below.

Succinylcholine

Succinylcholine is a depolarizing agent used for procedural and short-term paralysis. It has a rapid onset of action and, due to rapid degradation by pseudocholinesterase in the blood, it has a brief duration of action (<10 min). Following administration, the neuromuscular junction depolarizes releasing potassium from myocytes. Potassium levels can rise as much as 1 mEq/L in patients with rhabdomyolysis, multiple trauma, burns, neuromuscular disease, or peritonitis occasionally causing life-threatening hyperkalemia.[15] The administration of succinylcholine can also cause histamine release. Hypotension is particularly common in combination with barbiturates. Because of its rapid onset, succinylcholine is a useful agent for rapid sequence intubation. However, prolonged use results in vagal stimulation and bradycardia. Genetically susceptible patients may develop prolonged paralysis or malignant hyperthermia, a rare but potentially lethal condition characterized by intractable masseter spasm, hyperventilation, tachycardia, labile blood pressure, fever, severe metabolic acidosis, hyperkalemia, rhabdomyolysis, and muscular hypertonicity.[16] Although the paralytic effects of succinylcholine are pharmacologically irreversible, dantrolene may be useful in treating malignant hyperthermia. Hypothermia decreases metabolism of succinylcholine, resulting in sustained paralysis.

Benzylisoquinoliniums

As nondepolarizing NMBA, the benzylisoquinoliniums block postsynaptic acetylcholine receptors and thus prevent muscular contraction. Their effects are irreversible. The benzylisoquinolinium NMBA, in contrast to the aminosteroidal NMBA, can cause histamine release without significant vagolytic effects resulting in hypotension and bronchospasm.

Cisatracurium is an intermediate-acting benzylisoquinolinium NMBA that causes few cardiovascular effects, in part because it does not cause significant histamine release. It is degraded in the blood by Hoffman degradation and does not need to be adjusted for renal or hepatic function.

Like cisatracurium, atracurium is an intermediate-acting agent with minimal cardiovascular adverse effects. It is also degraded by Hoffman degradation. Atracurium can cause dose-dependent histamine release and thus the attendant risk of hypotension and/or bronchospasm. Atracurium is often used in patients with renal failure, because the drug is not cleared by the kidney; and in older patients, because its elimination is not impaired by advanced age. In patients who have liver failure or who have received high NMBA doses of atracurium, an active metabolite, laundanosine, may lower the seizure threshold or directly excite the brain.

Doxacurium is a potent, long-acting NMBA not associated with cardiovascular effects. Its use in elderly patients and those with renal failure may result in significantly prolonged duration of paralysis. The drug's long duration of action, longer time to onset, and excretion by the kidney, however, limit its clinical utility.

Aminosteroidals

The aminosteroidals share a similar mechanism of action with the benzylisoquinoliniums. The aminosteroidals agents are less likely to cause hypotension or bronchospasm and are more likely to result in tachycardia.

Pancuronium is a long-acting and relatively inexpensive aminosteroidal paralytic. It is almost uniformly vagolytic (>90% of ventilated patients have a rise in their pulse by ≥10 bpm).[17] The increased heart rate frequently results in avoidance of its use in cardiovascular ICUs. Pancuronium may also cause histamine release and has been associated with prolonged paralytic effects in patients with either renal or liver dysfunction due to production of active metabolites.

Vecuronium, an intermediate-acting aminosteroidal NMBA, is an analog of pancuronium but is devoid of its risk of tachycardia. Its brief onset of action and relatively short duration make vecuronium a popular drug for rapid sequence intubation. Accumulation of both the parent drug and active metabolites and poor clearance in renal failure make it less than ideal for long-term paralysis.

Rocuronium is an intermediate-acting agent. It has a more rapid onset and shorter duration of recovery than vecuronium, though its duration of action is prolonged in liver disease.

■ SUMMARY

Sedatives, analgesics, and neuromuscular blocking agents are key elements in the performance of ICU procedures. Specific knowledge of drug selection and dosing, proper patient monitoring, and awareness of potential drug side-effects is necessary for the effective and safe management of critically ill patients.

■ REFERENCES

1. Jacobi J, Fraser GL, Coursin DB, et al. Clinical practice guidelines for the sustained use of sedatives and analgesics in the critically Ill adult. *Crit Care Med*. 2002;30:119–141.
2. Nasraway SA Jr, Jacobi J, Murray MJ, et al. Sedation, analgesia, and neuromuscular blockade of the critically ill adult: revised clinical practice guidelines for 2002. *Crit Care Med*. 2002;30:117–118.

3. Practice guidelines for sedation and analgesia by non-anesthesiologists. *Anesthesiology.* 2002;96:1004–1017

4. Sessler CN, Gosnell MS, Grap MJ, et al. The Richmond agitation-sedation scale: validity and reliability in adult intensive care unit patients. *Am J Respir Crit Care Med.* 2002;166:1338–1344.

5. Riker RR, Picard JT, Fraser GL. Prospective evaluation of the sedation-agitation scale for adult critically ill patients. *Crit Care Med.* 1999;27:1325–1329.

6. Myles PS, Leslie K, Mcneil J, et al. Bispectral index monitoring to prevent awareness during anaesthesia: the B-aware randomised controlled trial. *Lancet.* 2004;363:1757–1763.

7. Desbiens NA, Wu AW, Broste SK, et al. Pain and satisfaction with pain control in seriously ill hospitalized adults: findings from the support research investigations. For the support investigators. Study to understand prognoses and preferences for outcomes and risks of treatment. *Crit Care Med.* 1996;24:1953–1961.

8. Puntillo KA, Wild LR, Morris AB, et al. Practices and predictors of analgesic interventions for adults undergoing painful procedures. *Am J Crit Care.* 2002;11:415-429. Quiz 430–411.

9. Sessler Cn, Jo Grap M, Ramsay Ma. Evaluating and monitoring analgesia and sedation in the intensive care unit. *Crit Care.* 2008;12(Suppl 3):S2.

10. Reading AE. A comparison of pain rating scales. *J Psychosom Res.* 1980;24:119–124.

11. Gelinas C, Johnston C. Pain assessment in the critically Ill ventilated adult: validation of the critical-care pain observation tool and physiologic indicators. *Clin J Pain.* 2007;23:497–505.

12. Puntillo KA, Morris AB, Thompson CL, et al. Pain behaviors observed during six common procedures: results from thunder project II. *Crit Care Med.* 2004;32:421–427.

13. Kamijo Y, Masuda T, Nishikawa T, et al. Cardiovascular response and stress reaction to flumazenil injection in patients under infusion with midazolam. *Crit Care Med.* 2000;28:318–323.

14. Dhonneur G, Kirov K, Slavov V, et al. Effects of an intubating dose of succinylcholine and rocuronium on the larynx and diaphragm: an electromyographic study in humans. *Anesthesiology.* 1999;90:951–955.

15. Gronert GA, Theye RA. Pathophysiology of hyperkalemia induced by succinylcholine. *Anesthesiology.* 1975;43:89–99.

16. Larach Mg, Rosenberg H, Larach Dr, et al. Prediction of malignant hyperthermia susceptibility by clinical signs. *Anesthesiology.* 1987;66:547–550.

17. Murray MJ, Coursin DB, Scuderi PE, et al. Double-blind, randomized, multicenter study of doxacurium vs. pancuronium in intensive care unit patients who require neuromuscular-blocking agents. *Crit Care Med.* 1995;23:450–458.

3

Airway Management

Patricia Reinhard and Irene P. Osborn

■ INTRODUCTION

Airway management is often a difficult but vitally important skill in the ICU. The first responsibility of a practitioner assessing a critically ill patient is to assess the airway, and if any compromise or potential compromise is found, it must be dealt with as a first priority. Unlike a relatively healthy patient undergoing elective surgery, ICU patients frequently have a wide range of comorbidities, which limit physiology reserve. Therefore, when intubation in the ICU becomes necessary, it is very important for the entire care team to have an effective plan that involves both knowledge of the patient's medical problems and understanding of the various techniques for airway management. Modern airway management has evolved with the introduction of novel supraglottic devices and newer techniques for facilitating endotracheal intubation. This chapter will focus on the management of the difficult airway (DA) and the role of alternative airway devices for managing failed ventilation and/or intubation. It will also discuss techniques for tube changes and extubation in the DA.

P. Reinhard (✉)
Attending Anesthesiologist, Munich, Germany
e-mail: patriciareinhard@web.de

H.L. Frankel and B.P. deBoisblanc (eds.), *Bedside Procedures for the Intensivist*,
DOI 10.1007/978-0-387-79830-1_3,
© Springer Science+Business Media, LLC 2010

■ DEFINITION OF A DIFFICULT AIRWAY

The incidence of difficult ventilation, difficult laryngoscopy, and difficult intubation are not well established. The American Society of Anesthesiologists (ASA) Task Force has defined a difficult airway as "The clinical situation in which a conventionally trained anesthesiologist experiences difficulty with mask ventilation, difficulty with tracheal intubation, or both." The Task Force further noted that the "difficult airway represented a complex interaction between patient factors, the clinical setting, and the skills and preferences of the practitioner." The principal adverse outcomes associated with the difficult airway include (but are not limited to): death, brain injury, myocardial injury, and airway trauma.[1]

■ AIRWAY ASSESSMENT, PREDICTION, AND PREPARATION

The initial step in the difficult airway algorithm (Fig. 3-1) is evaluation and recognition. It is estimated that 1–3% of patients who need endotracheal intubation have existing airway problems that make the procedure more difficult. Although a preprocedural general airway assessment is recommended, often this is not possible in the ICU. Historical information about airway risk may have been communicated prior to the need for intubation, but if not, one must proceed without it. The spontaneously breathing patient with only minimal distress should receive supplemental oxygen and continue to be assessed, while apneic patients require emergent airway management.

Airway evaluation of an ICU patient:

1. Urgency of airway management
2. Assessment of the ability to secure the airway
3. Risk of aspiration
4. Hemodynamics
5. Access to the patient

There are several physical signs that can alert one to the possibility or probability of a patient having a difficult airway (Fig. 3-2). The 6-Ds of airway assessment are one method used to evaluate the signs of difficulty:

1. Disproportion (tongue to pharyngeal size/Mallampati classification)
2. Distortion (e.g., neck mass, short muscular neck)
3. Decreased thyromental distance (receding or weak chin)
4. Decreased interincisor gap (reduced mouth opening)
5. Decreased range of motion of the cervical spine (atlanto-occipital joint assessment)
6. Dental overbite

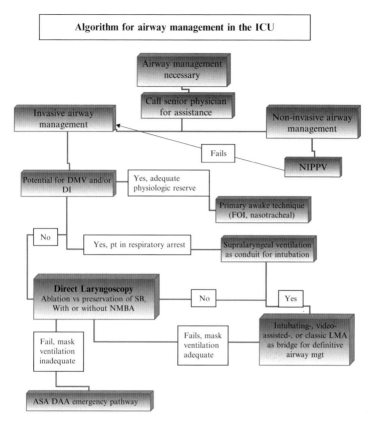

Figure 3-1. Algorithm for airway management in the ICU. NIPPV: Non-invasive positive pressure ventilation; FOI: fiberoptic oral intubation; DMV: difficult mask ventilation; SB: spontaneous breathing; DI: difficult intubation; NMBA: neuro-muscular-blocking-agent.

Difficult laryngoscopy can often be predicted at the time of the initial physical examination, but unexpected difficult laryngoscopy can occasionally occur. Having a prepared action plan for unforeseen difficulties during endotracheal intubation is a critical element in the airway management of ICU patients. The action plan may have to be developed "on the fly," but it begins by assembling all of the personnel and equipment that might be utilized.

Preparation for intubation:

1. The patient must be properly positioned in the "sniffing position" with the patient's head near the head of the bed and with the bed

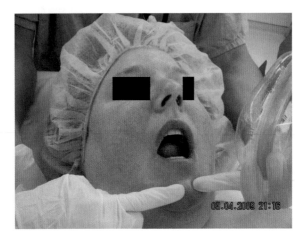

Figure 3-2. Patient with typical features of a potentially difficult airway.

at the proper height so that the operator does not have to bend over and reach.

2. Suction and airway equipment must be available. The location of the difficult airway cart should be ascertained prior to attempts at intubation of the patient.

3. At least one functioning I.V. line must be available for the administration of medications or I.V. fluids.

4. In any airway that is deemed truly difficult, a second experienced critical care physician and an anesthesiologist should be present, if feasible.

5. If the airway presents more than the usual degree of challenge, equipment and expertise for an emergency surgical airway must be immediately available.

6. All medications that might be needed for intubation (propofol, etomidate, neuromuscular blocking agents, phenylephrine, and ephedrine) must be at the bedside.

■ VENTILATION

The ability to ventilate and oxygenate a patient effectively using a bag-mask breathing system is a vital first step in securing the airway. Correct bag-mask ventilation is a lifesaving skill, the nuances of which are often underappreciated. When properly executed, it provides oxygenation with minimal adverse hemodynamic effects. However, if not performed properly it can lead to hypoxemia, gastric inflation, and aspiration. The maximum risk

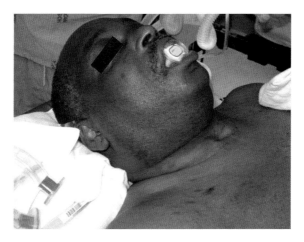

Figure 3-3. Proper head positioning for airway management with oral airway in place mask.

in airway problems arises in the "cannot intubate and cannot ventilate" situation. Therefore, it is very important to perform bag-mask ventilation properly and to have strategies to handle patients who are difficult to ventilate. Bag-mask ventilation is often made more effective with the use of an oral or nasal airway and with proper head positioning (Fig. 3-3).[2]

Predictors of difficult mask ventilation:

- Age over 55 years
- BMI exceeding 26 kg/m^2
- Presence of beard
- Lack of teeth
- History of snoring

To establish sufficient bag-mask ventilation each of the following should be addressed:

1. The patient should be placed in the "sniffing position". This is especially important in obesity.
2. Select the correct size of the facemask.
3. The facemask should be held with the "C-grip" technique. Begin adjusting the mask on the face from nose to mouth to create a good seal. The thumb and index finger should press the mask on to the face, and the rest of the fingers should grab the jaw and lift it (Fig. 3-4).
4. If the single hand technique doesn't provide a good seal, the physician should switch to the "double-C" technique and have an assistant to squeeze the bag.

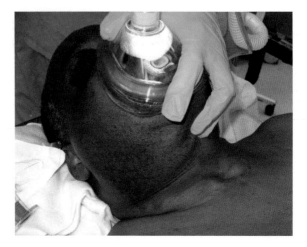

Figure 3-4. Mask ventilation using proper handgrip and jawlift.

5. To avoid gastric insufflation, the bag-mask ventilation should be performed carefully, with low pressure (<20 cm H_2O) and adequate volume.

Occasionally, the base of the tongue may fall back into the velopharynx and obstruct the airway. In this case, an oropharyngeal airway may be gently inserted. To quickly determine the appropriate size of the oropharyngeal airway, one can measure the distance from the corner of the mouth to the earlobe of the patient. Improper placement of the oropharyngeal airway may worsen airway obstruction by forcing the tongue backward. A tongue depressor can be used to facilitate placement of the oropharyngeal airway if placement is difficult.

If the bag-mask ventilation with an oropharyngeal airway fails, the intensive care physician should consider the placement of a supraglottic airway (SGA). The SGA represents a major advance in airway management and has been incorporated into difficult airway algorithms. The SGA allows ventilation and oxygenation with less stimulation than laryngoscopy and intubation, but it does not guarantee protection against aspiration. If patients are actively vomiting or known to have a full stomach then SGAs are not recommended. However, if ventilation is impossible and the patient is becoming hypoxic, then SGA placement and ventilation can be life-saving.

The laryngeal mask airway (LMA) is the most commonly used SGA. It acts as a cross between a facemask and endotracheal intubation (ET).[3] In general, a size 4 LMA is used for women and size 5 is used for men.

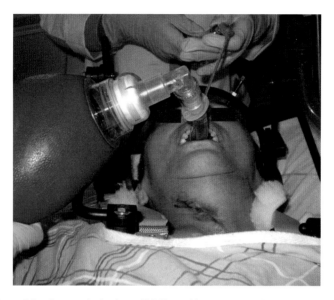

Figure 3-5. A supraglottic airway (SGA) used for rescue ventilation in a patient.

The insertion technique for most SGA's is best accomplished with patient's head in the "sniffing position." The device is pushed along the roof of the mouth and the posterior wall of the pharynx (the same route a bolus of food would follow), until it stops. The correctly positioned SGA tip lies at, and partially blocks, the upper esophagus. It is very important to avoid over-inflation of the cuff of any SGA device. This happens commonly in an effort to achieve a good seal and is often the source of problems. In general, a SGA can be used as a temporary ventilation device and can be removed for intubation (Fig. 3-5). Most SGAs can be used as conduits for fiberoptic intubation or bronchoscopy.[4] If the patient is known to be difficult to ventilate, use of the intubating LMA (ILMA) should be considered.

The ILMA consists of a mask attached to an anatomically shaped rigid stainless steel shaft that aligns the barrel aperature to the glottic aperature. The ILMA has a 13-mm internal diameter that can accommodate an 8.0-mm cuffed endotracheal tube, which can be inserted into the larynx either blindly or with fiberoptic assistance (see below). The device is short enough to ensure that the tracheal tube cuff extends beyond the vocal cords. The mask of the ILMA is similar to the classic LMA except that it does not have aperture bars but instead has an epiglottic-elevating bar, which facilitates tube placement. The device is best utilized with special

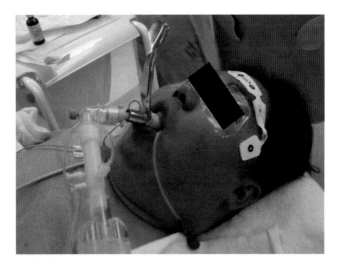

Figure 3-6. An intubating laryngeal mask airway (ILMA) in place with endotracheal tube inserted.

tubes that have a soft, blunt tip that can be exchanged for a regular ETT if mechanical ventilation is anticipated for several days or copious secretions exist (Fig. 3-6).

■ INTUBATION

The purpose of direct laryngoscopy is to provide adequate visualization of the glottis to allow correct placement of the endotracheal tube with minimal effort, elapsed time, and potential for injury to the patient. The Macintosh blade is generally recommended, since the tongue is easier to control.[5] Regardless of handedness of the operator, the laryngoscope is always held in the left hand near the junction between the handle and blade of the laryngoscope. The laryngoscopist opens the mouth with the right hand using "the scissor" technique. The blade is then inserted in the right side of the patient's mouth so that the incisor teeth are avoided and the tongue is deflected to the left, away from the lumen of the blade. Pressure on the teeth or gums must be avoided as the blade is advanced forward and centrally toward the epiglottis in the vallecula. The laryngoscopist's wrist is held firmly as the laryngoscope is lifted along the axis of the handle to produce the anterior displacement of the tongue and epiglottis that brings the laryngeal structures into view. The handle should not be rotated or flexed as it is lifted, as these maneuvers can cause injury to the

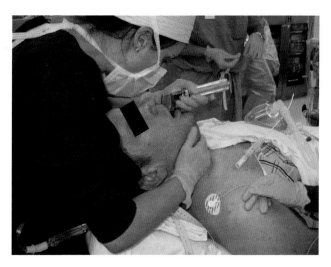

Figure 3-7. Direct laryngoscopy for intubation.

patient's upper teeth or gums (Fig. 3-7). In a difficult airway case, direct laryngoscopy may not provide an adequate view to safely place the endotracheal tube. There are several intubating stylettes on the market that can facilitate a difficult intubation. Ideally, an intubating stylette should be approximately 60-cm-long, 15-French sized, stiff yet malleable, and has a 40° curve approximately 3.5 cm from the distal tip to lift the epiglottis. In addition, newer models are hollow to permit jet ventilation if the operator is unable to pass the endotracheal tube. It has been used successfully in patients with a poor laryngoscopic view.[6] It is passed in the midline under the epiglottis and into the airway. A characteristic "clicking" may be felt as the stylette moves down the trachea over the tracheal cartilages. Once the stylette is in the trachea, the endotracheal tube is loaded over it and advanced into position and then the stylette is removed.

Intubation using an intubating stylette:

1. The laryngocopist must first visualize the glottis in the standard fashion.
2. The stylette should then be inserted with the "hockey stick" end first using the tip to lift the epiglottis and bring the vocal cords into view. The stylette should then be advanced in the midline gliding along the posterior surface of the epiglottis through the vocal cords and into the trachea. When properly placed, the tip of the stylette can often be felt skipping along the tracheal cartilages.
3. The laryngocopist must keep the view and hold the stylette while an assistant loads a lubricated ETT over the free end of the stylette.

4. The laryngoscopist must then move the stylette backwards until the free end sticks out beyond the end of the ETT and can be held by the assistant.
5. The stylette should be immobilized by the assistant while the ETT is advanced by the laryngoscopist into trachea under direct laryngoscopy. The endotracheal tube has to be grasped at its midpoint and rotated 90° counterclockwise so that the Murphy eye is anterior. This maneuver prevents the tube tip from hanging up on the right arytenoid. Hang-up occurs because the stylette falls posteriorly into the interarytenoid fissure. If the tube still hangs up, the tube has to be rotated another 90° counterclockwise. The endotracheal tube is advanced until the 22- or 23-cm mark on the tube is at the teeth.
6. The stylette can then be removed by the assistant while the ETT is held in place by the laryngoscopist.
7. The cuff of the ETT should be inflated, and oxygenation and ventilation through the ETT are confirmed by the use of SpO_2, $ETCO_2$, and breath sounds.

After an LMA has been placed to ventilate a patient, it can also be used as a conduit for a fiberoptic intubation. Fiberoptic intubation has become a common technique in the ICU practice, but it requires advanced fiberoptic skills and is therefore usually performed by pulmonologists, anesthesiologists, and ENT physicians. The technique can be performed nasally or orally in both awake and anesthetized patients. The first step is to decide whether to do a fiberoptic intubation with the patient anesthetized or awake. This decision depends on the ability to easily ventilate the anesthetized patient and the need to evaluate the awake patient after intubation. Furthermore, the physician must decide if the patient will be intubated orally or nasally. There are no specific contraindications to fiberoptic intubation, but under certain circumstances, such as major bleeding, copious secretions in the airway, and massive facial injury, successful fiberoptic intubation may be nearly impossible. Furthermore, awake fiberoptic intubation can be extremely difficult in uncooperative or combative patients.

The fiberoptic intubation through an LMA has two main advantages. With the help of a swivel adaptor, the ventilation of the patient can be continued while the LMA is used as a guide for the bronchoscope. This method is ideal for inexperienced bronchoscopists, since usually there is less that 5 cm to navigate the fiberscope from the LMA to the glottis. In addition, secretions and tissue are moved aside to allow a better view. This technique is also useful for bronchoscopy and airway inspection in the extubated patient. The LMA has been used to successfully intubate adults with a history of difficult tracheal intubation, limited mouth opening, or restricted neck movement.[7]

Fiberoptic intubation through an LMA:

1. Video bronchoscopy should be used whenever possible to enable all assistants to identify the next steps in the procedure.

2. If possible the bronchoscope and its cart should be placed on the left side of the patient to avoid crossing of cables; since the fiberoptic cables exit on the left side of the scope handle, it is properly held in the left hand. Make sure all cables are free of loops.
3. Lubricate the fiberoptic scope with a small amount of water-soluble lubricant, and apply defogging solution to the tip.
4. Choice of an appropriate endotracheal tube depends on the internal diameter of the LMA.
5. The endotracheal tube should be loaded all the way on to the scope and gently secured in position with tape.
6. A little lubricant should be smeared on to the cuff and distal end of the endotracheal tube.
7. The fiberscope should then be passed through LMA "guide," under epiglottis, until a clear view of glottis is obtained.
8. The fiberscope should be advanced well into trachea until the carina is in view.
9. The left hand is used to loosen the endotracheal tube connector from the bronchoscope handle. The fiberscope should be held immobile while the lubricated ETT is advanced over it, through LMA and into trachea. The endotracheal tube has to be grasped at its midpoint and rotated 90° counterclockwise so that the Murphy eye is anterior. This maneuver prevents the tube tip from hanging up on the right arytenoid. Hang-up occurs because the fiberoptic shaft falls posteriorly into the interarytenoid fissure. If the tube still hangs up, the tube has to be rotated another 90° counterclockwise.
10. The endotracheal tube is advanced into the trachea over the bronchoscope shaft until the 22- or 23-cm mark on the tube is at the teeth.
11. ETT and LMA should be immobilized when the fiberoptic scope is withdrawn.
12. The cuff of the ETT should be inflated, and oxygenation and ventilation through the ETT are confirmed by the use of SpO_2, $ETCO_2$, and breath sounds.
13. LMA should then be deflated and ETT secured to shaft of the device.
14. The entire unit (ETT and LMA) should remain in place until the ETT is exchanged over an exchange catheter.

To remove the LMA, an ETT change over an airway exchange catheter has to be performed:

LMA/ETT exchange using an airway exchange catheter:

1. To measure the depth of insertion that is required for the exchange catheter, the catheter should be held over the torso and the length from incisors to the mid-sternum noted.
2. A stiff 80 cm hollow airway exchange catheter should be passed through ETT well into the trachea to the measured length.
3. The airway exchange catheter should be fixed in place to permit removal of the LMA and ETT over airway exchange catheter.

4. The new ETT should then be loaded over the exchange catheter into trachea.
5. If the ETT hangs up on the vocal cords, it may have to be slightly withdrawn, rotated 90° and then readvanced as described above.
6. The ETT must be held securely to remove the airway exchange catheter.
7. The cuff of the ETT should be inflated, and oxygenation and ventilation through the ETT are confirmed by the use of SpO_2, $ETCO_2$, and breath sounds.
8. The ETT should then be secured.

In the absence of a video bronchoscope, operators may perform blind intubation passing a custom ETT through an ILMA by use of the "Chandy maneuver." The Chandy maneuver consists of two steps, which are performed sequentially. The first step, which is important for establishing optimal ventilation, is to rotate the ILMA slightly in the sagittal plane using the metal handle until the least resistance to bag ventilation is achieved. The second step is performed just before blind intubation and consists of using the metal handle to lift slightly (but not tilt) the ILMA away from the posterior pharyngeal wall.

Blind intubation through an ILMA (Fig. 3-8):

1. The ILMA must be advanced into the pharynx by following the natural curvature of the patient's upper airway.
2. With the patient breathing oxygen, the Chandy maneuver should be used to optimize the position of the ILMA.
3. The custom ETT should be inserted into the shaft of the ILMA. Slight resistance to advancing the ETT may be felt as the horizontal marking on the tube aligns with the proximal end of the ILMA.

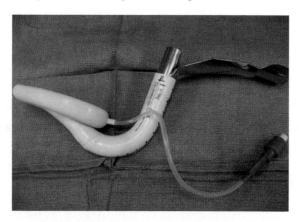

Figure 3-8. The intubating laryngeal mask airway (ILMA).

This position marks the depth at which the endotracheal tube impacts the epiglottic elevating bar in the bowl of the mask.

4. The custom ETT should then advance without resistance toward the glottis opening and the trachea.
5. After verification of endotracheal intubation, the cuff of the ILMA should be deflated, the 15 mm endotracheal tube connector disconnected, and the ILMA removed by using the stabilizing bar to push the endotracheal tube through the ILMA.
6. The 15-mm connector should be reattached to the breathing circuit and ventilation begun.

With proper patient preparation, fiberoptic intubation can be less stimulating than intubation performed under direct laryngoscopy. The timely administration of an antisialagogue, the application of topical anesthesia (Table 3-1), and the administration of light sedation (Table 3-2) greatly facilitate the procedure. Since all equipment to perform fiberoptic intubation may not be readily available in the ICU setting, proper preparation for the circumstances is necessary.

Fiberoptic intubation can be performed in an unconscious, spontaneously breathing patient with the use of an intubating oropharyngeal airway.

Table 3-1. Topical anesthetic agents.

Agent	Dosing and Administration	Comments
Benzocaine	Hurricaine® spray 60 mg/s Topex® metered dose spray 50 mg/spray	Toxicity observed with excessive spray
Cetacaine®	Apply spray for <1 s	Delivers 200 mg benzocaine/ butyl amino benzoate/tetracaine residue/second
Lidocaine	4% topical, direct spray 1–5 ml (40–200 mg) or nebulize 4–5 ml	Maximum adult dose 10 ml of 4% solution (400 mg). More effective after glycopyrrolate (0.2 mg IV or IM)
	2% viscous, gargle 15 ml solution	No greater than 8 doses in 24 h period
	2% jelly, apply to ETT shortly before use	No more than 600 mg or 30 ml of lidocaine jelly per 12 h period
Tetracaine	2% solution, apply with cotton pledgetts	Maximum dose 100–200 mg
	0.5% nebulized	Lower threshold for CNS symptoms compared to lidocaine
Cocaine	4% solution apply topically with cotton applicators	Maximum dose 1–3 mg/ kg (or 400 mg)caution in patients with sepsis or traumatized mucosa in area of application

Table 3-2. Agents for sedation.

Agent	Dose	Actions	Side Effects
Midazolam	1–4 mg (.075 mg/kg) slow intravenous bolus	Sedation, amnesia	Respiratory depression at high doses
Fentanyl	50–100 ug (1.0 µg/kg) slow intravenous bolus	Analgesia	Respiratory depression, antitussive
Ketamine	0.5–1 mg/kg slow intravenous bolus	Sedation, analgesia at higher doses	Salivation, hallucination
Remifentanil	0.05 µg/kg/min intravenous infusion	Analgesia, antitussive	Respiratory depression, bradycardia
Dexmedetomidine	1 µg/kg intravenous bolus over 10 min, followed by 0.7 µg/kg/h intravenous infusion	Slow onset sedation without coma, maintains respiration	Occasional hypotension

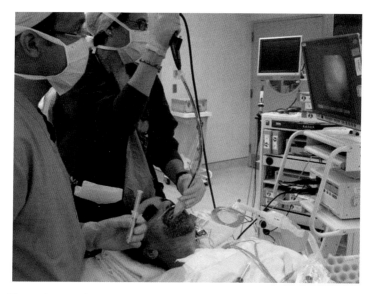

Figure 3-9 Intubation using the flexible fiberoptic bronchoscope.

Fiberoptic intubation in an unconscious spontaneously breathing patient:

1. As soon as the patient is prepared for the procedure an Ovassapian or other airway is inserted as a guide (Fig. 3-9).
2. The fiberoptic scope with ETT preloaded is advanced along the airway until the epiglottis can just be visualized.
3. The scope is guided under the epiglottis until you see glottis and cords.
4. The fiberoptic is advanced so far until the carina can be seen and the intubation is accomplished as described above.

Another technique for patients with limited mouth opening or respiratory failure is the fiberoptically assisted nasal intubation. The patient's nose is prepared as described and an ETT size 6.5–7.5 is gently advanced into the nostril until it meets resistance at the nasopharynx. At this point, the fiberoptic scope is advanced until the glottis structures are visualized. Topical lidocaine is administered if the patient is stable enough to wait for anesthetic effects to develop and then the fiberoptic scope is advanced into the trachea and the ETT inserted as described above. This is a useful maneuver when oral intubation has failed.

Videolaryngoscopy is the latest in an expanding array of airway devices for difficult and failed intubation. Videolaryngoscopes have a light source and either fiberoptic bundles or a video camera chip built directly into the tip of a range of different-sized Macintosh shaped blades. A magnified image from the tip of the blade is relayed to a video screen. This technology provides improved laryngeal views compared with direct laryngoscopy, both because the view is wide-angled (60° view vs. 10° view provided by direct laryngoscopy) and because the view is from the tip of the blade rather than through the incisors allowing the laryngoscopist to "look around the corner" (Fig. 3-10a). Additionally, the video image permits assistants to externally manipulate the larynx into better view and

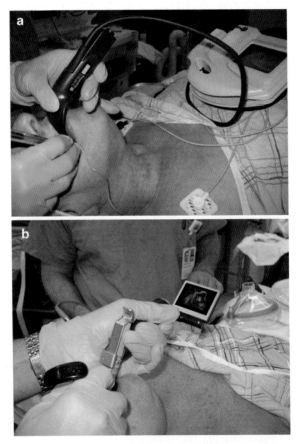

Figure 3-10. (a) GlideScope® Ranger videolaryngoscope. (b) McGrath® videolaryngoscope.

permits supervisors to watch the endotracheal tube passing through the cords allowing immediate and direct confirmation of successful intubation. It has been shown that the use of a videolaryngoscope frequently improves intubation success (Fig. 3-10b).

In order to benefit from this new technology, it is important to remember that the view on the screen is a "virtual view" of the glottis in contrast to the direct line-of-site view during direct laryngoscopy. Therefore, it is essential that you obtain the best view possible before advancing the ETT. If the epiglottis, vocal cords, and arytenoids cannot be seen in the same view, then the device should be slightly withdrawn until the epiglottis flips down and the full view is obtained. With videolaryngoscopy, it is often better to use an intubating stylette technique as described above to avoid obscuring the view with the ETT.

■ ETT CHANGES

If an ETT cuff is leaking, partially obstructed with concretions, or does not permit adequate ventilation because of a small size, then it should be changed. Tube changes can be particularly hazardous in critically ill patients especially if previously difficult to intubate. Performing a tube change with videolaryngoscopy is quite helpful. It permits inspection of the larynx and placement of the ETT under constant view, reducing the risk of laryngeal injury especially if the supraglottic structures are swollen. Furthermore assistants have the advantage of being able to visualize difficulties in tube advancement as they develop.

Endotracheal tube exchanges:

1. Preoxygenate and deeply sedate the patient, making sure that there is an adequate backup rate of ventilation if apnea ensues. Topical lidocaine instilled down the existing ETT can help reduce coughing. Often neuromuscular blockade will be required.
2. Determine the depth of insertion of the airway exchange catheter by measuring the length of the existing ETT with its connector and swivel adaptor and then adding the distance from the existing ETT to the carina.
3. The existing ETT should be untaped.
4. A laryngoscopist should expose the larynx as described above while holding on to the existing ETT.
5. A lubricated, stiff, hollow airway exchange catheter of >80 cm in length should be inserted down the existing ETT with side-ported end first to the predetermined depth by using the markings on the side of the catheter.
6. The ETT cuff should be deflated by an assistant and the old ETT removed while the assistant carefully holds the airway exchange catheter in place.

7. Maintaining position of the airway exchange catheter using the patient's mouth or nasal orifice as a landmark, the new ETT should then be loaded and advanced over the airway exchange catheter to the appropriate level.

8. If resistance is encountered, the ETT should be gently rotated and advanced as described above. In patients with very tenuous oxygenation, oxygen can be jetted through the hollow lumen of the airway exchange catheter during the exchange.

9. The balloon cuff of the new ETT should be inflated once it is in position and the airway exchange catheter removed by the assistant while the laryngoscopist holds the new ETT in place.

10. Confirmation of placement should be performed using standard methods.

■ EXTUBATION

The extubation of a critically ill patient with a difficult airway should be done only after careful assessment of gas exchange, ventilatory mechanics, hemodynamic stability, level of consciousness, effectiveness of cough, volume of secretions, upper airway patency, and need for deep sedation or general anesthesia in the near future. Several factors are associated with a relatively high incidence of failed extubation in intensive care: difficult intubation, obesity, prolonged intubation, neuromuscular disease, and surgical procedures of the head and neck.

Assessment of extubation criteria:

1. Underlying cause of respiratory failure improving (e.g., sepsis).
2. Spontaneous breathing trial with a frequency/tidal volume ratio of <100.
3. Negative inspiratory muscle force <20 cm H_2O.
4. SpO_2 ≥90%, FIO_2 ≤0.5, PEEP≤5 cm H_2O during spontaneous breathing trial.
5. Hemodynamically stable off of vasoactive drugs.
6. Patient verbally and physically responsive to simple commands.
7. Good head and neck control with good gag reflex and cough.
8. Positive cuff leak test (>10% of delivered tidal volume escapes through the mouth when the ETT cuff is deflated).

The ASA Task Force on Difficult Airway Management recommends that anesthesiologists and critical care physicians develop a preformulated strategy for extubation of patients with difficult airways including:

1. Evaluation for general clinical factors that may produce an adverse impact on postextubation ventilation.
2. Formulation of an airway management plan that can be implemented if the patient is not able to maintain adequate ventilation after

extubation, e.g., if a patient suffers airway obstruction following extubation, an oral airway may be needed.

3. Consideration of the short-term use of a small, stiff, hollow airway exchange catheter to be used as a guide for reintubation. The airway exchange catheter is inserted through the lumen of the ETT into the trachea before the ETT is removed.

■ CONCLUSION

The difficult airway continues to be an unexpected challenge in intensive care medicine. Having a plan for management can reduce complications and improve outcome. It is essential to first identify patients with potentially difficult airways. We have reviewed the guidelines for assessment, the necessary advanced airway skills, and a variety of devices available for difficult and failed intubation. Importantly, communication and teamwork among nursing staff and other professionals will facilitate the care of these patients.

■ REFERENCES

1. Practice guidelines for management of the difficult airway. An updated report by the American Society of Anesthesiologists Task Force on Management of the Difficult Airway. *Anesthesiology*. 2003;98:1269-1277.
2. Hillman DR, Platt PR, Eastwood PR. The upper airway during anaesthesia. *Br J Anaesth*. 2003;91(1):31-39.
3. Verghese C, Brimacombe JR. Survey of laryngeal mask airway usage in 11, 910 patients: safety and efficacy for conventional and nonconventional usage. *Anesth Analg*. 1996;82:129-133.
4. Ferson DB. Laryngeal mask airway. In: Hagberg CA, ed. *Benumof's Airway Management*. 2nd ed. Elsevier: Mosby; 2007:476-501.
5. Cassel W. Advantages of a curved laryngoscope. *Anesthesiology*. 1942;3:580.
6. Latto IP, Stacey M, Mecklenburgh J, Vaughan RS. Survey of the use of the gum elastic bougie in clinical practice. *Anaesthesia*. 2002;57:379-384.
7. Lee CM, Yang HS. Case of difficult intubation overcome by the laryngeal mask airway. *J Korean Med Sci*. 1993;8:290-292.

4

Ultrasound Physics and Equipment

Sarah B. Murthi, Mary Ferguson, and Amy C. Sisley

■ INTRODUCTION

The physics of ultrasound can seem both dry and complicated, but by understanding a few basic principles, essential lessons about its strengths and limitations become clearer. Additionally, concepts that can help optimize image acquisition will have a context and be more easily remembered.

Sound is simply the transmission of energy in the form of mechanical vibrations through a medium. The ultrasound signal is sent from the transducer at a set frequency. By interpreting the signal when it returns to the transducer after reflection from an object, an image is generated. While the rest of ultrasound physics can become very complex, it all arises from this simple concept. This chapter focuses on the mechanics of sound waves, image formation, the modes of ultrasound, ultrasound artifacts, and a review of basic instrumentation.

A.C. Sisley (✉)
Department of Trauma and Critical Care, R. Adams Cowley Shock Trauma Center, University of Maryland, Baltimore, MD, USA
e-mail: asisley@umm.edu

H.L. Frankel and B.P. deBoisblanc (eds.), *Bedside Procedures for the Intensivist*,
DOI 10.1007/978-0-387-79830-1_4,
© Springer Science+Business Media, LLC 2010

Physics

Sound Waves

Sound travels in sinusoidal waves (Fig. 4-1), which can be characterized in terms of amplitude, frequency, wavelength and velocity, or speed of propagation.

- The *amplitude* of an ultrasound wave refers to the strength of the signal and is measured in decibels (dB). In audible sound, amplitude is analogous to "loudness."
  - In generating a two-dimensional (2D) ultrasound image, the amplitude of the return signal is assigned a pixel value, which is displayed on the screen such that returning signals with higher amplitude appear brighter.
- The *frequency* of sound is measured as cycles per second or Hertz (Hz). Sound audible to the human ear is in the range of 20 Hz to 20 kHz.
  - Sound frequencies above the audible range are referred to as ultrasound. The range for diagnostic ultrasound is between 1 and 20 mega (million) Hertz (MHz).

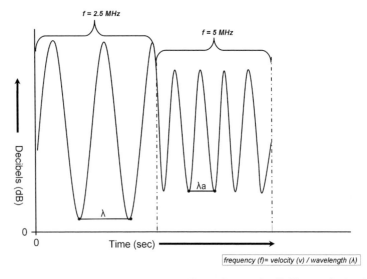

frequency (f) = velocity (v) / wavelength (λ)

Figure 4-1. A sinusoidal wave at two different frequencies (*f*). The amplitude of the wave is measured in decibels. The first wave (*left*) has a longer wavelength (λ) and thus a lower *f*. The second wave (*right*) has a shorter λ_a and a higher *f*. To the human ear, amplitude is heard as loudness whereas *f* is heard as pitch.

- – Doppler ultrasound displays the change in the frequency of the return signal (or Doppler shift). This is in contrast to 2D ultrasound, which is a visual display of the amplitude of the return signal.
- The *wavelength* of an ultrasound signal is inversely related to the frequency of the signal. The shorter the wavelength, the more cycles per second, the greater the frequency of the wave.
- The *velocity* of an ultrasound wave is proportional to the density of the tissue it travels through.
  - – The velocity through a low-density medium, such as air (330 m/s), is much less than the speed of propagation through a higher density medium such as liver (1,550 m/s).
  - – The clinical implications of this are simple: ultrasound does not transmit well through air. Hence, optimizing an ultrasound image involves positioning the patient and the transducer to avoid air-filled structures such as lung tissue or bowel.
  - – Most of the soft tissues in the human body as well as blood have similar densities and therefore a similar propagation speed of, on an average, 1,540 m/s.

The relationship between these variables is described by the equation:

$$\text{Velocity } (v) = \text{wavelength } (\lambda) \times \text{frequency } (f)$$

The importance of this relationship is its effect on the depth of penetration of the signal and on image resolution. A high-frequency signal with its shorter wavelength will interact with more (and smaller) molecules in the imaged tissue than a low-frequency wave. This provides for greater image resolution; however, it also results in more rapid degradation of the signal. Conversely, a low-frequency signal with a longer wavelength interacts with fewer molecules in the tissue. This results in poorer resolution but greater depth of penetration in the tissues. Unfortunately, this means that there is an inescapable trade-off between resolution and depth of penetration (Table 4-1).

Image Formation

An ultrasound image is obtained when a signal generated by the transducer propagates through the tissue and is reflected back to the transducer. The transducer both transmits and receives the ultrasound signal. This is possible because crystals in the transducer head rapidly expand and contract when an electric current is applied, producing vibrations in the form of ultrasound waves. The same crystals when impacted by the returning sound waves deform and generate an electric current.

Table 4-1. Comparison of high- and low-frequency transducers.

Ultrasound Modality	Common Clinical Applications	Uses	Property Displayed	Alignment of Transducer	Optimal Resolution
Two dimensional	FAST Thoracic ultrasound Echocardiography Guided procedures	Real-time anatomic assessment	Amplitude (dB)	Perpendicular	High frequency
M-mode	Echocardiography IVC diameter assessment	Detailed measurement of anatomic change	Amplitude (dB)	Perpendicular	High frequency
CW Doppler	Echocardiography	High-velocity blood flow	Frequency (kHz)	Parallel	Low frequency
PW Doppler	Echocardiography	Blood flow at a specific anatomic point	Frequency (kHz)	Parallel	Low frequency
CF Doppler	Echocardiography Vascular assessment	Direction of blood flow in a 2D image	Frequency (color)	Parallel	Low frequency

- This useful property is termed the piezoelectric effect, and the crystals, which include quartz and titanate ceramics, are called piezoelectric crystals.
- Lead zirconate titanate (PZT) is the crystal most commonly used in modern diagnostic ultrasound transducers.
- The number of crystals in the transducer is generally between 64 and 128.
- The signal frequency that the transducer emits is determined by the thickness of the crystal and the voltage applied to it.

This ability to both send and receive a signal allows the returning signal to be interpreted in terms of density and depth. A corresponding image is created, which provides a vast amount of clinical information.

- *Density*: The denser the structure visualized, the more intense the received signal to the transducer and the brighter the corresponding pixel on the screen. Thus bone is white, solid organs gray and fluid black.
- *Depth*: The amount of time that elapses between the emission and return of the signal, known as the "go-return" time, allows the depth of the structure to be determined using the range equation.
- Distance from transducer = ½[go-return time] × 1,540 m/s.
- This is the speed of propagation, multiplied by the time it takes to send and receive the signal divided by 2. This accounts for the time it takes for the signal to return, allowing for the depth of the original signal to be determined.

The piezoelectric crystals in the transducer emit brief pulses of ultrasound and then listen for returning signals. This is necessary in order for the range equation to be useful in assigning depth to the returning signal. If the transducer continuously generated ultrasound waves then ultrasound waves would be continuously returning. It would then be impossible to determine when any particular returning wave had been emitted.

To allow the crystal to listen for the return signal, the originating signal is pulsed followed by a pause; pulse-pause, pulse-pause (Fig. 4-2). The pause time is also called the dead time, and this is when the crystal receives or listens to the return signal.

- The pulse-pause time is called the pulse repetition period (PRP).
- The number of signals in a second, or frequency, is called the pulse repetition frequency (PRF).
- The time dedicated to the pulse is a small fraction of the PRP, only 0.1%. Since the "go-return" time is longer for deeper structures, lengthening the pause time can increase resolution of deeper structures such as the kidney and the heart. In ultrasound, listening is more important than transmitting.

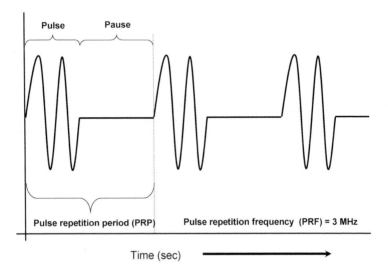

Figure 4-2. The pulse repetition period (PRP) includes the pulse of the ultrasound signal and the pause time. The signal is a sinusoidal wave. The number if PRP sent per second is the pulse repetition frequency (PRF).

Reflection

Image formation depends on the reflection of the ultrasound wave from the tissues back to the transducer. The amount of the ultrasound wave reflected depends in part on the differences in acoustic impedance between tissues.

- Acoustic impedance is the product of the density of the tissue and the velocity of the sound wave:
  - Acoustic impedance $(Z) = $ velocity $(v) \times$ density (ρ).
  - An acoustic impedance mismatch occurs when sound waves encounter a boundary between tissues of different density resulting in increased reflection of the signal. This means that ultrasound images enhance tissue boundaries and interfaces.
  - The border of a kidney appears bright because of an impedance mismatch between the liver and Gerota's fascia. The kidney and the liver have the similar densities. However, the fascia of the kidney is much denser and reflects the signal back more strongly.
- The amount of ultrasound that is reflected back to the transducer also depends upon the angle between the transducer and the object being imaged. In 2D ultrasound, a 90° angle (perpendicular) yields maximum reflection. This a key point to remember in obtaining ultrasound images. Continuously angling the transducer over the organ of interest will help to achieve this 90° angle and optimize the image.

Attenuation

As an ultrasound wave propagates through a medium, the signal strength degrades or becomes attenuated. The degree of attenuation depends on two factors: the frequency of the ultrasound wave and the distance it has traveled.

Attenuation (dB) = $\frac{1}{2}$ [frequency (MHz)]×[distance traveled (cm)]

This phenomenon is familiar to all of us in terms of audible sound. The farther away you are from the source of a sound, the more difficult it is to hear. Additionally, anyone who has stopped at a traffic light next to a fellow traveler blasting a car radio is aware that lower frequency sounds (bass) travel farther than the higher frequency sounds. The same characteristics are true of ultrasound. The question is, where does the signal go?

- Reflection of some of the ultrasound waves back to the transducer partially accounts for attenuation. While reflection is helpful in terms of forming an ultrasound image, it necessarily results in some signal loss.
- Absorption occurs when the ultrasound wave interacts with the molecules in the tissue and is converted to heat, and is also responsible for some signal loss.
- Finally, scattering refers to radiation of the ultrasound wave in all directions with only a small proportion reflected back to the transducer. This occurs when the ultrasound wave interacts with small structures (less than 1 wavelength).

High-frequency ultrasound waves undergo more attenuation than low frequencies and therefore penetrate less deeply into tissues. The depth of penetration of ultrasound is limited to approximately 200 wavelengths. Beyond this point, attenuation results in too much degradation of the signal to return useful information to the transducer.

- Since higher frequency waves have shorter wavelengths, the depth of 200 wavelengths is less than that for lower frequency waves with longer wavelengths.
- The depth of tissue penetration for a 1-MHz transducer is approximately 30 cm, while that for a 5-MHz transducer is 6 cm and a 20-MHz transducer only 1.5 cm.

The process of displaying the return signal as a visual representation of the data is complex and beyond the scope of this chapter. In short, the return wave is converted into a voltage signal and then into digital data. Both the voltage signal and the digital data are processed and enhanced, so that a meaningful image is produced on the screen. This is done through electronics, circuitry, and computer analysis in the transducer head and in the ultrasound machine itself.

Table 4-2. Modalities of ultrasound.

Frequency (MHz)	Wavelength (l)	Resolution	Penetration (cm)
Low (2.5)	Long	Low	High
High (10 MHz)	Short	High	Low

Modes of Ultrasound

There are three primary modes of ultrasound: two-dimensional (2D), M-mode, and Doppler. Each mode provides important clinical information and has distinct clinical applications (Table 4-2).

2D Ultrasound

To create a moving 2D image, multiple piezoelectric crystals work in concert. An array of 64–128 crystals is used to produce a beam. To see movement over time, the beam must be repeatedly swept across the field of interest.

- A beam is a collection of scan lines, each scan line produced by one crystal. The more scan lines there are, the more data provided and the better the resolution of the image.
- The higher the density of scan lines, the longer it takes the beam to sweep a given area.
- The length of time allocated for the sweep is the frame rate. The frame rate and the number of scan lines are inversely proportional.

For moving structures such as the heart, a high frame rate is needed to create a smooth moving image. This is referred to as temporal resolution, which is the ability to accurately track movement of a structure. To illustrate this concept, consider that the aortic valve can move from completely closed to completely open in 0.04 s. If the frame rate is 30 frames per second, it would take 0.03 s for each sweep. The valve would very likely appear open in one frame and closed in the next. The details of leaflet motion would be lost. As with all things ultrasound, there is a trade-off. In this case, the cost of a higher frame rate is a decrease in scan line density and poorer image resolution.

M-mode Ultrasound

M-mode, one of the earliest methods of ultrasound, sends a signal along a narrow slice of the image, sometimes called an "ice pick" view (Fig. 4-3). Because the field is much smaller, the temporal or time-related resolution is greatly improved. A much narrower field is seen, but it is seen continually.

- M-mode allows for exact measurements of wall diameter changes and valvular function. This makes it a valuable tool in the intensive care unit (ICU).

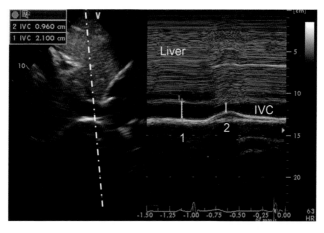

Figure 4-3. The *dotted line* (cursor) on the *left* defines the "ice pick" or M-mode image on the *right*. The diameter of the IVC during tidal ventilation is denoted by the numbers 1 and 2. Note the >50% compression of the vessel during inspiration, indicating hypovolemia (see text).

- Example: Using M-mode is one of the best ways to determine if a pericardial effusion is causing tamponade.
- If the right ventricular wall collapses in diastole, it is evidence that the pericardial effusion is obstructing flow into the heart and confirms that tamponade physiology is present.
- M-mode is also useful in quantifying the diameter change in the inferior vena cava with respiration, which can help determine if a patient may respond to volume with an increase in cardiac output (Fig. 4-3).
- M-mode may seem difficult to interpret at first, because it is not as intuitive as 2D ultrasound. However, its applications in the ICU are relatively straight forward and can be readily mastered with practice.

Doppler Ultrasound

The *amplitude* of the return signal is displayed in 2D ultrasound; this is analogous to loudness. Conversely, the *Doppler shift* (f_{dop}) is displayed in Doppler ultrasound. The Doppler shift can be used to measure the velocity of blood flow.

- The Doppler shift is the familiar change in pitch (frequency) heard when a speeding train approaches and then passes a stationary listener: as the train approaches, the pitch of the engine becomes higher and then drops just after the train passes.

- A stationary object will reflect the original signal at the same frequency at which it was sent, so that $f_0 = f_r$, where f_0 is the frequency of the original signal and f_r is the return signal. The frequency of the ultrasound transducer is f_0.
- An object in motion, relative to the transducer, will reflect a signal back to the transducer with a different frequency.
- If the object is moving toward the transducer, f_r will increase; if it is moving away, f_r will decrease. The magnitude of that change is called the Doppler shift (f_{dop}).
- Because f_0 is known, as it is a property of the transducer, and f_r can be measured, f_{dop} can be easily obtained by subtracting out f_0.
- The range for f_{dop} is much lower than f_0, in the 5–10 kHz range, and easily heard by the human ear.
- Example: If a 5-MHz transducer emits a signal that impacts blood flowing toward the transducer at a velocity such that f_r increases to 5.01 MHz, then for blood flowing away at the same velocity f_r will decrease to 4.09 MHz. In this case, the f_{dop} is 0.01 MHz or 10 kHz.

The relationship between the Doppler shift and blood flow velocity can be expressed as:

$$f_{dop} = \left[(2f_0 v) / c \right] \times (\cos \theta)$$

where v is the velocity of blood, c is a constant, and θ is the angle of the ultrasound beam hitting the flow of blood, which termed the angle of acquisition. Because the f_0 is fixed for a given transducer, and c is constant, this equation can be restated more simply as:

$$f_{dop} \, \alpha \, v (\cos \theta)$$

Note that the Doppler shift (f_{dop}) is directly proportional to the blood velocity (v).

- The peak of a Doppler waveform provides a measure of the velocity of blood at that time point.
- In calculating blood velocity, the angle of acquisition is critically important.
- When the ultrasound beam is aligned *parallel* to blood flow, the angle of acquisition is 0°. Note that the cosine of 0 is 1.
  - As the angle of acquisition increases from 0 to 90°, the cosine decreases from 1 to 0.
- The measurement of velocity can be significantly underestimated if the Doppler beam is not *parallel* to flow since at any angle greater than 0 (parallel), $\cos \theta$ is less than 1.

- The highest flow on repeated measurements is the most likely to be correct.
- Interestingly, in Doppler Ultrasound, lower frequency transducers are better able to assess higher velocity blood flow than high-frequency transducers.
  - This is in distinction to 2D, where high-frequency transducers provide better resolution.
- In Doppler ultrasound, it is also best to have the transducer parallel to the blood flow.
  - Conversely, in 2D ultrasound, it is best to have the transducer perpendicular to the imaged structure.

Types of Doppler Ultrasound

There are three types of ultrasound Doppler: pulsed wave (PW), continuous wave (CW), and color flow (CF). In both PW and CW Doppler, a pixel value is assigned to the frequency of the return signal expressed around a base line. If f_{dop} is positive, because blood is flowing toward the transducer, it is shown above the baseline, whereas if it is negative it will appear below the baseline (Fig. 4-4).

- Continuous Wave Doppler
  - CW Doppler simultaneously transmits and receives the signal using two crystals.
  - CW is able to accurately measure high-velocity blood flow along the entire sampled area.
  - Advantage: CW is valuable when accessing regurgitant and stenotic heart valves in which blood flow velocity is extremely high.
  - Disadvantage: Because there is no pause time in the signal, depth cannot be determined with CW Doppler.
  - In the ICU, CW Doppler can be used to estimate the pulmonary artery (PA) pressure.
    - (a) Since most patients have some element of tricuspid regurgitation, the peak of the jet measured with CW can be used to estimate the PA systolic pressure.
  - As is true for all forms of Doppler, it is important to place the transducer parallel to blood flow to prevent underestimation of the flow's velocity.
    - (a) Sonographers will often measure a high-velocity tricuspid jet from several acoustic windows and select the highest reading as the most accurate.
- Pulsed Wave Doppler
  - PW Doppler intermittently receives and transmits using one crystal.
  - Advantage: PW allows for detailed assessment of flow over time at a precise depth or point on the image.

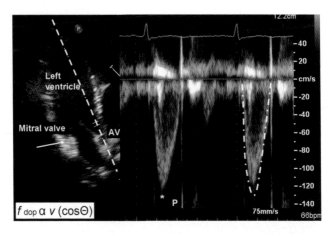

Figure 4-4. The *dotted line* (cursor) on the *left* defines the Doppler ultrasound displayed on the right. The cursor passes directly through the aortic valve (AV), parallel to flow, to bring angle of acquisition to 0 (cosθ = 1). AV flow is away from the transducer and is expressed below the baseline. The peak (*P*) is the highest velocity flow through the valve (120 mm/s). The area under the curve is the total blood flow.

- Disadvantage: There is a limit to the maximum flow that can be assessed with PW Doppler.
  - (a) This is primarily an issue when accessing stenotic and regurgitant jets, where PW is unable to accurately measure the high-velocity flow.
- PW Doppler can be used in the ICU to measure:
  - (a) Total flow through the aortic valve.
    - This can be used to calculate the cardiac output and index.
    - CW Doppler can also be used for this application.
  - (b) Mitral valve flow at the tip of the leaflets.
    - This can provide detailed assessment of diastolic function.

    - Color Flow Doppler
- CF Doppler is a pulsed wave signal with a color value assigned to the received signal, which is superimposed on a 2D image.
- A higher frequency flow toward the transducer is expressed in shades of red and lower frequency flow away from the transducer in shades of blue.
  - (a) The color scheme has no connection to arterial or venous flow.
- CF is very useful in accessing overall valvular flow in the heart. It is also important in vascular assessment for guided procedures.

– CF can be used in the diagnosis of abnormal blood flow
between two structures including ventricular septal defects
(VSD), atrial septal defects, and aortic venous fistulas
(Fig. 4-5).

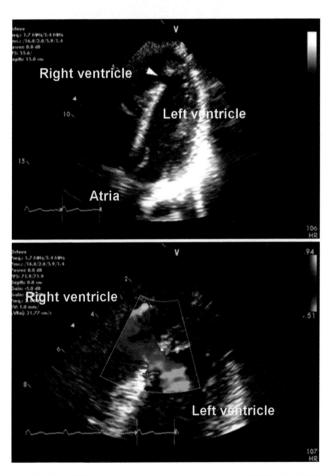

Figure 4-5.   The 2D image on the *upper panel* shows a VSD in the distal septum of a trauma patient who was hypotensive following a motor vehicle crash.
In the image on the *lower panel*, CF Doppler confirms abnormal blood flow
through the defect.

Aliasing

Aliasing is an artifact that is particular to Doppler. Both pulsed wave and color flow, which is a form of pulsed wave, are limited by the maximal velocity that can be imaged accurately. When maximum velocity is exceeded, aliasing occurs.

- The threshold for aliasing is expressed by the Nyquist equation; $f_{dop} = PRF/2$.
- If the velocity of blood flow is high, it can generate an f_{dop} that is more than half PRF at which point aliasing will occur. This is because the PRF determines how often the f_{dop} is sampled. If the sampling rate is too slow, sampling error will occur.
- The same phenomenon occurs when car wheels appear to move backwards on film. The frame rate of the film is less than twice the rotation speed of the wheel so the whole turn is not captured.
- This can complicate the measurement of gradients created by regurgitant and stenotic jets (Fig. 4-6).
- CW Doppler does not alias, which is why it can be used to measure high-velocity flow.
- Aliasing is not an issue for 2D ultrasound because the amplitude and not the frequency of the return wave is measured.

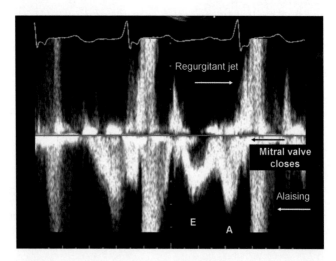

Figure 4-6. A TEE PW Doppler at the mitral leaflets. Diastolic flow is away from the esophageal transducer, shown below the baseline. E and A waves are labeled. Immediately after the mitral valve closes, there is a high-velocity jet flowing to the transducer. Because the PRF of the PW wave is less the two times the f_{dop}, there is aliasing of the jet seen below the baseline.

Artifacts

To avoid misinterpretation of ultrasound images, it is important to understand some common artifacts. An artifact occurs when a structure seen on an ultrasound image does not correspond to an actual structure in the tissue being imaged. Certain assumptions are "built in" to an ultrasound machine. When one of these assumptions is violated, an artifact is generated.

Assumptions:

- The speed of ultrasound in tissue is always 1,540 m/s.
- The longer it takes for a signal to return to the transducer, the deeper the structure lies.
- The ultrasound waves travel in a straight line from the transducer to the imaged object and back to the transducer.

Acoustic Shadowing

Acoustic shadowing occurs when an ultrasound beam encounters tissue that is extremely dense (i.e., with very high acoustic impedance) such as a gallstone or bone. Virtually, the entire signal is reflected back to the transducer. Since no signals are returning from deeper structures, the ultrasound machine shows the area as black (Fig. 4-7).

Examples:

- Rib shadowing obscuring the hepatorenal fossa, which can interfere with the detection of intra-abdominal fluid in the FAST examination.
  - Obtaining an alternative acoustic window by angling or moving the transducer slightly can mitigate this artifact.
- Cardiac imaging due to calcified or prosthetic valves.
  - A different transthoracic window may be adequate to correct the shadow but if prosthetic valves are the issue, TEE may be required.

Shadowing may also occur because of excessive refraction of the ultrasound signal. Refraction occurs when an ultrasound wave is deflected from a straight path. Typically refraction artifacts result in displacement of the imaged object on the ultrasound screen. However, when an ultrasound beam encounters a strong reflector with a highly irregular surface, refraction occurs in multiple directions simultaneously and the entire signal from deeper tissues is lost.

Acoustic Enhancement

Acoustic enhancement occurs when the attenuation of the sound wave is less than anticipated (Fig. 4-7). The deeper tissues appear overly bright

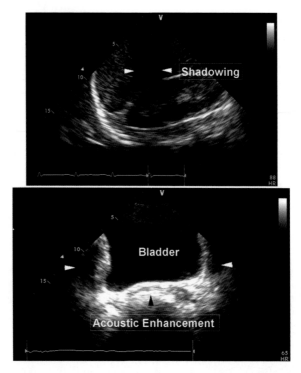

Figure 4-7. The image on the *upper panel* demonstrates acoustic shadowing (between *arrows*) caused by a rib. The image on the *lower panel* shows acoustic enhancement demonstrated in the pelvis.

on the ultrasound image. As a result, other structures may appear relatively dark. This most commonly occurs when imaging fluid-filled structures such as cyst or the urinary bladder.

- Ultrasound waves passing through fluid undergo relatively little attenuation because fluid is a very efficient transmitter.
  - The ultrasound machine assumes a constant rate of attenuation of the signal as it passes through tissues.
  - Structures behind fluid appear brighter than they should.
- An example of this artifact can be seen in the pelvic view of the FAST examination in which the tissues deep to the urinary bladder show acoustic enhancement.
- The area behind the bladder appears very bright while adjacent structures appear relatively dark.
  - (a) If unrecognized, this artifact can lead to darker adjacent structures being misinterpreted as free fluid in the abdomen.

Reverberation

A reverberation artifact occurs when the ultrasound beam bounces back and forth between two strong interfaces. When this occurs, the ultrasound beam traverses the same path multiple times. Since each round trip takes twice as long as the one before it, it is interpreted by the ultrasound machine as being twice as far away.

- This results in a set of false echoes, which appear as sequential bright lines such as rungs on a ladder.
- Example: Ultrasound beam strongly reflected from a tracheal ring to the transducer and back again creating a set of false echoes that appear to be in the tracheal lumen (Fig. 4-8).

Comet Tail

Comet tails are a type of reverberation artifact in which the ultrasound beam bounces back and forth so rapidly that the sequential bright lines

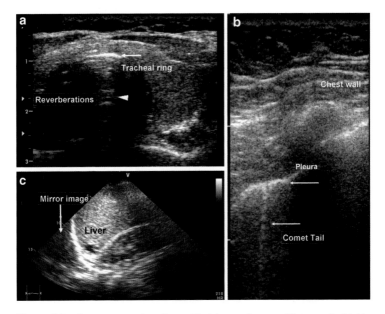

Figure 4-8. *Image a*: reverberation artifact in an ultrasound image of a highly reflective tracheal ring. *Image b*: comet tail or ring-down artifact at the interface between pleura and lung caused by very rapid reverberations between a specular reflector (air bubble) and the transducer. *Image c*: mirror image artifact in the right upper quadrant of the thoracoabdomen showing an image of the liver superimposed on the lung.

generated on the ultrasound image appear to fuse into a nearly solid beam (Fig. 4-8).

- This occurs when the ultrasound signal strikes a strong reflector with a smooth surface, most commonly a gas bubble.
  - The reflector behaves like a bell and the ultrasound wave like a clapper, "ringing" repeatedly.
    - (a)   Another name for the comet tail artifact is ring-down artifact.

Like many ultrasound artifacts, comet tails can actually be helpful in providing clinical information. In the ultrasonographic examination of the chest for pneumothorax, the presence of comet tail artifacts is indicative of normal lung while their absence indicates the possibility of pneumothorax.

Mirror Image Artifact

Smooth tissue boundaries, which are curved rather than flat, can act as specular or "mirror-like" reflectors. The ultrasound beam is reflected multiple times in various directions before finally returning to the transducer. The diaphragm and urinary bladder are specular reflectors.

- Since the reflections take longer to reach the transducer, they are assumed to be farther away and are placed deeper on the image.
- The mirror image artifact is commonly seen just above the diaphragm (Fig. 4-8).
  - The air-filled lungs are poor transmitters of ultrasound waves, so there are virtually no signals returning from the area.
  - There are, however, signals still returning from the diaphragm as re-reflected waves.
  - The "lung" tissue seen just above the diaphragm is not lung at all, but rather a mirror image of the liver.

Harmonic Imaging

Throughout this chapter, a recurrent theme has been the difficulty in imaging deeper structures due to the seemingly inescapable trade-off of resolution for depth of penetration. Tissue harmonic imaging directly addresses this issue.

- Harmonics are created when an ultrasound signal interacts with molecules in the tissues causing them to vibrate.
- The vibrations include the original signal frequency (fundamental frequency) as well as frequencies that are multiples of the original.
  - These frequencies are called harmonics.
- Both the fundamental frequency and the harmonic frequencies are reflected back to the transducer.

- Subtracting out the fundamental frequency leaves only the harmonic frequencies.
- The harmonic frequencies are all higher than the fundamental frequency.
- Harmonic imaging enables us to send out a low-frequency sound (good penetration) and receive a higher frequency sound (improved resolution).
- Advantages: Subtracting out the fundamental frequency improves resolution of deeper structures, reduces near field noise, and decreases reverberation artifact.
- Disadvantage: Harmonic imaging can make deeper structures, such as valve leaflets appear thicker than they are, and cause false measurements.

■ INSTRUMENTATION

Ultrasound is a technology-dependent tool, with a complex set of instruments that can be used to acquire and enhance the information-rich images presented on the screen. The most important tools available to the sonographer are transducers and the control panel of the ultrasound machine.

Transducer Frequency

The balance between resolution and penetration dictates the transducer frequency selected. To optimize resolution, select the highest frequency transducer that will still provide the necessary depth of penetration required to image the desired structure. Newer transducers allow for adjusting the frequency within one transducer to obtain the best image in a particular patient (Table 4-3).

- Example#1: Abdominal scanning.
  - For the standard adult abdomen, a 3.5-MHz transducer is ideal.
  - For a child or a thin adult, a 5-MHz transducer may provide better images by improving the resolution of the image while still providing the necessary depth of penetration.

Table 4-3. Ultrasound transducer selection.

Application	Transducer Frequency (MHz)
Vascular	10–12
Transesophageal ECHO	7–8
Transthoracic ECHO	2.5–3.5
Abdomen	
Child, thin adult	5
Average adult	3.5
Obese adult	1–2.5

- In an obese patient, a 2.0-MHz transducer may be required for adequate penetration, but this will come at the cost of poor resolution.
- Example #2: Transthoracic versus transesophageal echocardiogram in the same patient (Fig. 4-9).

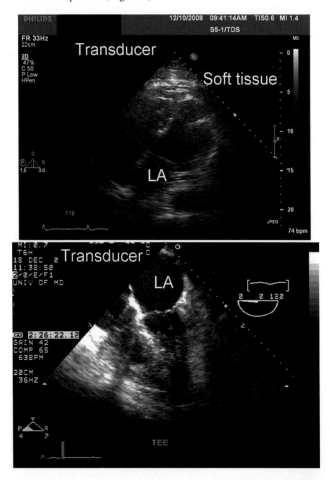

Figure 4-9. TTE (*upper panel*) and TEE (*lower panel*) in the same patient; *T* transducer, *LA* left atrium. The LA is at the *bottom* of the screen on the *upper panel*, and the *top* on the *lower panel* image. Because the 7-MHz TEE signal only passes through the thin esophageal wall there is little attenuation of the wave. TTE requires a 3.5 signal to penetrate the soft tissue.

– In transthoracic echocardiography (TTE), a 2.5- to 3.5-MHz transducer is employed. The skin, fat, chest wall, and lung separate the transducer from the heart. To penetrate the tissues, a lower frequency transducer is required.

– In transesophageal echocardiography (TEE), a 7-MHz transducer is employed. Since only the thin wall of the esophagus separates the transducer from the heart, a higher frequency transducer can be used, resulting in greater image resolution.

Control Panel

Unlike most diagnostic modalities, ultrasound is extremely user-dependent. The quality of the images obtained depends a great deal on the technique used to obtain them. An important part of image optimization is developing a familiarity with the control panel of an ultrasound machine which contains a variety of knobs and switches, which can be used to enhance ultrasound images (Fig. 4-10).

- *Gain*: The gain increases the amplitude of the return signal, expressed on the screen by brightness of the corresponding pixels (Fig. 4-11). Turning up the gain will make the whole image brighter. This can allow for better visualization; however, if too much gain is applied, it will white out the area of interest.

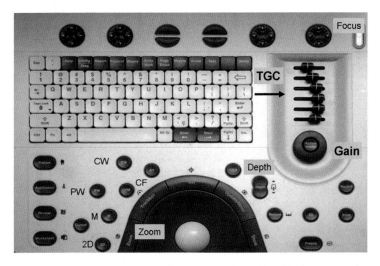

Figure 4-10. The control panel of an ultrasound machine. The buttons on the *left*, correspond to the mode of ultrasound used, CW (CW Doppler), PW (PW Doppler), CF (CF Doppler), M (M-mode), and 2D (two-dimensional).

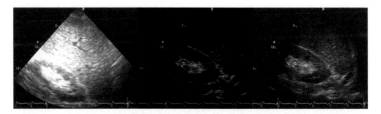

Figure 4-11.   The first image (*left*) shows overuse of gain. The second image (*center*) is too dark from lack of gain. The third image (*right*) shows appropriate use of gain.

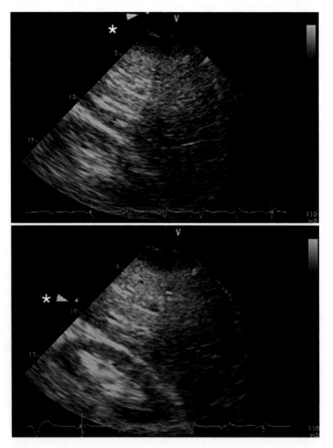

Figure 4-12.   The (*asterisk*) on the *upper panel* shows a focal point that is set too high, making the area beneath it blurry. The (*asterisk*) on the *lower panel* shows a focal point set correctly, thus the kidney liver boarder more defined.

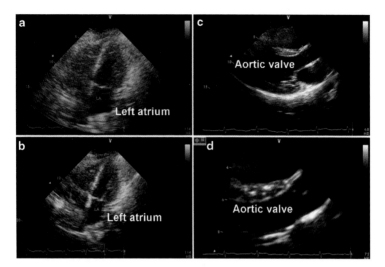

Figure 4-13. Images **a** and **b** on the *left* illustrate increasing the depth of field. The left atrium becomes more defined and the resolution improves, the left ventricle appears smaller. Images **c** and **d** on the *right* show the effect of zoom on the aortic valve.

- *Time gain compensation (tgc)*: The tgc is controlled by a vertical row of toggles. Time gain compensation allows the gain to be adjusted differently at different depths. Remember that the depth is determined by the time it takes the signal to return to the transducer, which is why it is called *time* gain compensation. Hence, the amount of gain in the near field might be decreased to darken areas of soft tissue, while increasing the gain in the far field to brighten the deeper structure of the heart, making it appear clearer on the screen.
- *Focus*: The focal point of an ultrasound signal is the narrowest part of the beam. The focus button on the ultrasound console allows the focus of the signal to be adjusted in the near field on structures of interest (Fig. 4-12). This will improve resolution of the signal at that point; however, the rate of signal dispersion in the far field is greater. This can make deeper structures appear more grainy.
- *Depth*: Like focus, depth of the ultrasound signal is usually controlled by a labeled button on the console. Adjusting the depth will make deeper structures appear clearer and more defined; however, shallower structures will appear smaller (Fig. 4-13).
- *Zoom*: The zoom feature allows the sonographer to see a structure in detail. It does not change the resolution of the image, so structures may appear more grainy. It is useful for caliper measurements of 2D images (Fig. 4-13).

No matter how talented the sonographer or how sophisticated the system, the realities of the patients' body habitus may impede image acquisition. Often, maneuvering the patients' position will help obtain optimal acoustic windows. For example, placing the patient in the left lateral decubitus position will bring the heart closer to the chest wall and to the transducer. Knowing how to angle, tilt, and rotate the transducer is also a key component of image acquisition. This skill can only be acquired with practice and perseverance.

■ CONCLUSION

An understanding of the basic physics principles underlying ultrasound is a prerequisite to developing the ability to acquire and correctly interpret ultrasound images. Although ultrasound physics can seem complex, mastery of a few simple principles will enable the sonographer to maximize the potential of this versatile modality.

■ SUGGESTED READING

Feigenbaum H, Armstrong WF, Ryan T. Physics and instrumentation. In: Feigenbaum H, Armstrong WF, Ryan T, eds. *Echogardiography*. 6th ed. Philadelphia, PA: Lippincott Williams and Wilkins; 2005:11–45.

Fry WR, Smith RS. Ultrasound physics and principles. In: Machi J, Staren ED, eds. *Ultrasound for Surgeons*. 2nd ed. Philadelphia, PA: Lippincott Williams and Wilkins; 2005:9-21.

Oh JK, Seward JB, Tajik AJ. Transthoracic echocardiography. In: Oh JK, Seward JB, Tajik AJ, eds. *The Echo Manual*. 2nd ed. Philadelphia, PA: Lippincott Williams and Wilkins; 1999:7–22.

Otto CM. Prinicipals of echocardiographic image acquistion and Doppler analysis. In: *Textbook of Clinical Echocardiography*. 3rd ed. Philadelphia, PA: Elsevier Saunders; 2004:1–29.

5

Ultrasound-Guided Vascular Access Procedures

Christian H. Butcher and Alexander B. Levitov

■ INTRODUCTION

Vascular access procedures are extremely common in the critical care unit. Central venous catheter (CVC) placement alone accounts for upward of five million procedures annually.[1] Arterial catheters are also commonplace and are an important tool in the management of many ICU conditions, including shock, severe hypertension, and other circumstances in which blood pressure management are important. Peripherally inserted central venous catheters (PICCs) and peripherally inserted catheters sited in a midline position (midlines) have gained increased popularity as an alternative to CVCs in the care of selected patients because of their ease of insertion, longevity, and low rate of early complications.

A.B. Levitov (✉)
Departments of Pulmonary and Critical Care Medicine, Carilion Clinic,
Virginia Tech Carilion School of Medicine, Roanoke, VA, USA
e-mail: alevitov@carilion.com

H.L. Frankel and B.P. deBoisblanc (eds.), *Bedside Procedures for the Intensivist*,
DOI 10.1007/978-0-387-79830-1_5,
© Springer Science+Business Media, LLC 2010

Table 5-1. Complications of central venous access according to site.

	Pneumothorax (%)	Arterial puncture (%)	Failed attempt (%)
Internal jugular	0–1	5–10	15–20
Subclavian	2–3	3–5	5–15
Femoral	N/A	5–15	15–40

Although there is little data available as to the actual number of CVC, arterial, and PICC line procedures performed per annum in the USA, the number is likely enormous. Therefore, even though vascular access procedures are associated with a relatively low rate of serious complications,[1] the absolute number of complications is likely to be high. An improved understanding of complications and why they occur may assist the critical care physician in reducing their risk.

Complications of central venous catheterization have been well described and may be categorized in several different ways. Immediate complications are those that occur as a consequence of the procedure itself (also known as mechanical complications) and include multiple venous punctures, arterial puncture and/or cannulation, hematoma, hemothorax, pneumothorax, thoracic duct injury with or without chylothorax, and catheter tip malposition. Delayed complications occur later in the hospital course and include catheter-related bloodstream infection, thrombosis, and vessel/heart chamber perforation (especially with left sided catheters). The risk of catheter-related bloodstream infection is substantially decreased by utilization of full barrier precautions. Thrombosis may be reduced by assuring that the catheter tip position is in a high-flow area (distal third of the superior vena cava) and is not in direct contact with a vessel wall. The risk of catheter-related complications as a function of insertion site is shown in Table 5-1.

Another method of categorization divides complications based on certain patient or operator characteristics that are known, or presumed, to increase risk. Large body habitus, presence of coagulopathy, prior surgery with distortion of the superficial or deep anatomy, and vascular anatomic variation are patient-associated risk factors. Operator factors include level of experience, presence of fatigue, and use (or nonuse) of ultrasound for guidance.

Arterial catheter placement can be complicated by venous puncture, multiple arterial punctures, hematoma formation, failed placement, and limb ischemia. Although annoying for the practitioner and possibly uncomfortable for the patient, with the exception of limb ischemia, arterial line complications are rarely clinically significant. PICC and midline placement are also associated with hematomas and are sometimes inserted arterially. One of the most common complications of PICC line placement is catheter tip malposition into the ipsilateral internal jugular vein, or coiling in the subclavian vein or a thoracic branch such as the thoracodorsal vein (Fig. 5-1).

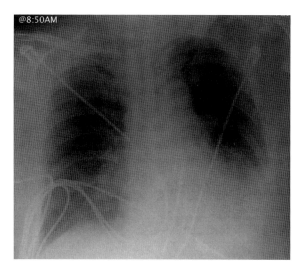

Figure 5-1. Peripherally inserted central catheter (PICC) with tip in the ipsilateral internal jugular vein.

Complications from these procedures are likely to be associated with excess direct costs derived from prolonged hospital and ICU lengths of stay (LOS) and additional procedures, such as chest tube insertion or hematoma evacuation, to treat the complications. For example, a single episode of iatrogenic pneumothorax has an attributable LOS of 3–4 days.[2] Indirect costs, such as additional provider time and patient suffering, are also important issues to consider. It is important to understand, however, that this has not been adequately studied in a systematic fashion.

■ ULTRASOUND USE FOR ACCESS

In 1984, Legler et al. published a report describing the use of Doppler ultrasound to locate the internal jugular vein prior to cannulation.[3] Two meta analyses investigating the use of ultrasound for CVC placement,[4,5] several review articles and standardized procedure guidelines,[6,7] and the SOAP-3 trial have since been published.[8] These and other studies demonstrate that the use of 2-D ultrasound during central venous access is associated with fewer complications, fewer attempts before successful cannulation, shorter procedure times, and fewer failed procedures when compared to a landmark-based approach. As a result, the Agency for Healthcare Research and Quality (AHRQ) and the British National

Institute of Clinical Excellence (NICE) have issued statements advocating ultrasound guidance in central venous access procedures.[9,10]

Despite these evidence-based guidelines, some providers continue to resist and do not use ultrasound at all, or use it only in potentially "difficult to cannulate" patients such as the morbidly obese or in cases of failed cannulation.[11] However, predicting, with any degree of certainty, which patients will be difficult to cannulate and the recognition of a failed attempt, as may arise from an occluded vessel, can only be viewed retrospectively after the failure has occurred.[12] Therefore, the utilization of ultrasound in all central venous access procedures is recommended in an effort to improve safety.

An additional consideration in the decision to use ultrasound is the concept of preventable medical error (PME). PME refers to either outright mistakes or poor outcomes that could potentially have been prevented in some way. Hospital-acquired conditions (HAC), which are medical problems not present on admission, may be a form of PME. There is significant interest on the part of insurers and the federal government (CMS) to identify cases of PME and HAC, which may lead to changes in compensation patterns in the future.

■ REVIEW OF ULTRASOUND

Transducer Selection

Transducers come in a variety of frequencies, each with different properties and clinical applications. Two important concepts need to be reviewed here. First, the relationship between ultrasound frequency and the depth of tissue penetration is an *inverse* relationship. This implies that low-frequency ultrasound (1–3 MHz) penetrates more deeply than high-frequency ultrasound (7–10 MHz). Second, the relationship between frequency and image detail, or resolution, is *proportional*. This means that low-frequency ultrasound has poorer resolution than high frequency ultrasound. Therefore, high-frequency ultrasound provides a very-detailed image of superficial structures, to a depth of approximately 5 cm, but cannot penetrate into deeper tissues. Alternatively, lower frequency ultrasound is capable of reaching into deeper structures but provides a less-detailed image. These relationships form the basis for transducer selection. For percutaneous vascular access, which is a procedure that is superficial, higher frequency transducers (in the 5–7 MHz range) are ideal though lower frequency probes may be necessary in obese patients.

Modes

B-mode ultrasound uses an ultrasound probe with many active elements aligned in a specific orientation, or "array," to create a recognizable

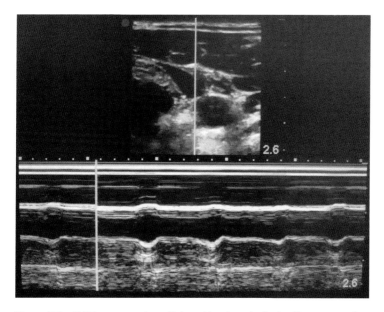

Figure 5-2. 2-D transverse view of internal jugular vein (*top*), with corresponding m-mode image (*bottom*).

two-dimensional image (Fig. 5-2, *top*); this is the most common mode currently employed in diagnostic medical ultrasound. There are many different "arrays" available (linear, phased, etc.). For vascular cannulation, linear array probes are most suited.

M-mode ultrasound uses information obtained with B-mode to create an image that demonstrates the movement of structures over time (Fig. 5-2, *bottom*). The most common ICU applications of M-mode are to assess valve leaflet movement and wall motion in cardiac ultrasound, as well as to assess changes in IVC diameter with respiratory variation in an effort to gauge volume status in hemodynamically unstable patients.

Doppler mode exists in several forms. The simplest produces no image; there is only an audible signal that varies in intensity with the velocity of the structure being studied (e.g., blood). A commonly used example is the continuous wave "Doppler wand" present on many code carts, which is used to confirm the presence or absence of a pulse during code situations. The more technically sophisticated equipment that has become available recently allows Doppler to be used in combination with B-mode, to both create an image and give information ab out velocity (Fig. 5-3). Color Doppler takes velocity information obtained by the Doppler shift and

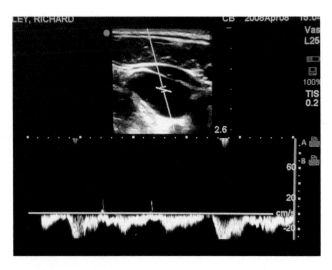

Figure 5-3. 2-D transverse view of internal jugular vein (*top*), with corresponding Doppler waveform (*bottom*).

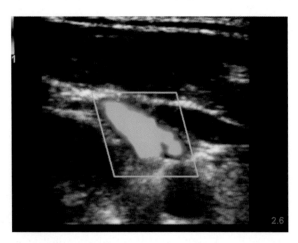

Figure 5-4. 2-D transverse view with color Doppler through the internal jugular vein, as it joins with the subclavian vein.

applies color to it, which is then superimposed on the B-mode image (Fig. 5-4). Color Doppler is very commonly used in vascular applications, including vascular access.

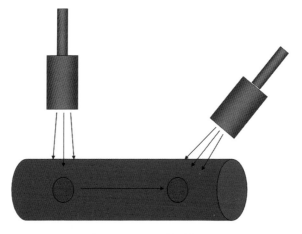

Figure 5-5. Relationship between angle of incidence and strength of the Doppler signal. An angle of 0° would be ideal. However, since that is not possible (unless the transducer was intravascular), an angle of 45–60° is acceptable. An angle of 90° results in no flow toward or away from the transducer, with a markedly diminished Doppler signal. When the angle between the incident beam and the target vessel approaches 0 (parallel), the Doppler signal becomes stronger. At 90°, the signal is weakest, since blood is not flowing toward or away from the transducer.

There are some important concepts to understand in regard to Doppler ultrasound that may help avoid costly mistakes. First, the strength of the Doppler signal is related to the velocity of the target tissue (e.g., blood) and the angle of incidence. The best estimate of velocity occurs at an angle approaching 0 (Fig. 5-5), which would be parallel to the blood vessel. If the same vessel is imaged at 90°, there is no perceived motion of blood either toward or away from the transducer, and the Doppler signal fades. An angle of about 60° is both adequate to produce a strong Doppler signal and is technically feasible. Second, when the angle of incidence changes from one "side" of the 90° mark to the other "side," the color of the blood within the target vessel changes (from red to blue). This is very important and a potential source of error when a beginner is becoming familiar with orientation and selecting a vessel for cannulation.

■ TECHNIQUES OF ULTRASOUND GUIDANCE

- Ultrasound is not a substitute for a thorough knowledge of the landmark-based technique for central venous cannulation. Frequently,

Table 5-2. Dynamic versus static guidance.

Static	Dynamic
Localization only	Localization and cannulation
Cannulation is not image-guided	Precise; "real time" cannulation
Time delay between marking and cannulation	No time delay; cannulation is image-guided
Less difficult to maintain sterility	More difficult to maintain sterility
Less technically demanding	Requires significant technical skill

the beginner may focus on the image on the screen and be inattentive to anatomic landmarks and the position of the needle.

- Ultrasound-guided procedures can be categorized as static or dynamic.
- Static guidance refers to the use of ultrasound to localize and mark a site on the skin to facilitate a subsequent percutaneous procedure, much like a traditional landmark-based approach. B-mode or Doppler ultrasound is used to locate the internal jugular vein, assess its patency, and mark a suitable site on the skin for cannulation. The cannulation itself is not performed with ultrasound.
- Dynamic guidance refers to performing the procedure in "real time" with ultrasound imaging viewing the needle puncturing the vessel wall.
- For vascular access, static guidance appears to be inferior to dynamic, but still better than the landmark-based technique alone. This is due to the time interval between marking with static guidance and the puncture during which patients may move or marks removed during skin preparation, both of which can lead to complications.
- Table 5-2 provides a comparison between static and dynamic guidance techniques. Dynamic guidance is more technically demanding since it requires significant hand-eye coordination.

Planes and Views

- There are two planes to be considered: transverse and longitudinal. These refer to the orientation of the ultrasound transducer (and, thus, the image), to the vessel axis.
- A transverse view is a cross-section and provides the operator with information about structures that lay adjacent to the vessel of interest. For example, a cross-sectional view of the internal jugular vein will enable visualization of the adjacent common carotid artery and, perhaps, the vagus nerve, thyroid gland, and trachea (Fig. 5-6).
- A longitudinal view will depict structures anterior and posterior to the vessel of interest and may allow for visualization of the entire needle during cannulation, but does not allow simultaneous visualization of structures lateral to the vessel (Fig. 5-7).

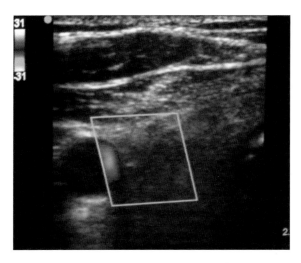

Figure 5-6. Transverse view through carotid with color Doppler. Note the presence of surrounding structures, in this case the right thyroid lobe and the trachea.

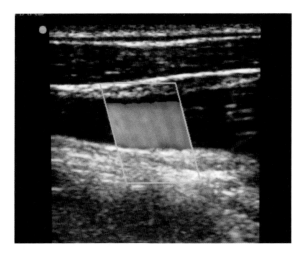

Figure 5-7. Longitudinal view of internal jugular with color Doppler. This view allows identification of structures anterior or posterior to the vessel, but not laterally.

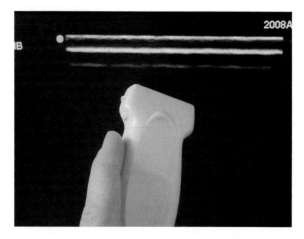

Figure 5-8. The most important step is to ensure proper orientation. Most systems have a notch on the transducer that corresponds to a mark on the screen.

- All commonly utilized central venous and peripheral arterial sites can be visualized in either orientation.
- In our experience, transverse views tend to be easier for the novice to learn ultrasound-guided cannulation.

Methods of Orientation

Orientation is probably the most important step to a successful procedure.

- Most transducers have an identifiable mark, known as a "notch," on one side. This corresponds to a mark displayed on one side of the image, and allows right-left, or lateral, orientation (Fig. 5-8).
- In rare instances, where the orientation is uncertain, a finger can be rubbed on one side of the transducer surface to produce an image and confirm the orientation (Fig. 5-9).

Problems with orientation can largely be prevented by ensuring proper patient, transducer, and ultrasound console positioning adjacent to each other.

- The operator, transducer, and console should be arranged in a straight line, (Fig. 5-10). In this way, the vessel to be cannulated and the image screen will be in the direct line of sight of the operator.
- When accessing the internal jugular vein, the console should be on the *same* side as the vessel to be cannulated, usually at the level of the patient to ensure transducer orientation: the right side of the

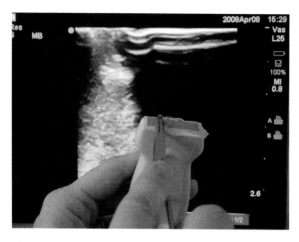

Figure 5-9.   A fingertip or instrument can also be used to gain orientation.

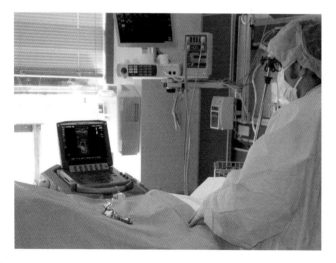

Figure 5-10.   The cannulation site, transducer, and screen should all be in the operator's direct line of vision; this minimizes any excess movements that could interfere with the cannulation.

transducer, the right side of the patient, and the right side of the image are all aligned.

- When cannulating the subclavian or axillary vein, the console should be on the *opposite* side of the patient, directly across from the operator, again, in the direct line of vision of the operator. In this example, the right side of the transducer corresponds to the inferior aspect of the patient, but everything else is the same.

Once the proper orientation is assured, the area of interest is scanned and the operator needs to be able to differentiate an artery from vein, which can be done in several ways.

- First: Assess vessel compressibility by applying downward pressure with the transducer while visualizing the vessel on the screen. Veins will typically compress at a lower applied pressure than arteries, unless a clot is present.
- Second: Assess for the influence of respiratory variation on vessel diameter. Veins usually have easily identifiable respiratory variation as compared to arteries.
- Third: Apply standard Doppler or color Doppler to the vessel and listen to the audible signal or observe the character of the color "pulsation," both of which give an estimation of blood velocity inside the target vessel.
- *Remember*: The color (red versus blue) of the blood in the vessel is dependent on the incident angle of the ultrasound beam. It is useful to compare color Doppler signals of all vessels in the area of interest; with a little practice arterial flow is easily differentiated from venous flow.
- Large, rapid fluctuations in intrathoracic pressure can create very high venous blood flow velocities that can mimic arterial flow, which may require the use of the other two methods of respiratory variation and compressibility to help differentiate the vessel type.
- Occasionally, the vein cannot be visualized. The most common reason for this is hypovolemia with associated venous collapse, which can be remedied by placing the patient in the Trendelenburg position or applying a vagal maneuver or fluid administration. Other less common causes are agenesis, chronic occlusion or scarring of the vessel, and clot that is completely occluding the lumen.
- Clot may be difficult to distinguish from the surrounding tissue and appears similar to that of an absent vessel. In this case, a thorough examination of the proximal and distal parts of the vessel should be performed and a formal venous Doppler should be performed to evaluate for deep venous thrombosis prior to any attempted central venous cannulation. If access is critical and vessel presence or patency cannot be assured, a different vessel should be cannulated.

■ HOW TO PERFORM ULTRASOUND-GUIDED CANNULATION

Internal Jugular Vein

- The first step in successfully cannulating the internal jugular vein is proper positioning of the patient.
- The head should be rotated slightly contralaterally, with the neck extended.
- Severe rotation of the neck and head should be avoided, since this may lead to significant distortion of the anatomy, and may increase the amount of overlap of the carotid artery and jugular vein.
- The bed should be placed in Trendelenburg position and the ultrasound machine should be placed by the ipsilateral side of the bed, at about the level of the patient's waist.
- An initial examination of the landmarks, without ultrasound, should be performed, followed by selection of an insertion site.
- The site should then be confirmed with ultrasound. There are two reasons for this:
  - Immediate feedback regarding landmark-based positions
  - Facilitates teaching both the landmark-based approach and ultrasound-guided approach
- During this process, proper orientation, both transverse and longitudinal, should be ensured.
- The target vessel and surrounding structures should be identified and the patency of the vessel should be confirmed and subsequently documented in the procedure note.
- The patient's skin can now be prepped and full barrier precautions should be used to maintain sterility and reduce the incidence of catheter-related infections.[13]
- A sterile ultrasound sheath should be placed on the sterile field for when an assistant hands you the ultrasound transducer.
- After the patient is prepped and draped, the catheter is set up as per normal routine.
- The components needed for catheter insertion, including needles, wire, dilator, scalpel, and catheter, should be arranged in an orderly fashion and within easy reach.
- The assistant holds the transducer, with ultrasound gel applied (can be nonsterile gel), in a position such that the operator can both acquire the transducer and place it in the sterile sheath in one motion (Fig. 5-11).
- Note that instead of utilizing an assistant, the transducer can be "picked up" by the operator, whose hand is inside the sterile sheath. The sheath is then extended to cover the transducer cord, and sterile rubber bands are applied to secure the sheath in place.

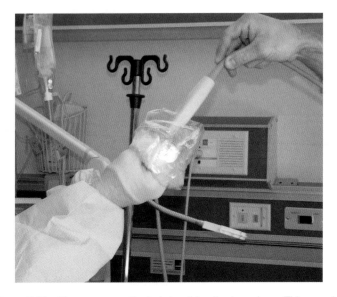

Figure 5-11. Two-person method of sheathing the transducer. This can also be done solo by "picking up" the transducer instead of having an assistant hold it for you.

- Before cannulation, a second ultrasound examination should be performed to ensure that the original insertion site is still viable.
- Orientation needs to be re-acquired any time the probe is removed from the patient and set down.
- During cannulation, always use the same insertion site and needle trajectory that you would if you were using the landmark-based approach (lateral, medial, etc.).
- Center the vessel lumen on the screen (when visualizing in the transverse plane); remember that if the vessel is centered on the screen, it is directly underneath the middle of the transducer head.
- Perform a "mock poke" to confirm your proposed insertion site relative to the underlying vessel. This is done by laying the needle on the skin surface, then applying the transducer to it (Fig. 5-12). The acoustic shadow produced by the needle should directly overly, or be superimposed on, the target vessel (Fig. 5-13).
- The skin puncture should be approximately 1 cm proximal to the transducer, which in most cases will result in visualization of the needle tip entering the vessel without having to move the probe much.
- If the needle tip cannot be visualized indenting either the subcutaneous tissue overlying the vessel or the vessel itself, move the probe along

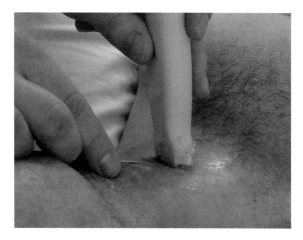

Figure 5-12. Technique of performing a "mock poke." A needle is placed over the proposed insertion site, and the site is then imaged to confirm proper positioning. This can be done before creating a sterile field (as in this case) or after.

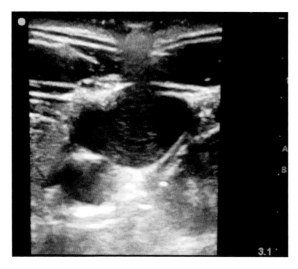

Figure 5-13. If the needle is positioned directly over the underlying vein, the acoustic shadow that is produced will bisect the vein in the image.

the axis of the vessel while slightly "agitating" the needle; this will accentuate the image of the needle and tip.

- The point of the "V" caused by indenting the subcutaneous tissue above the vein with the needle tip should be directly over the vessel.
- Be sure to visualize the tip of the needle at all times; it is very easy to misinterpret the shaft of the needle as the tip; be sure to move the probe axially along the vessel frequently to maintain imaging of the tip.
- If done properly, the needle tip should be seen entering the lumen at about the same time as the flash of blood is obtained in the syringe.
- Once the vessel has been successfully cannulated, the transducer can be set aside and the procedure can proceed normally with wire placement.
- Intravascular position of the needle can be confirmed with ultrasound (Fig. 5-14); save a picture for documentation in the medical record.

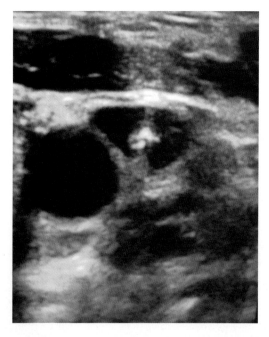

Figure 5-14. During the cannulation attempt, needle progress can be seen on the screen. You may have to adjust the transducer position to keep the needle tip in view. In this example, an echogenic needle is seen within the lumen of the internal jugular vein.

• Once the line is in place, a quick ultrasound examination of the anterior chest wall can be performed to evaluate for a pneumothorax by looking for bilateral "sliding pleura"; this should be included in the procedure note.

Subclavian Vein

• The subclavian vein is more difficult to visualize ultrasonographically than either the internal jugular, axillary, or femoral veins due to its position under the clavicle.
• Proper imaging requires significant angulation and manipulation of the transducer, especially when a transverse view is attempted.
• Two additional challenges are the difficulty visualizing the vein in some obese patients using an infraclavicular view and the inability to compress the vein with the transducer, which makes it difficult to assess the vein for clot.
• In our experience, it is usually easier to visualize the subclavian with a longitudinal, supraclavicular view in obese patients and a subclavicular view in thin patients.
• However, considering the ease with which the internal jugular and axillary veins are visualized, we have largely abandoned the subclavian vein in our practice, except for specific clinical situations, such as for long-term TPN administration or for emergency central venous access.
• Figure 5-15 shows the typical transducer placement for imaging the subclavian vein, and Fig. 5-16 provides the ultrasound image.
• Cannulating the subclavian under dynamic guidance is associated with a longer learning curve because of transducer manipulation and the use of the longitudinal view; however, the procedure itself is largely the same as that outlined under "Internal Jugular Vein" cannulation.

Axillary Vein

• Using the axillary vein for central venous access has many unique advantages over other sites[14–17]:
  – Since the insertion site is on the anterior chest, the axillary approach likely shares a low incidence of catheter-related infections with the subclavian approach.
  – Unlike the subclavian vein, axillary vein cannulation may be associated with fewer complications, such as pneumothorax, hemothorax, and chylothorax.
  – The axillary vein is easier to compress than the subclavian vein which allows easier recognition of clots.
  – Unlike the standard subclavian approach, axillary cannulation could potentially cause a brachial plexus injury, particularly if a far lateral puncture is performed.[17]

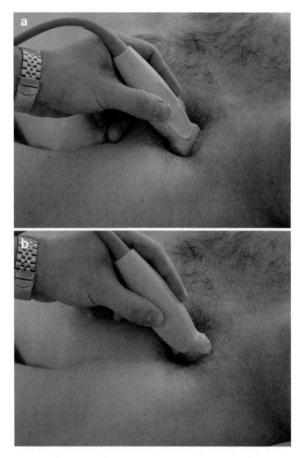

Figure 5-15. (a) Proper position of the transducer to image the subclavian vein longitudinally. Note the angulation under the clavicle (cranial aspect of the patient is to the right). (b) A transverse view of the subclavian vein is more difficult, due to a combination of probe position and angulation; it can also cause pain in awake patients.

- One distinct disadvantage of the axillary approach is the unique dependence on ultrasound to ensure localization and subsequent cannulation; landmark techniques are not as effective as with the other common sites used to access the central venous system.
- Figure 5.17 shows proper transducer placement for viewing the axillary vein transversely.

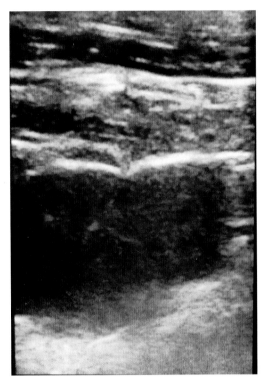

Figure 5-16. Longitudinal view through the subclavian vein. Dynamic guidance of SCV cannulation is more cumbersome than that of IJV cannulation, largely due to difficulty in maintaining a good image during the respiratory cycle as well as probe angulation.

Femoral Vein

- Femoral cannulation has a relatively low incidence of life-threatening complications.
- Several clinically important complications may occur that lead to significant morbidity.
  - Accidental (or intentional) femoral arterial cannulation, especially in coagulopathic patients, may cause life-threatening retroperitoneal hemorrhage and hematoma.
  - Inadvertent puncture of the femoral nerve during needle cannulation can cause severe pain.
  - A puncture site that is too proximal can result in inadvertent puncture of intraperitoneal structures (bowel).

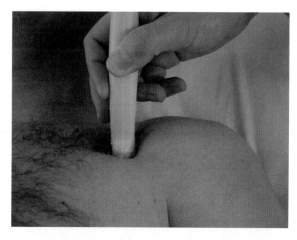

Figure 5-17. Proper probe position used to image the axillary vein. Sometimes it is easier to find the axillary vein by finding the subclavian, then slowly changing probe position while keeping the vein in view (on the screen). Using the axillary vein has several advantages over the subclavian or internal jugular veins (see text).

- Like internal jugular, subclavian, and axillary cannulation, the first step in successful femoral access is achieving proper orientation.
- The ultrasound machine should be placed on the contralateral side of the patient, directly across from the operator.
- The entire area should be scanned, with identification of all vascular structures, including the femoral artery, common femoral vein, and saphenous or profunda femoris vessels if possible.
- Once the vein is identified, it should be evaluated for the presence of clot.
- Additionally, a longitudinal view of the vein should be obtained as it dives under the inguinal ligament, and the ligament itself should be marked on the skin. This ensures that an intraperitoneal puncture will not occur (Fig. 5-18).
- All other steps are similar to internal jugular or subclavian puncture.

■ ARTERIAL CATHETER PLACEMENT WITH ULTRASOUND GUIDANCE

- Arterial catheterization is exceptionally common in the ICU and, although theoretically simple, can occasionally be all but impossible to perform successfully, especially in hemodynamically compromised patients.

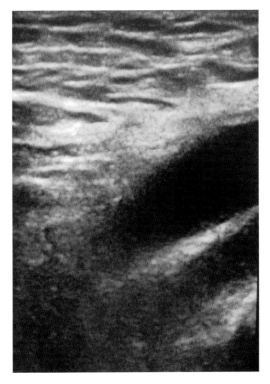

Figure 5-18. Femoral vein (*top*) and artery (*bottom*) as they "dive" under the inguinal ligament (*bright white*). Using this view when choosing an insertion site can reduce accidental intraperitoneal sticks (above the inguinal ligament).

- Reasons to consider using ultrasound:
  - Small caliber of most target vessels.
  - Patients are usually hypotensive with diminished palpable pulses.
  - Yokoyama and colleagues demonstrated anatomic variations using ultrasound in 11 of 115 (2.6%) patients scheduled to undergo percutaneous coronary intervention via a radial artery approach. These findings confirm that although anatomic variations exist, ultrasound guidance can identify many of these in anticipation of the procedure.[18]
- The principles and techniques of ultrasound guidance for CVC insertion can be easily adapted to the placement of arterial catheters since, from an ultrasound guidance perspective, the procedures are very similar.

- The most commonly cannulated arteries include the radial, axillary, and femoral, with the radial approach significantly exceeding the others in terms of popularity.
- Advantages of the radial artery are:
  (a) Easy accessibility of the wrist.
  (b) The presence of a dual circulation of the hand (in most patients).
  (c) The wrist is a relatively clean site (when compared to the femoral).
  (d) It is important to understand, however that radial artery catheterization is not risk free.
- The brachial artery may be associated with catastrophic limb ischemia if thrombosed; however, this continues to be debated.
- The femoral approach is commonly used, usually due to failure (or predicted failure) of radial placement.
- In 1929, Edgar van Nuys Allen described Allen's test, designed to ascertain the duality of the circulation of the hand, so that if one of the arteries was obstructed (from thrombus or spasm after puncture), the palmar circulation would not be compromised.
- There is some debate as to the value of Allen's test in predicting who is at risk of hand ischemia; however, the test continues to be performed on a routine basis, especially in the setting of radial artery harvesting for coronary bypass grafting.
- Ultrasound use may improve the accuracy of Allen's test, which was first reported in 1973.[19]
- The steps are as follows:
  - Use Doppler ultrasound to localize the palmar arteries.
  - Occlude the radial artery with finger or thumb.
  - If there is adequate dual circulation, the color flow usually reverses, indicating a change in direction of blood flow in the palmar arch (Fig. 5-19).
  - This suggests that radial artery cannulation or harvesting is safe.
- Unsuccessful attempts at radial artery catheterization can be associated with hematoma formation, usually insignificant and without clinical consequence.
  - However, hematomas can seriously impair further attempts at cannulation by obscuring the arterial pulsation during palpation, prolonging procedure times, increasing pain, and increasing risk of failure.
  - Using either static guidance to mark a suitable site for cannulation or cannulation under dynamic guidance has been shown to reduce the number of unsuccessful attempts.[20–22]
  - If a hematoma occurs while using ultrasound, arterial flow is still readily apparent with application of Doppler or color Doppler to the 2-D image, enabling subsequent attempts.
- The technique is essentially the same as that for central venous access.

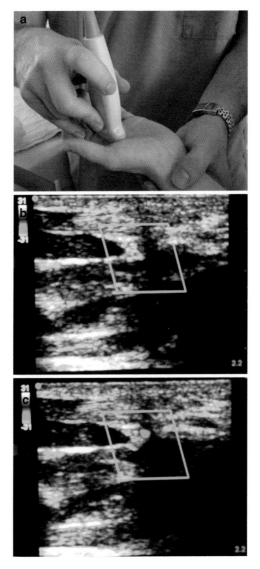

Figure 5-19. (**a**) Technique of imaging the palmar arch. Note that the angle of incidence in this example is close to 90°; the transducer can be manipulated to change the incident angle to yield a better Doppler signal. (**b**) Color Doppler image of the superficial palmar arch before occlusion. (**c**) Color Doppler image of the same vessel after occlusion of the radial artery. Note continued, although reversed, blood flow.

■ PICC LINES/MIDLINES

- PICC lines have gained significant popularity in recent years, presumably because of a low incidence of complications from insertion, improved patient comfort as compared to standard CVCs, safety and ease of care in the outpatient setting, and a relatively low incidence of catheter-related infections.[23,24]
- First described as an alternative to CVCs placed in the internal jugular, subclavian, or femoral veins, PICCs are placed in peripheral veins of the upper extremities and "threaded" into the central venous system (Fig. 5-20).
- Common complications include:
  - Thrombosis
  - Catheter-related infection
  - Catheter tip malposition or migration
  - Vessel or heart chamber perforation
  - Deep venous thrombosis
  - Malfunction[23–26]

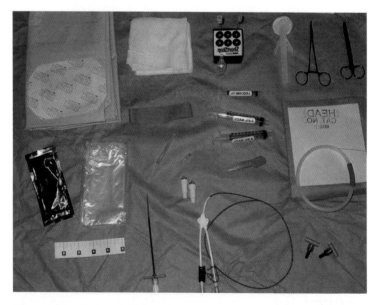

Figure 5-20. Typical PICC line kit. Note that this is a Seldinger-type system, with needle, guidewire, and dilator/peel-away introducer. The catheter itself is seen at the *bottom, center.*

- Thrombosis risk is increased from:
  - Large catheter size
  - Cephalic vein placement
  - "Peripheral" placement (outside of the vena cava)
  - Long duration of catheterization
  - Presence of underlying solid-tumor malignancy or hypercoagulation disorders[25]
- The best catheter tip position is the distal third of the superior vena cava at the superior vena cava-right atrial junction. This position causes the catheter tip to "float" within the lumen, which is associated with a lower incidence of thrombus formation.[26] Also, the superior vena cava has a higher flow rate compared to the axillary, subclavian, or brachiocephalic veins, which has implications for thrombus formation and damage to the vessel from infusion of caustic substances.[26]
- The risk of catheter-related infection with PICCs is substantially lower than that of CVCs, but is still a significant problem. Factors associated with higher infection rates are:
  - Use of any skin prep other than 2% chlorhexidine.
  - Lack of full barrier precautions (cap, mask, gown, gloves, and large drape).
  - The use of catheters with more than a single lumen (the more lumens, the higher the risk).
  - Antimicrobial PICC lines may reduce this risk, but the evidence at this point is inconclusive.
- There are several PICC line kits on the market. It is important to review the needs of your particular patient when selecting a catheter.
  - A PICC that is capable of handling high-pressure infusions, such as may be used with intravenous contrast agents, may be indicated.
  - PICCs come with one, two, or three lumens.
- There are two basic methods of PICC placement:
  - First, a Seldinger technique, where the vessel is cannulated with a needle, a wire is threaded through the needle followed by needle withdrawal, and a dilator/tear-away introducer is then inserted. The dilator is removed from the introducer, and the PICC is inserted to the appropriate position, followed by removal of the introducer.
  - The second method requires cannulation with a device similar to an angiocath, where the vessel is cannulated by a needle/catheter combination, and then the catheter is advanced over the needle into the vessel. The PICC is advanced through this catheter, which is then "torn away." This method tends to be more cumbersome.
- An institutional algorithm that governs IV access taking into consideration indications, patient factors, and alternatives when deciding on the type of vascular access device may avoid excessive and inappropriate PICC line use. The algorithm used at our institution is shown in Fig. 5-21.

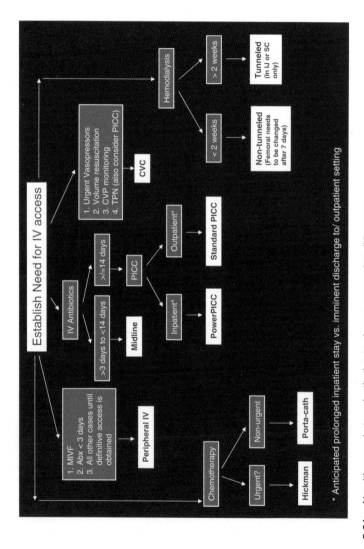

Figure 5-21. Algorithm used at our institution to choose appropriate IV access.

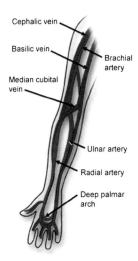

Figure 5-22. Cartoon depiction of the venous anatomy of the upper extremity. The basilic vein is usually larger in adults and, thus, is a better option than the cephalic vein.

- For PICC line insertion, 2-D and color Doppler ultrasound is used to "map" the extremity of interest. All superficial vascular structures of the distal brachium are identified, paying particular attention to differentiating the artery from the vein and assessing vein size. Figure 5.22 shows the typical venous anatomy of the upper extremity. After mapping is complete, a candidate vein is selected for insertion and marked. Patency should be assessed, by ensuring compressibility, as well as venous flow.
- Once all the necessary equipment is ready, the patient is positioned and sterilely prepped and draped.
  - The right arm is preferable due to the higher incidence of catheter tip malposition when inserted in the left arm.
  - The patient is positioned supine, the shoulder is abducted 90° and slightly externally rotated, and the elbow is flexed 90° (Fig. 5-23). The arm is secured with tape or restraints. This allows easy access to the basilic vein and may help reduce catheter tip malposition by forming a straight line from the insertion site to central venous system. If the arm is left at the patients' side, the catheter tip must negotiate a turn when entering the subclavian; this increases the

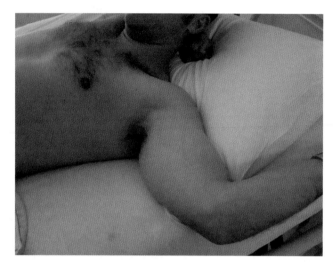

Figure 5.23. Proper position of the patient during PICC insertion. Note that the shoulder is abducted and externally rotated, and the elbow is flexed to 90°. This position allows easy access to the basilic vein.

risk of the catheter either entering the ipsilateral internal jugular vein or coiling in the subclavian.

– The risk of air embolization with PICC or midline placement is unknown, but likely to be negligible and roughly the same as that with peripheral IV insertion. Trendelenburg position, therefore, is probably not necessary.

• The desired PICC kit is opened and the line itself is prepared. Usually, these lines have a long metallic obturator that provides stiffness during insertion; this should be partially withdrawn to allow for catheter trimming.

• The desired catheter length is estimated by measuring the distance from the proposed insertion site to the glenohumeral joint, adding the distance from the glenohumeral joint to the sternal notch, then adding about 6 cm to allow for proper positioning in the distal superior vena cava.

• Once this distance is determined, the catheter should be trimmed to length. *Do not cut the obturator, as this will produce a sharp point capable of puncturing the vessel.*

• Re-scan the area and confirm the position of the target vein.

• Cannulate the vessel under dynamic guidance as described above in the CVC section. When access to the vein is obtained, remove any dilators that may be present with the introducer and advance the catheter slowly to the hub. Quickly advancing the catheter increases the risk of catheter tip malposition. By slowing the rate of advancement, the catheter becomes more "flow directed" and follows the flow into the correct position. Remember, the catheter was trimmed to an appropriate length already, so advancing the hub will ensure correct tip position.

- When the catheter is fully advanced, remove the inner stylette or obturator, attach a syringe, and aspirate blood to confirm an intravascular position.
- Ultrasound can also be used to evaluate for catheter tip malposition by scanning the ipsilateral internal jugular vein and contralateral subclavian, if possible.
- The line can then be secured by a suture, or one of several commercially available adhesive devices and dressed appropriately. Of course, a portable chest radiograph should be obtained to confirm correct placement.
- One of the most common reasons cited for placing PICC and midline devices is difficulty obtaining adequate peripheral access. This can, in part, be avoided by providing nursing and support personnel with ultrasound guidance principles for peripheral IV access.

■ SUMMARY

- Ultrasound guidance for vascular access can make the procedures easier, quicker, and safer.
- Once the technique of dynamic guidance is mastered, it can be applied to almost any procedure, even outside the realm of vascular access (thoracentesis, paracentesis, percutaneous biopsy procedures, etc.).
- Ultrasound use should *never* be used as a substitute for proper understanding of the landmark-based technique.
- Use ultrasound to teach landmark-based vascular access; compare the landmark approach with that of ultrasound in every patient to reinforce your landmark skills.

■ REFERENCES

1. McGee DC, Gould MK. Preventing complications of central venous catheterization. *N Engl J Med.* 2003;348:1123–1133.
2. Light RW. *Pleural Diseases.* 5th ed. Philadelphia: Lippincott Williams and Wilkins; 2007.
3. Legler D, Nugent M. Doppler localization of the internal jugular vein facilitates central venous cannulation. *Anesthesiology.* 1984;60:481–482.

4. Randolph AG, Cook DJ, Gonzales CA, Pribble CG. Ultrasound guidance for placement of central venous catheters: a meta-analysis of the literature. *Crit Care Med*. 1996;24:2053–2058.
5. Hind D, Calvert N, McWilliams SR, et al. Ultrasonic locating devices for central venous cannulation: meta-analysis. *BMJ*. 2003;327:361.
6. Feller-Kopman D. Ultrasound-guided internal jugular access. *Chest*. 2007;132:302–309.
7. Maecken T, Grau T. Ultrasound imaging in vascular access. *Crit Care Med*. 2007;35:s178-s185.
8. Milling TJ Jr, Rose J, Briggs WM, et al. Randomized, controlled clinical trial of point-of-care limited ultrasonography assistance of central venous cannulation: the third sonography outcomes assessment program (SOAP-3) trial. *Crit Care Med*. 2005;33:1764–1769.
9. NICE guidelines. <http://www.nice.org.uk/nicemedia/pdf/Ultrasound_49_GUIDANCE.pdf>. Accessed 20.12.07.
10. AHRQ evidence based practice. <http://www.ahrq.gov/clinic/ptsafety/pdf/chap21.pdf>. Accessed 20.12.07.
11. Muhm M. Ultrasound guided central venous access (letter). *BMJ*. 2002;325:1374-1375.
12. Forauer A, Glockner J. Importance of US findings in access planning during jugular vein hemodialysis catheter placements. *J Vasc Interv Radiol*. 2000;11:233-238.
13. Mermel LA. Prevention of intravascular catheter-related infections. *Ann Intern Med*. 2000;132:391-402.
14. Sandhu NS. Transpectoral ultrasound-guided catheterization of the axillary vein: an alternative to standard catheterization of the subclavian vein. *Anesth Analg*. 2004;99:183–187.
15. Mackey SP, Sinha S, Pusey J. Ultrasound imaging of the axillary vein-anatomical basis for central access (Letter). *Br J Anaesth*. 2003;93:598–599.
16. Galloway S, Bodenham A. Ultrasound imaging of the axillary vein-anatomical basis for central venous access. *Br J Anaesth*. 2003;90:589-595.
17. Sharma S, Bodenham AR, Mallick A. Ultrasound-guided infraclavicular axillary vein cannulation for central venous access. *Br J Anaesth*. 2004;93:188–192.
18. Yokoyama N, Takeshita S, Ochiai M, Koyama Y. Anatomic variations of the radial artery in patients undergoing transradial coronary intervention. *Catheter Cardiovasc Interv*. 2000;49:357–362.
19. Mozersky DJ, Buckley CJ, Hagood CO Jr, Capps WF Jr, Dannemiller FJ Jr. Ultrasonic evaluation of the palmar circulation. A useful adjunct to radial artery cannulation. *Am J Surg*. 1973;126:810–812.
20. Maher JJ, Dougherty JM. Radial artery cannulation guided by Doppler ultrasound. *Am J Emerg Med*. 1989;7:260–262.
21. Levin PD, Sheinin O, Gozal Y. Use of ultrasound guidance in the insertion of radial artery catheters. *Crit Care Med*. 2003;31:481–484.
22. Shiver S, Blaivas M, Lyon M. A prospective comparison of ultrasound-guided and blindly placed radial artery catheters. *Acad Emerg Med*. 2006;13:1275–1279.

23. Schmid MW. Risks and complications of peripherally and centrally inserted intravenous catheters. *Crit Care Nurs Clin North Am.* 2000;12:165–174.
24. Maki DG, Kluger DM, Crnich CJ. The risk of bloodstream infection in adults with different intravascular access devices: a systematic review of 200 published prospective studies. *Mayo Clin Proc.* 2006;81:1159–1171.
25. PICC line evidence based practice recommendations. Carilion Clinic Institutional Policy.
26. National Association of Vascular Access Networks (NAVAN). Tip location of peripherally inserted central catheters. NAVAN position statement. *J Vasc Access Devices.* 1998;3:9–10.

6

Ultrasound-Guided Drainage Procedures for the Intensivist

Kathryn M. Tchorz

■ INTRODUCTION

Ultrasound-guided procedures in the ICU have increased due to critical-care providers' interest and expertise, the portability of newer ultrasound machines, and the availability of user-friendly percutaneous catheter kits. In addition, with the increasing demands for proper documentation – both for patient safety and financial reimbursement – ultrasound has emerged as an ideal imaging modality for several reasons. First, ultrasound is a portable imaging modality; with the advent of compact, hand-held machines, ultrasound is user-friendly and readily available, especially when caring for critically ill and injured patients. Second, ultrasound provides safe and painless imaging that may be readily utilized in pediatric and pregnant

K.M. Tchorz (✉)
Department of Surgery, Wright State University – Boonshoft School of Medicine, Dayton, OH 45409, USA
e-mail: Kathryn.tchorz@wright.edu

H.L. Frankel and B.P. deBoisblanc (eds.), *Bedside Procedures for the Intensivist*,
DOI 10.1007/978-0-387-79830-1_6,
© Springer Science+Business Media, LLC 2010

patients. Third, ultrasound imaging is easily repeatable; for example, residents, fellows, and nonphysician health-care providers (physician assistants and advanced practice nurses) within an academic environment can image, record, and submit copies for operator critique. The same idea holds true for a physician practicing in the private sector. Given our commitment to life-long learning in medicine, educational alliances with identified, local ultrasound experts may prove to be extremely rewarding.

In light of the desire for expeditious clinical diagnosis, therapeutic intervention, and minimization of complications, the role of ultrasound at the ICU bedside is expanding.[1,2] Critically ill and injured patients depend on a multitude of tubes and invasive catheters to monitor a myriad of dynamic metabolic and physiologic changes. In these patients, transport away from the safe and protective ICU environment for various diagnostic and therapeutic procedures may prove disastrous because monitoring devices may be easily dislodged or disconnected. In an effort to prevent these untoward events, critical-care specialists have begun to perform several diagnostic and therapeutic procedures at the patient's bedside.

When performing bedside procedures, especially during an emergency situation, astute clinical judgment and attention to technical detail must be employed. First, given the infectious risks of exposure to bodily fluids, attention to patient and bedside health-care provider safety is vital and requires the provider to wear full barrier protection. Second, patient protection and safety requires documentation of patient (or surrogate) discussion and informed consent, coupled with ultrasound images of the pre and postprocedures. Third, a "time-out" for patient identification and a procedure plan should be performed for all ICU procedures. Finally, all ultrasound-guided procedures should be documented in an ICU database and outcomes examined by the critical care physicians. This will allow for the best clinical practices to emerge and financial review to ensue.

Although many bedside ultrasound procedures may be performed for diagnosis and/or therapeutic intervention, this chapter focuses on three common ICU clinical scenarios and provides corresponding comments regarding indications, contraindications, and equipment preparation. After discussion of essential ultrasound physics principles and practices, three ultrasound-guided bedside drainage procedures will be presented: thoracentesis, pericardiocentesis, and paracentesis.

■ ESSENTIAL ULTRASOUND PHYSICS AND IMAGING PRINCIPLES

The practice of ultrasound in the ICU mandates the understanding and application of essential ultrasound physics principles to imaging. Although ultrasound frequencies are inaudible to humans, this sound energy has the capacity to perform work. During ultrasound imaging, the mechanical energy of electricity and sound are interconverted within the piezoelectric crystals of the transducer, and these electric impulses press the crystals to vibrate. The transducer, when placed on human tissue such as skin, emits ultrasound waveforms. In general, the thickness of the piezoelectric crystals is the main determinant of resonance frequency: thin piezoelectric crystals emit high frequencies and thick crystals emit low frequencies. When operating the newer broad-bandwidth transducers, the sonographer simply selects the type of clinical ultrasound examination to be performed, and the pre-set configurations of the ultrasound machine determine the frequency emitted. Regardless of the frequency resonance, the waveforms emitted are propagated through the tissues. Because most of the emitted ultrasound energy becomes attenuated due to scattering, reflection, and absorption of the energy, less than 1% of the ultrasound waves that are originally emitted return to the piezoelectric crystals to then form the image produced on the ultrasound monitor. The piezoelectric elements are electrically stimulated to emit sound waves for a precise period of time (per second), referred to as the pulse repetition frequency (PRF). However, to produce the image on the monitor, the piezoelectric crystals must be silent to be able to receive the returning echoes from the tissue. This is referred to as the pulse-echo principle.

During ultrasound imaging, the power of the ultrasound machine is kept at a minimal level, known as the principle of As Low as Reasonably Achievable (ALARA). As human tissues absorb ultrasound energy, sound energy is converted into heat energy. Tissue injury, namely cavitation, may be a consequence of thermal injury; however, this does not occur with current ultrasound imaging because, as one of the key safety regulations that ultrasound machine manufacturers observe, the machines are pre-set to the lowest possible power. Therefore, in order to observe the ALARA principle and ensure patient safety, the best diagnostic images are created using automated digital postimaging programs.

The average speed of ultrasound through soft tissues is 1,540 m/s. However, ultrasound travels slowest through air and fastest through bone. Therefore, it is the medium that determines the speed by which ultrasound travels. Due to this, ultrasound machines are programmed to make assumptions regarding the speed of tissue propagation, which result in numerous imaging artifacts. When ultrasound waves traverse a fluid-filled structure, such as the bladder or a blood vessel, posterior acoustic enhancement is noted inferior to that structure. The posterior acoustic enhancement appears as if the ultrasound waves traveled very quickly though the fluid-filled structure and "slowed-down" inferiorly to the bladder. Likewise, when ultrasound waves strike a highly dense tissue structure, such as the diaphragm or a gallstone, the result is posterior acoustic shadowing. This artifact appears as if the ultrasound beam is completely reflected from the structure, hence the dark shadowing. In many instances, these artifacts can actually assist with the clinical diagnosis.

Ultrasound images are described with regard to echogenicity, which refers to the strength of the returning echo. Fluid, such as blood, bile, or serous fluid, returns no echo and is described as anechoic. An image that appears more brilliant than surrounding tissues is referred to as hyper-echoic, a less brilliant image is described as hypoechoic, and an image that appears to have the same echodensity as surrounding tissues, such as a liver tumor, is isoechoic. In this instance, accurate diagnosis may require additional imaging modalities. In addition to echogenicity, images are homogenous or heterogenous: homogenous describes the contents of a distended, anechoic bladder image, while heterogeneous describes the contents of a subcutaneous abscess. Within this structure, one could image liquid, solid, and semisolid materials emitting various degrees of echogenicity. Brightness mode (B-mode) imaging will be demonstrated in this chapter and differences in echogenicity will be noted.

For the intensivist–sonographer, the three most important elements of ultrasound imaging include: (1) proper transducer selection, (2) proper transducer orientation, and (3) proper image plane orientation. Because low-frequency transducers emit long wavelengths and have deep tissue penetration, they are effective for deep tissue imaging such as that used to detect a pleural effusion, hemopericardium, or hemoperitoneum. Conversely, for imaging structures that are superficial to the skin, such as the internal jugular vein or a soft-tissue mass, a high-frequency transducer is used; these transducers emit short wavelengths, produce excellent image resolution, but have poor tissue penetration.

After selecting the proper transducer, the operator must select the proper transducer orientation. Although many ultrasound machine companies have knobs or "dots" imprinted on the transducer for ease of orientation, a physician-sonographer should always test for orientation. This is performed by holding the transducer in the transverse plane and simply touching the left edge of transducer. A coupling agent, such as hypoallergenic aqueous ultrasound gel, should be plentiful on the footprint of the transducer. In this orientation, tapping the transducer should correspond to real-time tapping on the monitor image, which should display toward the left side of the screen. This way, when placing the transducer in the transverse orientation of the body, left-sided images on the monitor correspond to the organs on the patient's right side; for example, if the patient is in the supine position and the low-frequency transducer is placed in the supraumbilical transverse orientation, the patient's aorta will pulsate on the right side of the image on the monitor facing the sonographer. This is tremendously important because not checking for proper transducer orientation can result in an erroneous diagnosis of situs inversus.

Finally, proper image-plane orientation is crucial to imaging the body structures. The sagittal plane divides the body into right and left sides (Fig. 6-1). The coronal view separates the body into anterior and posterior divisions (Fig. 6-2). Finally, the transverse view divides the body into superior and inferior portions, much like a computed tomography (CT) scan (Fig. 6-3). These imaging planes can be applied with regard to the body or to an individual organ; therefore, it is clinically important

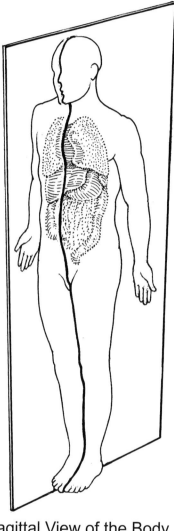

Sagittal View of the Body

Figure 6-1. Sagittal view of the body.

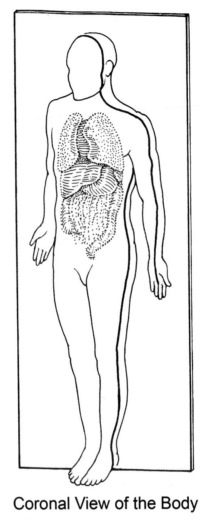

Coronal View of the Body

Figure 6-2. Coronal view of the body.

to apply two-dimensional viewing planes to three-dimensional organs. Remember, the imaging planes correspond to the point of interest and must be stated as such. For example, to obtain a sagittal (or longitudinal) view of the gallbladder, the transducer should be placed in a transverse view of the body in the right upper quadrant.

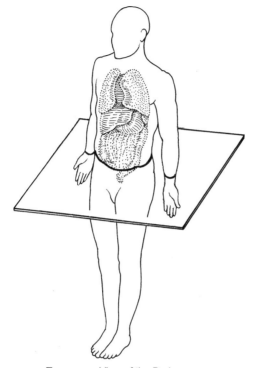

Transverse View of the Body

Figure 6-3. Transverse view of the body.

■ ULTRASOUND-GUIDED BEDSIDE DRAINAGE PROCEDURES

Thoracentesis

By applying the essential ultrasound physics principles to clinical imaging of critically ill and injured patients, fluid (or blood) can be readily noted in the dependent portions of the thoracic and abdominal cavities (Fig. 6-4). In the ICU setting, pleural effusions commonly occur in critically ill and injured patients; this may be due to exacerbation of preexisting disease states, postresuscitation efforts leading to fluid sequestration, acute lung injury, or infection, especially in mechanically ventilated patients. A pleural effusion is a collection of fluid within the hemithorax that surrounds the lobes of the lung. The right hemithorax contains three lobes: the upper,

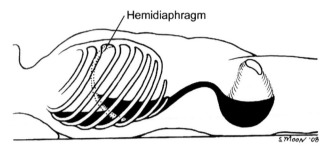

Dependent portions of thoracic and peritoneal cavities

Figure 6-4. Fluid in the dependent portions of the thoracic and abdominal cavities.

middle, and lower. The left hemithorax contains two lobes: the upper and lower lobes. Ultrasound imaging of a pleural effusion can characterize size and determine whether it is free-flowing or loculated, perhaps the two most important considerations when contemplating bedside thoracentesis. In addition, a quantitative assessment can be readily made using bedside ultrasound.[3,4] Chest radiographs are notoriously inaccurate with respect to pleural volume assessment.[3–6] For a patient with a scarless hemithorax, free-flowing effusions are usually demonstrated. In a patient with previous thoracic surgery or tube thoracostomy placement, a loculated effusion may be present as a result of adhesion formation within the chest cavity. A loculated effusion may also be present in a patient with emphysema or pulmonary empyema. During imaging, loculations appear as hyperechoic septae separating pockets of fluid. If these intrathoracic septae appear as flimsy or wispy white threads under real-time ultrasound imaging, percutaneous thoracentesis and tube thoracostomy are not absolute contraindications. If the hyperechoic septae do not move with respiration, or the lobe of the lung within the effusion does not demonstrate a floating or waving motion, thoracentesis should not be attempted due to the potential for serious parenchymal injury and inability to halt intrathoracic bleeding. In these patients, thoracic surgery consultation may be required for diagnostic or therapeutic intervention. Finally, limitations of ultrasound imaging of the thoracic cavity include subcutaneous emphysema, morbid obesity, massive resuscitation with soft-tissue fluid sequestration and emphysematous lung disease.

The technique for performing ultrasound-guided thoracentesis requires adequate setup by the sonographer and bedside assistance for conscious sedation by the ICU nurse. There are several commercially available percutaneous thoracentesis kits which can be purchased by hospitals. The thoracentesis kit currently purchased by my hospital is Cardinal Health Thoracentesis Tray with Catheter, Latex-free. (Cardinal Health, McGaw

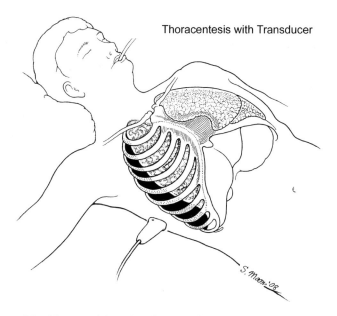

Figure 6-5. Ultrasound detection of pleural effusion.

Park, IL 60085, USA.) Alternatively, if continuous drainage over several days is planned, then a thoracentesis tray containing a locking pigtail catheter may be purchased (Cardinal Health Safe-T-Centesis™ Catheter Drainage Tray, Latex-free, Cardinal Health, McGaw Park, IL 60085, USA). Although many ICU care providers have utilized central line kits for thoracentesis, commercially available catheter drainage kits are complete with easy-to-follow directions, drapes, local anesthetic, catheters, and closed gravity drainage bags.

This procedure is performed with the patient in the supine position (Fig. 6-5). Place the low-frequency transducer in the coronal view of the body to image the right hemithorax (Fig. 6-6). Note a nonloculated, large pleural effusion in the right hemithorax (Fig. 6-7). Place a mark on the skin at the site of imaging needle insertion. After the intensivist dons sterile full barrier protection, the patient's chest should be prepped and draped in a sterile fashion. When performing a thoracentesis on a male patient, include the nipple in the sterile field as it is usually a constant landmark (Fig. 6-8). For female patient, the needle insertion site should be in the infra-mammary fold, never through the breast or axilla. Once local anesthetic is used at the skin site, a small nick of 2–4 mm should be made to facilitate catheter placement. Inject additional local anesthetic onto the periosteum of the rib, usually the fifth, and advance the needle over the top of the rib into the

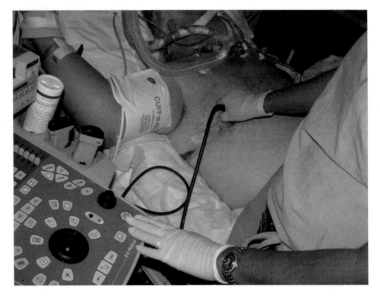

Figure 6-6. Placement of transducer on patient to view pleural effusion.

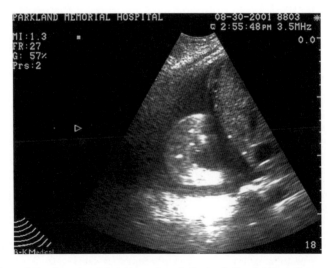

Figure 6-7. A nonloculated, large pleural effusion in the right hemithorax.

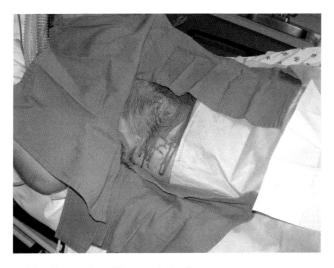

Figure 6-8. Preparation of thoracentesis site.

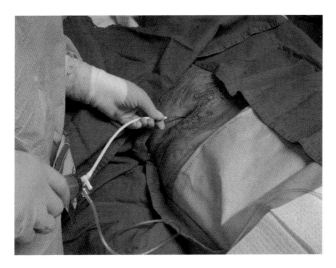

Figure 6-9. Placement of thoracentesis catheter into thoracic cavity.

thoracic space. Quite commonly, pleural fluid and/or several air bubbles return into the syringe. After administering adequate local anesthetic, place an introducer needle containing the catheter through the skin

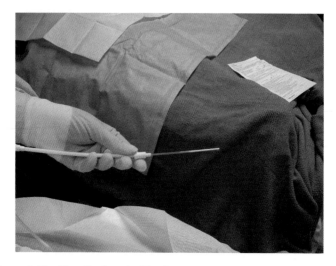

Figure 6-10. Visualization of white thoracentesis catheter after retraction of needle.

and soft tissue and then over the rib into the pleural space (Fig. 6-9). After withdrawing pleural fluid from the attached syringe, withdraw the inner cannula; the thoracentesis catheter automatically slides over the needle (Fig. 6-10). The thoracentesis catheter is placed to drainage, and a sample of the fluid can be collected for laboratory analysis. Both gravity drainage, supplied in the thoracentesis kit, and suction canister evacuation of the pleural effusions can be used (Figs. 6-11 and 6-12).

Once the catheter is removed, postprocedure ultrasound imaging will show removal of the pleural effusion with the low-frequency transducer and the absence of pneumothorax with the high-frequency transducer. Place the high-frequency transducer on the anterior chest wall in the second to third mid-clavicular space and in the sixth to seventh anterior axillary line space. The presence of comet-tail artifacts, coupled by to-and-fro motion of visceral pleura against the parietal pleura of the thoracic cavity, indicates the absence of a pneumothorax. Image the contralateral chest wall as a control. At this time however, standard ICU practices require a postprocedure chest radiograph for documentation.

When utilizing the pigtail catheters for extended drainage of the pleural effusions, these catheters are uncoiled as they are placed over a long trocar (Fig. 6-13). After introduction of the whole unit into the thoracic cavity, the sharp tip of the trocar automatically retracts once inside the pleural space. The trocar is removed as the pigtail catheter is advanced into the pleural cavity and sutured in place to the skin (Fig. 6-14).

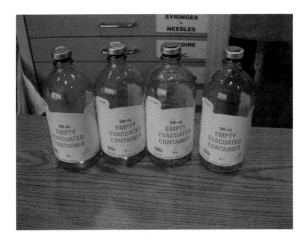

Figure 6-11. Vacuum containers for thoracentesis.

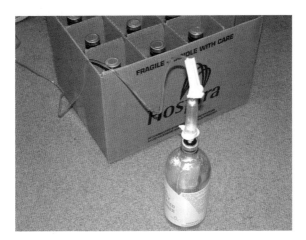

Figure 6-12. Attachment of thoracentesis catheter tubing to vacuum container for evacuation of pleural effusion.

The most recent data suggest that ultrasound-guided thoracentesis is safe. Although rare, complications from percutaneous thoracentesis include resulting pneumothorax, injury to lung parenchyma causing hemothorax, and re-perfusion pulmonary edema. In a recent retrospective study of ultrasound-guided radiology resident-performed thoracentesis,

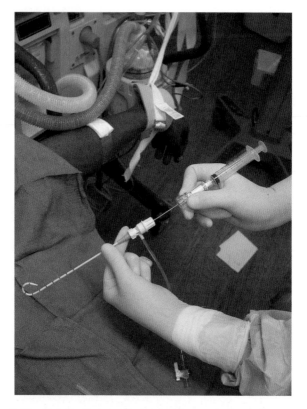

Figure 6-13. Pigtail catheter and retracted thoracentesis needle.

212 patients had 264 procedures.[7] The mean volume removed from each hemithorax was 442 ml. Twenty-nine of these patients had >1,500 ml of fluid removed and none developed re-expansion pulmonary edema.[7] The incidence of pneumothorax occurred in 4.2% of study patients. Although this study was not performed in the ICU, none of the mechanically ventilated patients developed a postprocedure pneumothorax.[7] Interestingly, the authors did not find justification in performing postprocedure chest radiograph.[7] In another recent retrospective study of ultrasound-guided thoracentesis by European radiologists, there was a 2.8% pneumothorax rate.[8] The mean volume evacuated from the hemithorax was 823 ml.[8] Furthermore, there were no cases of re-expansion pulmonary edema or hemodynamic abnormalities in any of the patients, even in those having bilateral thoracenteses performed. The authors also concluded that a postprocedure

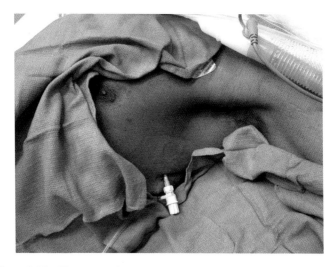

Figure 6-14. Placement of pigtail catheter into patient's left thoracic cavity.

chest radiograph was not warranted.[8] Finally, in a prospective study of febrile medical ICU patients with pleural effusions who had bedside ultrasound-guided thoracentesis, empyema was diagnosed in 16% of the patients.[9] Ultrasound characteristics of an empyema included presence of complex septated effusions with hyperechoic densities. Most transudates were anechoic and nonseptated on ultrasound. Hemothorax, at a rate of 2%, was the only complication, and 81% of these consecutive ICU study patients were mechanically ventilated.[9] Recently, a prospective study of mechanically ventilated patients demonstrated a pneumothorax rate of 1.3%.[10] In this study conducted at a tertiary referral teaching hospital, two ultrasound-trained intensivists supervised medical house-staff with the procedure.[10] Two hundred thirty-two ultrasound-guided thoracenteses were performed on 211 serially ventilated patients with the clinical diagnosis of a pleural effusion.[10] Massive obesity prevented successful thoracentesis in 1.3%, most likely a factor of catheter length. Interestingly, most patients in this population were receiving PEEP and/or vasopressor therapy at the time of thoracentesis, and there was no correlation between illness acuity and rate of complications.[10]

Pericardiocentesis

Bedside pericardiocentesis may be lifesaving in select critically ill and hemodynamically abnormal ICU patients. Prompt recognition and urgent drainage of the pericardium is required once the diagnosis of cardiac tamponade is made. In the ICU setting, this diagnosis of hemopericardium is easily made with bedside ultrasonography. Prior to the advent of ultrasonography, cardiac tamponade was clinically diagnosed.[11] However, the presence of Beck's triad (neck vein distention, hypotension, and muffled heart tones) and pulsus paradoxus is noted in only 10–40% of cases.[12] Interestingly, at least 200 ml of fluid must accumulate within the pericardium before the cardiac silhouette is altered on chest radiograph.[12] The volume of fluid causing tamponade is due to the rate of accumulation and inversely related to pericardial compliance.[13] Therefore, bedside ultrasound has led to prompt recognition and diagnosis of pericardial effusions causing cardiac tamponade.

In penetrating cardiac injuries, surgeon-performed ultrasound in the trauma bay has led to rapid diagnosis and quicker transfer to the OR for patients with penetrating precordial wounds presenting with subclinical cardiac tamponade.[14] During this 1-year study, 247 patients with penetrating thoracic trauma presented to a Level I urban center.[14] Surgeon-performed ultrasound demonstrated an accuracy of 100% for hemopericardium and the median time from ultrasound to OR was 12 min.[14] Operative findings confirmed hemopericardium and all injuries were repaired. In this small series, all patients had meaningful survival and were discharged from the hospital.[14] Likewise, in the emergency department setting physician-performed ultrasound has changed how patients presenting with pulseless electrical activity (PEA) or PEA-like conditions are managed.[15] In a small study of 20 nonsequential physician-selected patients, 40% had PEA due to death, and 60% of patients presented with minimal cardiac motion due to pericardial effusion from aortic dissections, metastatic cancers, and renal failure. Three of these patients underwent emergent pericardiocentesis or surgical intervention. Therefore, early diagnosis of life-threatening pericardial effusions from correctible conditions may improve patient outcome.

Intensivist-performed urgent ultrasound-guided pericardiocentesis can diagnose and manage chronic effusions in ICU patients can be performed safely. Our hospital supplies this paracentesis tray for patient use: Boston Scientific PeriVac™. (Boston Scientific, One Boston Scientific Place, Natick, MA 01760, USA.) Using a low-frequency transducer placed in the sagittal view in the subxiphoid regions, rotate the transducer clockwise toward the left shoulder (Fig. 6-15). This ultrasound image was taken from a patient with acute tamponade from a knife injury to the right ventricle (Fig. 6-16). Using sterile techniques, place a commercially available sterile sheath over the transducer. With the patient in the supine position, prep and drape the subxiphoid region in a sterile fashion and infuse local anesthetic to the left of the xiphoid process. Then, incise the dermis about 2–4 mm for ease of catheter placement. Under real-time guidance, the radiopaque introducer is placed through the skin incision made between the xiphoid and the left costal arch. While using continuous aspiration, direct the needle at a 45° angle to midline toward the left shoulder (Fig. 6-17).

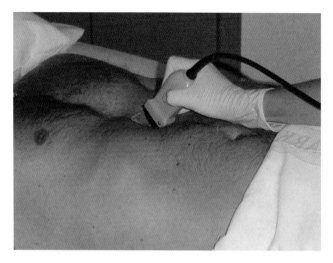

Figure 6-15. Placement of transducer to view pericardial effusion.

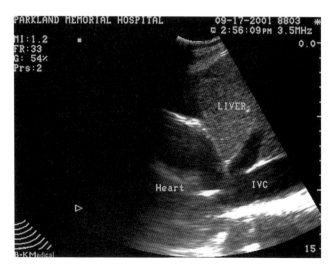

Figure 6-16. Ultrasound image of acute pericardial effusion causing cardiac tamponade.

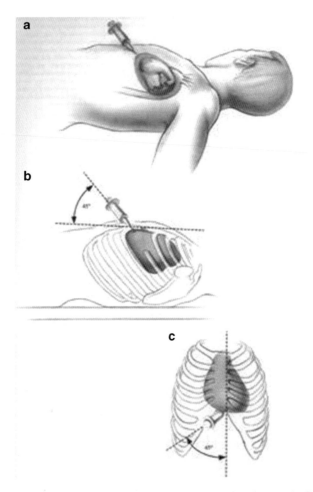

Figure 6-17. Angle of needle placement for urgent pericardiocentesis. From: Carrico, Thal, Weigelt. Operative Trauma Management: An Atlas. Stamford, Ct.: Appleton & Lang; 1998:25. Used with permission.

Hemodynamic improvement occurs with relief of pericardial fluid, and a wire can be placed through the needle using the Seldinger technique. The catheter or pigtail catheter can be placed within the pericardial sac for continuous drainage. A three-way stop cock on the end of the tubing helps facilitate continuous drainage. Completion ultrasound imaging can evaluate residual pericardial effusion and cardiac function.

One of the largest and longest studies to date on urgent ultrasound-guided pericardiocentesis is from the Mayo Clinic. During an 18-year period (1979–1997), 92 echocardiographic-guided urgent pericardiocenteses were performed in 88 patients for the treatment of clinically significant effusions resulting from cardiac perforation during catheter-related procedures.[16] Over 95,000 diagnostic and/or therapeutic cardiac procedures were performed during this time, and the estimated overall incidence of cardiac perforation was 0.08%.[16] On subset analysis, the highest rate of cardiac perforation resulting in tamponade was 1.9%.[16] This complication was associated with valvuloplasty. Conversely, the lowest rate of perforation requiring urgent pericardiocentesis was associated with cardiac catheterization 0.006%.[16] Of those 92 patients who required pericardiocentesis, there were no deaths and only a 3% rate of complications, which included pneumothorax, intercostal vessel injury, and isolated right ventricular laceration. In a subsequent study of the Mayo Clinic Echo-guided Pericardiocentesis Registry by the same authors, 1,127 consecutive therapeutic pericardiocenteses performed over a 21-year period (1979–2000) were reviewed.[17] In this database review, 70% of these procedures were performed for pericardial malignancy or catheter-related cardiac perforations. The overall complication rate was 4.7%, with major complications occurring in 1.2%.[17] This complication rate did not change during the time period, but the average age of the patient had increased over the study period.[17] A statistically significant change in practice was the use of pigtail catheters for extended drainage periods, which decreased the rate of surgical management.[17]

With regard to intensivist-performed ultrasound-guided thoracentesis, obtaining competence in focused echocardiography is a current topic of great interest. Recently, a World Interactive Network Focused on Critical Ultrasound (WINFOCUS) proposed several levels of competency, including means for verification for the intensivist.[18] Outlines of proposed levels of competence are complete with knowledge base and practical training requirements for each level of echocardiography expertise.

Paracentesis

In a critically ill patient, the bedside ultrasound diagnosis of peritoneal fluid can be ominous. Although fluid sequestration from massive resuscitation may occur, the etiology of this is usually pathologic. Common indications for ultrasound-guided percutaneous paracentesis in a patient with a scarless abdomen include: (1) intraabdominal hypertension with massive fluid present, (2) persistent metabolic acidosis despite aggressive resuscitation efforts, (3) involuntary guarding in mechanically ventilated patients, and (4) massive ascites in a critically ill patient. In each of these clinical scenarios, paracentesis or diagnostic peritoneal lavage (DPL) can be performed for diagnostic indications or therapeutic interventions. Furthermore, this procedure can be repeated at a later time if the patient fails

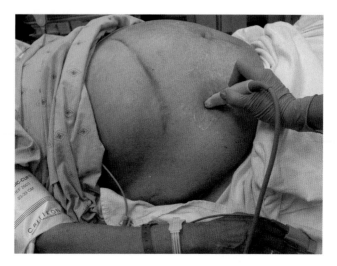

Figure 6-18. Ultrasound imaging of patient with ascites.

to clinically improve. In patients with previous midline abdominal scars, the peritoneal fluid may be sampled in select regions of the abdomen; however, CT-guided drainage may be indicated to prevent inadvertent bowel injury. In a patient with a previous midline or upper abdominal incisions, use of the high-frequency transducer placed laterally to the rectus muscles can be beneficial for imaging superficial pockets of peritoneal fluid (Fig. 6-18). Percutaneous paracentesis should only be performed when ultrasound can diagnose anechoic regions and free-floating loops of bowel within the peritoneal cavity. Percutaneous paracentesis should not be performed in a critically ill patient with a recent laparotomy scar, and consultation with the operating surgeon for re-exploration of the abdomen may be warranted. However, upper quadrant and periumbilical scars are not an absolute contraindication (Fig. 6-19).

With the patient in the supine position, the dependent portions of the abdominal cavity are located with the low-frequency transducer. If free-floating loops of bowel are imaged within the peritoneum, percutaneous paracentesis may be performed via the scarless midline. However, if septae are present, diagnosed as hyperechoic strands within the peritoneal cavity, matted loops of small bowel may be nearby.[1,19] In fact, this finding may suggest the presence of exudative ascites.[1] This peritoneal lavage tray is available in my hospital: Latex-free Peritoneal Lavage Kit 8F catheter (Arrow International, Inc. Reading, PA, USA).

The infraumbilical region of the abdomen is prepped and draped in a sterile fashion. Local anesthetic is infused into the dermis and through the

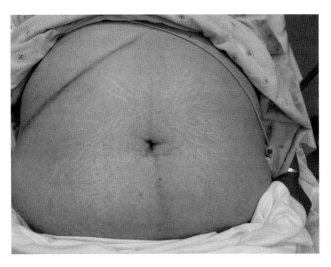

Figure 6-19. Right upper quadrant (Kocher) incision from cholecystectomy and periumbilical incision from laparoscopy.

linea alba approximately 2–3 cm inferior to the umbilicus or in the lower quadrant. If placed in the lower quadrant, the insertion site should be lateral to the rectus muscle, medial to the anterior axillary line, and inferior to the umbilicus. A small vertical incision, approximately 2–4 mm, is made in the skin for ease of catheter insertion. The introducer needle is placed perpendicular to the abdominal wall through the skin incision and the fascia and peritoneum are entered (Fig. 6-20). In performing this part of the procedure, it is important to keep the introducer needle perpendicular to the fascia at all times. In addition, successful placement of the introducer needle into the peritoneum is acknowledge with the sound and sensation of "two pops": one "pop" through the fascia and one "pop" through the peritoneum. The J-wire within the peritoneal lavage or paracentesis kit is placed through the introducer needle (Fig. 6-21). If the J-wire has "bouncing back" or is not advancing easily, the wire is most probably in the preperitoneal space, especially when performing this procedure through the linea alba. Therefore, the wire is removed and the introducer needle is re-inserted to obtain entry into the peritoneal cavity. Once the J-wire is successfully in place within the peritoneal cavity, the 8F long catheter, with numerous distal perforations, is placed over the wire and directed inferiorly (Fig. 6-22). The ideal location for the catheter should be in the dependent portion of the abdominal cavity. Fluid can easily be aspirated for diagnostic purposes and the catheter placed to suction vacuum containers. Inspection of fluid and laboratory analysis can help determine the etiology of the ascites.

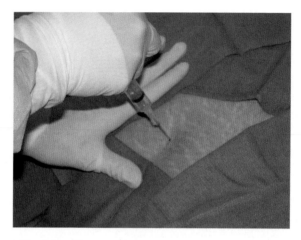

Figure 6-20. Perpendicular placement of introducer needle into peritoneal cavity. The site of needle insertion was marked by ultrasound in Fig. 6-18.

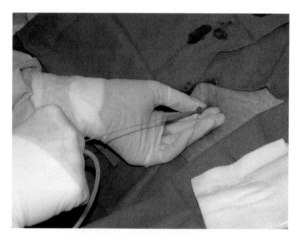

Figure 6-21. Placement of J-wire through introducer needle into peritoneal cavity.

Although paracentesis has been performed blindly in the past with minimal complications,[20] real-time ultrasound guidance of the radiopaque introducer needle can be observed entering the peritoneal cavity. Complications may include injury to the bowel, solid organs or mesentery with

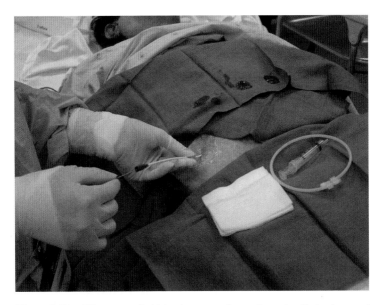

Figure 6-22. After removal of introducer needle, peritoneal catheter is paced over the J-wire. The J-wire is subsequently removed and the catheter is placed to gravity or vacuum suction for fluid drainage.

resultant peritonitis or hemoperitoneum. In patients with liver dysfunction, ultrasound assists with identification and avoidance of injury to the inferior epigastric vessels. Also, due to extensive collateral blood supplies seen in patients with cirrhosis, ultrasound may help the physician avoid large, tortuous venous complexes located in the abdominal wall. In the morbidly obese population, the traditional anatomic landmarks may not be helpful for catheter placement and therefore careful preprocedure imaging becomes critical to patient safety. Furthermore, when imaging the lateral aspects of the abdominal cavity, great care should be observed to keep the needle introduced medially to the anterior axillary line. The retroperitoneal attachments of the ascending and descending colon vary considerably and therefore, to avoid injury to the colon, ultrasound imaging remains invaluable.

The role of intensivist-performed ultrasonography in the ICU is rapidly becoming standard practice. With proper training and proctoring, efficient and effective bedside ultrasound-guided procedures can be readily performed with minimal patient risk. By performing serial, focused bedside ultrasound examinations of critically ill patients during ICU rounds, early diagnosis and possibly prompt intervention may enhance patient outcomes.

■ REFERENCES

1. Nicolaou S, Talsky A, Khashoggi K, Venu V. Ultrasound-guided interventional radiology in critical care [review]. *Crit Care Med.* 2007;35(suppl 5): S186–S197.

2. Habib FA, McKenney MG. Surgeon-performed ultrasound in the ICU setting. *Surg Clin N Am.* 2004;84:1151–1179.

3. Vignon P, Chastagner C, Berkane V, et al. Quantitative assessment of pleural effusion in critically ill patients by means of ultrasonography. *Crit Care Med.* 2005;33(8):1757–1763.

4. Roch A, Bojan M, Michelet P. Usefulness of ultrasonography in predicting pleural effusions >500 mls in patients receiving mechanical ventilation. *Chest.* 2005;127:224–232.

5. Sisley AC, Rozycki GS, Ballard RB, Namias N, Salomone JP, Feliciano DV. Rapid detection of traumatic effusion using surgeon-performed ultrasonography. *J Trauma.* 1998;44:291–296.

6. Rozycki GS, Pennington SD, Feliciano DV. Surgeon-performed ultrasound in the critical care setting: its use as an extension of the physical examination to detect pleural effusion. *J Trauma.* 2001;50:636–642.

7. Pihlajamaa K, Bode MK, Puumalainen T, Lehtimäki A, Marjelund S, Tikkakoski T. Pneumothorax and the value of chest radiography after ultrasound-guided thoracocentesis. *Acta Radiol.* 2004;45(8):828–832.

8. Mynarek G, Brabrand K, Jakobsen JA, Kolbenstvedt A. Complications following ultrasound-guided thoracocentesis. *Acta Radiol.* 2004;45(5):519–522.

9. Tu C-Y, Hsu W-H, Hsia T-C, et al. Pleural effusions in febrile medical ICU patients: chest ultrasound study. *Chest.* 2004;126:1274–1280.

10. Mayo PM, Goltz HR, Tafreshi M, Doelken P. Safety of ultrasound-guided thoracentesis in patient receiving mechanical ventilation. *Chest.* 2004;125:1059–1062.

11. Beck C. Two cardiac compression triads. *JAMA.* 1935;104:714–716.

12. Spodocl DH. Acute cardiac tamponade. *N Engl J Med.* 2003;349:648–690.

13. Seferovic PM, Ristic AD, Imazio M, et al. Management strategies in pericardial emergencies. *Herz.* 2006;31:891–900.

14. Rozycki GS, Feliciano DV, Schmidt JA, Cushman JG, Sisley AC, Ingram W. The role of surgeon-performed ultrasound in patients with possible cardiac wounds. *Ann Surg.* 1996;223:737–746.

15. Tayal VS, Kline JA. Emergency echocardiography to detect pericardial effusion in patients in PEA and near-PEA states. *Resuscitation.* 2003;59(3): 315–318.

16. Tsang TS. Rescue echocardiography guided pericardiocentesis for cardiac performance complications catheter-based procedures: the Mayo Clinic Experience. *J Am Coll Cardiol.* 1998;32:1345–1350.

17. Tsang TS, Enriquez-Sarano M, Freeman WK, et al. Consecutive 1127 therapeutic echocardiographically guided pericardiocentesis: clinical

profile, practice patterns, and outcomes spanning 21 years. *Mayo Clin Proc*. 2002;77:429–436.

18. Price S, Via G, Sloth E, World Interactive Network Focused on Critical UltraSound ECHO-ICU Group, et al. Echocardiography practice, training and accreditation in the intensive care: document for the World Interactive Network Focused on Critical Ultrasound (WINFOCUS). *Cardiovasc Ultrasound*. 2008;6:49.
19. Hanbidge AE, Lynch D, Wilson SR. US of the peritoneum. *Radiographics*. 2003;23:663–685.
20. Mallory A, Schaefer JF. Complications of diagnostic paracentesis in patients with liver diseases. *JAMA*. 1978;239:628–630.

7

Focused Echocardiography in the ICU

Steven A. Conrad

■ INTRODUCTION

Technological advancements in portable ultrasound units have helped bring high-quality imaging to the bedside of the critically ill patient. The ability to obtain images of a quality that approaches traditional echocardiography imaging systems, including Doppler measurements, has enabled clinicians to obtain dynamic information about cardiac function and cardiopulmonary interaction that was not previously possible. Ultrasound examination, including focused echocardiography, has now become an integral part of care in many critical care units. The availability of transesophageal transducers for portable units has extended the utility of this diagnostic tool in critically ill patients.

The use of ultrasound by intensivists differs in many ways from that of traditional echocardiographers. The traditional approach is to record a

S.A. Conrad (✉)
Department of Medicine, Emergency Medicine, Pediatrics and Anesthesiology,
Louisiana State University Health Sciences Center – Shreveport, 1541 Kings Hwy,
Shreveport, LA 71103, USA
e-mail: sconrad@lsuhsc.edu

H.L. Frankel and B.P. deBoisblanc (eds.), *Bedside Procedures for the Intensivist*,
DOI 10.1007/978-0-387-79830-1_7,
© Springer Science+Business Media, LLC 2010

comprehensive imaging study, as a snapshot in time, in a proscribed and systematic fashion, typically obtained in advance by echocardiographic technicians for later interpretation. The intensivist, on the other hand, is problem focused, goal directed, and dynamic, providing immediately useful information, and is repeated throughout resuscitation to assess response to therapy. The extent of the exam varies, due to both the availability of adequate images in the challenging environment of critical illness and the amount of information necessary to answer the intensivist's question. Although goal directed, the intensivist must be able to evaluate a range of potential abnormalities of cardiac structure and function. Importantly, however, the intensivist does not need the full breadth of echocardiographic skills to begin using this highly useful technology. One can begin with 2D and M-mode imaging, which alone provides substantial information, then progressing to color flow and pulsed Doppler imaging as technical skill is acquired.

Cardiac imaging in the critically ill patient is challenging and often incomplete. Positioning of the patient may be limited to the supine position; positive pressure ventilation interposes the lung between the heart and chest wall; surgical incisions and bandages limit available acoustic windows; and ongoing procedures such as cardiopulmonary resuscitation restrict access. Despite these challenges and limitations, focused echocardiography provides information that frequently results in major alterations in therapy.

The application of ultrasound in the evaluation of the acutely unstable patient in shock or other circulatory dysfunction by the intensivist can take a two-phased approach,[1] in the form of primary and secondary surveys as performed in trauma resuscitation. The primary survey consists of transthoracic 2D imaging to gain an initial rapid assessment of the cause(s) of circulatory dysfunction. After initiation of resuscitation based on these findings, the secondary survey with Doppler and other techniques by transthoracic and/or transesophageal approaches is used to gain more insight into the hemodynamic status of the patient.

This chapter approaches cardiac ultrasound from a problem-focused perspective. First a brief introduction to ultrasound physics and the technical aspects of image acquisition will be provided. A section on functional assessment will follow. Lastly, a section on structural assessment will introduce the evaluation of some anatomical abnormalities that are not infrequently noted to contribute to cardiovascular dysfunction. A glossary is provided for a more in-depth definition of terms used throughout the chapter.

■ ULTRASOUND PHYSICS

Medical ultrasound employs frequencies in the range of 1–20 MHz. Selection of an imaging frequency is a trade-off between depth of penetration (lower frequencies penetrate deeper into tissue) and resolution (higher frequencies give a better resolution of cardiac structures). Cardiac ultrasound transducers in the adult patient give the best images with frequencies in the 2.5–3.5 MHz range, while pediatric patients can benefit from the higher resolution at frequencies up to 5 MHz or more.

Medical ultrasound waves are *compression waves* that interact with tissue in one of several ways (Fig. 7-1). The level of interaction is low enough as to not cause tissue damage, but of sufficient magnitude to be detected by a transducer. Waves are reflected from interfaces between and within tissues that differ in *acoustic impedance*, an inherent property of a given substance. *Reflection* forms the basis for ultrasound imaging and Doppler measurements, since it is primarily these reflected waves that are detected at the transducer following a transmitted pulse. *Scattering* results when the ultrasound signal interacts with small structures (<1 mm), in which ultrasound energy is radiated in all directions, of which only a very low amplitude component may return to the transducer. *Refraction* refers to the deflection of the signal from surfaces that are tangential to the beam direction. This component of the beam continues deeper at an angle, which can then be reflected from other tissues, forming a well-known artifact that causes objects to appear a distance away from their actual position. *Attenuation* refers to the loss of ultrasound signal strength as the beam penetrates further into tissue, and is the result of absorption by tissue as well as signal loss due to reflection, scattering, and refraction.

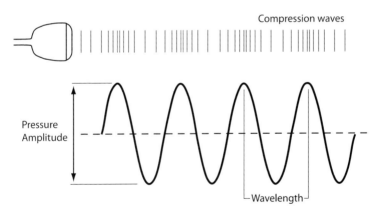

Figure 7-1. Schematic diagram of the propagation of ultrasound. Compression waves are mechanical vibrations that alternate compression with refraction. The wavelength is the distance that one compression cycle travels in tissue, and is related to the frequency of the signal and the speed of sound in tissue. The amplitude is the strength of the signal, with a greater amplitude inducing greater interaction with tissue.

Ultrasound transducers are provided in several configurations for different applications (Fig. 7-2). Transthoracic cardiac ultrasound requires a transducer with a small footprint to fit between ribs, and a sector image format that can include the dimensions of the heart. The sector format is achieved by a small array of crystals that can focus and steer the beam by way of adjusting the phase of each transducer in the pulse sequence. This methodology is known as *phased-array* scanning.

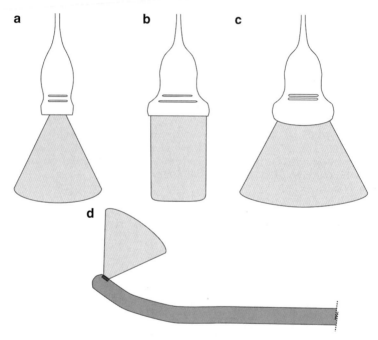

Figure 7-2. Diagram of the types of transducers used in ultrasound. A typical transthoracic echocardiographic transducer (**a**) provides for sector scanning, which permits penetration between the ribs near the transducer, with a wider scan area at a further distance. This is accomplished by a phased array of crystals, and yields a decreasing resolution with increasing depth. A linear array (**b**) has a larger number of crystals and provides a constant resolution with depth, but has a larger footprint and is used in vascular and other nonechocardiographic studies. A large sector scanner (**c**) has a larger number of crystals and thus better resolution but not suitable for echocardiography. It is used primarily in examination of abdominal and retroperitoneal structures. A transesophageal transducer (**d**) is a sector scanner that is small enough to be mounted on an esophageal probe.

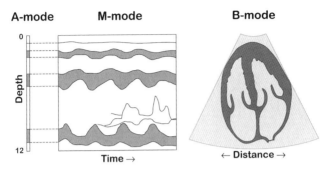

Figure 7-3. An A-mode (amplitude) scan is a one-dimensional scan representing a single line into tissue, with brightness representing signal strength. Although not used clinically, when traced against time, a M-mode (motion) scan results that shows a temporal graph enabling one to accurately measure distances and time intervals. Sweeping the A-mode scan along a distance rather than time yields the familiar two-dimensional B-mode scan.

Transesophageal transducers are also phased-array, but are smaller in size to fit in the esophagus.

Diagnostic ultrasound is available in several imaging modes. *A-mode* (amplitude mode) provides one-dimensional intensity vs. depth information, and is largely of historical interest. *M-mode* (motion mode) adds time information to A-mode in which the intensity is displayed as brightness on the vertical axis against time on the horizontal axis (Fig. 7-3). M-mode is ideal for looking at changes in structures in one-dimension over the course of time. In cardiac ultrasound, it is used to follow chamber and valve motion during the course of the cardiac cycle. *B-mode* adds spatial orientation and results in a two-dimensional image that can be updated frequently enough to give real-time images, hence its designation as real-time 2D ultrasound (Fig. 7-3).

The introduction of Doppler techniques has added another dimension of information, allowing the assessment of blood flow and hemodynamic function, and thus is of great utility to the intensivist. Pulse-wave Doppler allows the measurement of blood (or tissue) velocity at a precisely determined location within the heart (e.g., the inflow into the left ventricle), allowing measurement of volume flows (e.g., stroke volume) and pressure gradients across cardiac structures. Velocity is determined by measuring the Doppler frequency shift, in which a reflected wave shifts to a higher or lower frequency when the interface is moving toward or away from the transducer. Velocity is related to the frequency shift according to the equation:

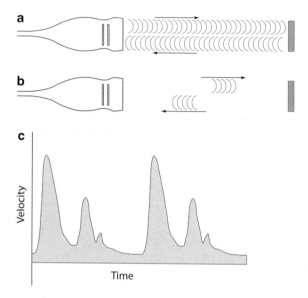

Figure 7-4. Comparison of continuous wave (**a**) and pulsed wave (**b**) Doppler interrogation methods. In continuous mode, a signal is constantly emitted and received, yielding a signal that represents a mixture of velocities along the entire path of the signal. When plotted against time, the familiar spectral display (**c**) is obtained. Continuous wave is unable to discern the depth of a particular velocity, and is most useful for studies that require high-fidelity sampling of the maximum velocity along a path. Pulsed wave Doppler sends a pulse into tissue, which can then be sampled at a particular time corresponding to a desired distance, allowing Doppler assessment in a small region of interest.

$$V = \frac{c \cdot (f_{rec} - f_{tran})}{2 \cdot f_{tran} \cdot \cos\theta},$$

where c is the speed of sound in tissue (1,540 m s^{-1}), f_{tran} the transmitted frequency, f_{rec} the received frequency, and θ the angle between the direction of the beam and the angle of the moving tissue ($\cos\theta = 1$ if they are collinear).

Two Doppler modes are available. In *continuous-wave Doppler*, the transducer continuously transmits and receives signals. The resulting velocity profile represents the aggregation of frequencies along the axis of the transmitted signal. It is most useful for finding the maximum velocity along the path without regard to depth, such as for finding the maximum velocity across a cardiac valve. *Pulsed Doppler* permits the interrogation of velocity within a small window along the signal path by transmitting a short pulse and receiving the signal following a predetermined delay. Since the speed of ultrasound is nearly constant in tissue, this delay maps into a specified depth. By rapidly repeating the interrogation of Doppler frequency, the velocity can be plotted in real-time, yielding a Doppler scan (Fig. 7-4). It is imperative to make Doppler velocity measurements along the axis of blood flow, or within 20° of it, otherwise the velocity will be underestimated. Some ultrasound units permit the inclusion of the angle θ to avoid this underestimation.

A second mode is Doppler *color flow imaging*. This technology extends pulsed Doppler by evaluating velocity over a two-dimensional area (scan area) using a phased array or linear transducer, rather than at one spot along the axis. The velocity is mapped to a color and overlaid onto the 2D real-time image, providing spatial orientation of velocity information (Fig. 7-5). Color flow imaging is particularly

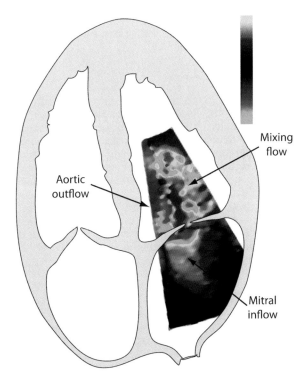

Figure 7-5. Schematic of color flow Doppler, which extends the pulsed Doppler technique from sampling at a single time in a single line to sampling over an interval of time (depth) and special orientation, depicting velocity as a color on a 2D color map. The color map indicates the strength and axial direction of the sampled flow.

useful for locating valvular regurgitant jets (for subsequent Doppler measurements) and intracardiac shunts.

■ IMAGE ACQUISITION

Instrument Settings

Portable ultrasound machines possessing capabilities for cardiac imaging usually include real-time 2D imaging, M-mode, color flow imaging, and continuous and pulsed Doppler modes. The ability to record images to a printer, hard drive, optical drive, USB drive, or compact flash card is important for documentation, and available with portable machines.

Imaging controls on portable machines provide considerable control over image acquisition and quality. Although differing slightly in implementation, these machines have a basic set of common controls that will be discussed in more detail. These are listed in a possible order that one may approach image adjustment.

Image Depth

The depth of the image shown on the display is manually adjustable. The depth is indicated on the display using a linear marker, and should be adjusted to bring the area of interest into full view on the screen. Each of the different views (discussed later in this chapter) will require a different depth. Example depths for adult transthoracic echocardiography will be about 15–16 cm for the parasternal view, and 19–20 cm for the apical view. Use of a greater depth reduces the *frame rate,* which can affect the real-time capabilities of the system. It also reduces the *pulse repetition frequency*, which can affect the velocities that can be detected with Doppler. Caution must be exercised to avoid missing deeper structures that may be helpful, so that starting an exam deeper for an initial survey and then switching to an appropriately shallower depth for the area of interest is a good practice.

Gain and Time-Gain Compensation

Gain refers to the amplification of the received ultrasound signal, resulting in a given level of overall image brightness. Time-gain compensation (TGC) is a built-in feature that automatically increases the gain of signals from deeper structures, since these will have traversed more tissue and lost power from attenuation. Without it, the deeper parts of the image will appear darker. A master gain control is present on ultrasound machines that adjust the brightness of the entire image. Recent portable machines include an auto-gain feature that when activated automatically adjusts the overall gain. Also present is the ability to fine-tune the TGC, either through separate near gain and far gain controls, or a series of sliders that allows more granular control of the signal at multiple depths. Note that some systems allow you to adjust the brightness of the display screen, which is separate from the gain control.

Tissue Harmonic Imaging

Portable ultrasound units now include *tissue harmonic imaging* (THI) for 2D modes. This modality incorporates the analysis of tissue harmonics (sideband frequencies) that are generated as a result of interaction with tissue. This feature reduces artifacts, enhances resolution, and improves the discrimination of interfaces, such as the endocardium.

Dynamic Range

The dynamic range refers to how the manufacturer maps the signal intensity to shades of gray on the display screen. It can adjust the number of gray shades displayed, and allows for adjustment of contrast. While standard settings are usually acceptable, adjusting the dynamic range may visually improve image quality. Some machines include a list of preset maps that are easily selectable.

Scan Area

In 2D imaging, the *scan area* refers to the physical width over which the beam is scanned. Wider images result in a lower frame rate and thus lesser image quality, but also reduce the field of view. In most portable machines, the scan area cannot be adjusted (expect for the depth). In color flow Doppler mode, the 2D velocity information is overlaid as a color overlay on a 2D image. Since processing Doppler over the entire image requires processing a larger amount of information (limiting pulse repetition frequency and velocity range), the area in which color flow is active is reduced in size to portion of the image. The Doppler scan area can be moved to a desired location on the screen, and its size can be altered. It is a best practice to reduce the scan area to the smallest size that interrogates the area of interest so that imaging fidelity is maximized.

Doppler Controls

In pulsed wave and continuous wave Doppler, the lateral location of the signal path and the depth of the interrogation area can be adjusted to lie over the area of interest on the 2D image. When the spectral signal is activated, controls are available for location of the baseline, pulse repetition frequency, and others. The use of these controls will be more evident during discussion of Doppler techniques.

Signal Power Output

The energy delivered by the ultrasound signal on portable ultrasound machines is usually not directly adjustable but is an indirect result of the mode and depth chosen. Increased depth, decreased frame rates, and lower pulse repetition frequencies will reduce the amount of delivered energy and also the duration of the exam. Manufacturers incorporate operating limits so that dangerous amounts of energy are not delivered, but the principle of ALARA (As Low As Reasonably Achievable) should always be considered.

Imaging Artifacts and Pitfalls

The influence of reflection, refraction, and attenuation can lead to imaging artifacts that can either confuse the ultrasonographer or be used to her advantage. Some of these artifacts will be described briefly. *Acoustic shadowing* is the appearance of a diminished signal behind highly reflective, refractive, or attenuating structures. It simply is the result of loss of signal power, and appears as a darker sector extending the remaining depth deep to the structure. A *ghosting* artifact can result when the beam encounters reflective or refractive surfaces that are nearly coincident with the beam. The beam is redirected at a slight angle, and thus deeper objects appear to be shifted to the left or right of their actual position. Imaging from different angles helps identify this artifact. *Reverberations* can result from a pair of parallel highly reflective surfaces, in which the signal can 'echo' back and forth, simulating a series of deeper reflective structures. Again, changing the angle of interrogation can help identify these artifacts.

■ THE ECHOCARDIOGRAPHIC EXAM

The traditional echocardiogram is obtained by a systematic approach to image and Doppler acquisition in each of the standard windows. If time permits in the critically ill patient, such a systematic approach is appropriate. In the focused evaluation of the patient in shock, however, the exam may be limited to one or two views that provide the most information for the primary survey, followed by a more complete examination for the secondary survey (as time permits).

Since the transthoracic exam can be performed rapidly and usually provides sufficient information, it is preferred for initial exam. A transesophageal exam can be performed if visualization by the transthoracic approach is too limited, or examination of structures seen better by transesophageal approach is better.

The traditional transthoracic exam is performed with the patient in the left lateral position, which brings the heart closer to the anterior chest wall and may improve the ability to obtain good images. The focused exam in the critically ill patient is frequently approached with the patient in the supine position, but it bears remembering that repositioning the patient, albeit difficult, may be rewarding. In the patient who must remain supine, the subcostal view may be the most revealing.

Transthoracic

The transthoracic exam is performed through three windows, the parasternal, apical, and subcostal windows. The location of each is approximate, so that some repositioning of the transducer is required to gain the best image.

Parasternal

The parasternal views are obtained just to the left of the sternum at or near the fourth intercostal space. Alignment of the plane of the transducer with the long axis of the heart gives the *parasternal long axis* view (Fig. 7-6). The structures visible include the left ventricle with inflow and outflow structures (left atrium, mitral valve, aortic valve, and left ventricular outflow tract). The left ventricle (LV) septal and inferior walls are visible, as well as a limited view of the right ventricle (RV). This view allows evaluation of LV dimensions, partial evaluation of LV wall motion, and mitral and aortic valve motion and blood flow. It also reveals a portion of the RV, and gives a crude estimate of RV distension.

Rotating the transducer 90° clockwise gives the *parasternal short axis* view (Fig. 7-7). By tilting the transducer away from and toward the apex gives a series of images is obtained. The LV and RV are seen in cross section from the apex through the mitral apparatus. Tilting further toward the base brings into view the aortic valve (cross section), the base of the RV with tricuspid valve, and the pulmonary outflow tract with pulmonary valve. From these views, an evaluation of LV size and contractility, RV size, and pulmonary velocities can be obtained.

Apical

The apical views are obtained by placing the transducer in an intercostal space near the apex, which is usually near the fifth intercostal space in the mid-clavicular line, and aiming at the base of the heart. In the coronal plane, all four chambers are imaged, resulting in the *apical four-chamber* view (Fig. 7-8). This view allows estimation of relative chamber sizes, LV septal and lateral wall function, and velocities associated with the mitral and tricuspid valves. Mitral annular velocity can be determined if tissue Doppler capability is present. Pulmonary venous inflow velocities can also be measured.

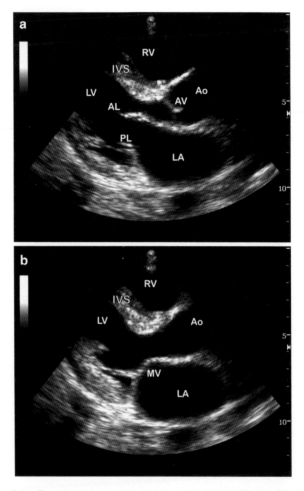

Figure 7-6. Transthoracic parasternal long axis views in diastole (**a**), with the mitral valve open and aortic valve closed, and in systole (**b**) with the converse valve positions. Some of the structures that can be identified include the left ventricular chamber (LV) in coronal section, left atrium (LA), the anterior (AL) and posterior (PL) leaflets of the mitral valve (MV), the aortic valve (AV), and the root of the aorta (Ao). The interventricular septum (IVS) is interposed between the LV and the right ventricle (RV), which is only partially seen in this view.

Angulation of the distal beam more anteriorly will bring in the LV outflow tract, yielding what is commonly called the *apical five-chamber view.*

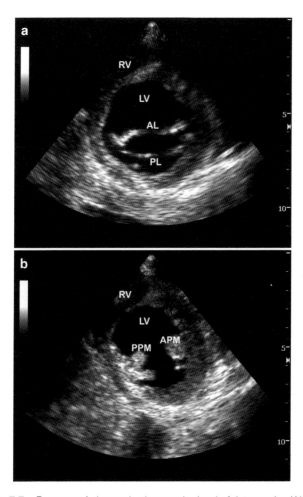

Figure 7-7. Parasternal short axis views at the level of the anterior (AL) and posterior (PL) mitral valve leaflets (**a**). The left ventricular (LV) chamber is seen in cross section. The right ventricle (RV) is incompletely seen. When the view is moved below the valve (**b**), the anterior (APM) and posterior (PPM) papillary muscles can be seen.

Rotating the transducer 60–90° clockwise brings the aortic outflow tract into view while the RV rotates out, resulting in the *apical two-chamber* view. This view can be used for further LV contractility assessment as

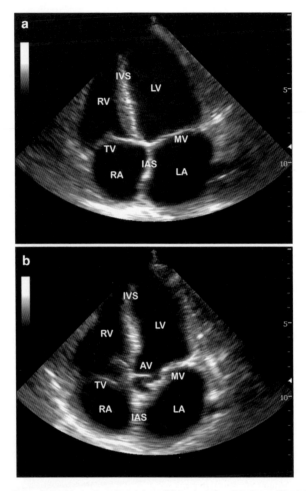

Figure 7-8. Apical four-chamber (**a**) and five-chamber (**b**) views. The left (LV) and right (RV) ventricles are easily identified, as are the left (LA) and right (RA) atria. The tricuspid (TV) and mitral (MV) valves are closed in these images during early systole. The five-chamber view allows viewing of the aortic outflow tract and the aortic valve (AV).

well as velocity measurements in the LV outflow tract. It is the view that is orthogonal to the four-chamber view for calculation of biplane stroke volume and ejection fraction.

Subcostal

The subcostal view gains additional importance in the critically ill patient, in whom the supine position and use of positive pressure ventilation and PEEP may limit information from the parasternal and apical views. The transducer is placed in the epigastrum just below the xyphoid process, aiming the transducer toward the patient's left shoulder. With the plane of the transducer in the coronal orientation, the *subcostal long-axis* view is obtained (Fig. 7-9). This view is similar to the apical four-chamber, but rotated such that the apex is to the right rather than under the transducer. It allows assessment of RV and LV size and contractility, but cannot be used for ventricular inflow or outflow velocity measurements. It is also a good view for evaluating the interatrial septum.

Rotating the transducer 90° clockwise gives the *subcostal short-axis view,* a cross-sectional view similar to the parasternal short axis, but largely limited to the ventricles.

Changing the orientation of the transducer so that it is aimed posteriorly in the sagittal plane allows evaluation of the inferior vena cava and velocity measurements of RV inflow in the hepatic veins.

Transesophageal

The transesophageal approach yields views that are comparable to the transthoracic views, except that they are oriented from the opposite direction. One has the option of inverting the image on the screen to provide a more familiar orientation. The structures at the base of the heart, especially the cardiac valves, are better seen from this approach. The TEE exam is limited by the fixed position of the esophagus, nonetheless by varying insertion *depth,* image plane *rotation* for multiplane transducers, and *angulation* or flexion a wide range of view orientations is possible.

Esophageal

Insertion of the TEE probe to the depth of the left atrium allows several important views. The *esophageal four-chamber view* is achieved at 0° rotation (horizontal plane) with slight angulation posteriorly, which corresponds to the apical four-chamber view (Fig. 7-10). Angulating anteriorly brings in the LV outflow tract similar to the apical five-chamber view.

Rotating the multiplane control to 60° results in the *esophageal two-chamber* view for assessment of inferior and anterior walls of the LV, and is used with the four-chamber view for biplane ejection fraction measurements.

Further rotation to 120° results in the *esophageal long-axis* view, which is comparable to the parasternal long-axis view.

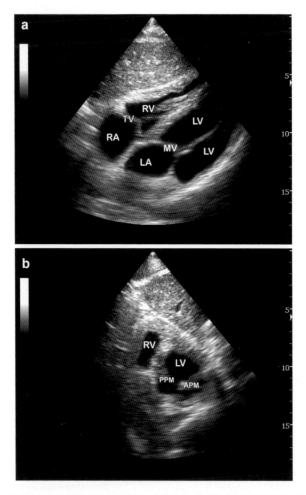

Figure 7-9. Subcostal long-axis (**a**) and short-axis (**b**) views demonstrating the left (LV) and right (RV) ventricles, and the left (LA) and right (RA) atria. Both the tricuspid (TV) and mitral (MV) valves are visible in the long-axis view. The short axis view allows both ventricles to be imaged, as well as valvular structures such as the anterior (APM) and posterior (PPM) papillary muscles as seen in (**b**).

The *esophageal short-axis* views, which are comparable to the parasternal short-axis with tilting toward the base, are obtained by angulating anteriorly with the multiplane at 0° (for atrial appendage) to about 30° (for aortic valve).

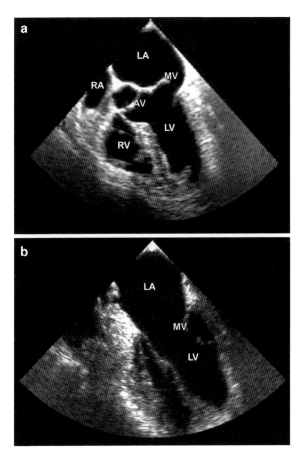

Figure 7-10. Esophageal five-chamber (**a**) and two-chamber (**b**) views. The five chamber view includes the aortic valve (AV) as well as the mitral valve (MV), the left (LV) and right (RV) ventricles, and the left (LA) and right (RA) atria.

Transgastric

Insertion of the probe into the stomach with anterior angulation places the transducer at the inferior wall of the heart. Rotating to 0° then gives the *transgastric short-axis* views, comparable to the parasternal short-axis. Adjusting the angulation allows viewing of the mitral apparatus in a fashion analogous to tilting the parasternal transducer to sweep the ventricle. Rotating to 90° provides the *transgastric two-chamber* view, comparable to the parasternal long-axis TTE view.

Transgastric Apical

Insertion further into the gastric fundus with anterior angulation places the transducer at or near the apex in most individuals. At 0° positioning, a *transgastric apical four-chamber* view can usually be obtained that is comparable to the apical four-chamber view.

■ FUNCTIONAL ASSESSMENT

Goal-directed therapy of the hemodynamically unstable patient requires assessment of intravascular volume, cardiac performance, and afterload. An algorithmic approach to resuscitation in sepsis has demonstrated improved outcomes,[2] and likely benefits all types of shock. Bedside echocardiography can provide hemodynamic measurements for goal-directed therapy that can be obtained quickly, and repeated frequently during the resuscitation phase to assess response to therapy.

This section will introduce the use of echocardiography for hemodynamic assessment, in the order that resuscitation is usually approached, e.g., assessment of preload and identification of preload responsiveness for volume resuscitation, followed by assessment of ventricular function for inotropic support, and assessment of afterload for vasopressor or vasodilator support. In contrast to most textbooks, no major distinction will be made between the transthoracic and transesophageal approaches; rather the emphasis will be on the approach. Information available from 2D and M-mode imaging will be presented before Doppler information, since the novice usually acquires skill in 2D imaging before moving on to Doppler interrogation.

Preload

Echocardiography is perhaps the most direct way at the bedside to measure preload, which represents the end-diastolic chamber volume and degree of myocardial stretch (Table 7-1). Invasive measurements such as

Table 7-1. Measurements for estimation of preload.

Measurement	Normal Value	Interpretation
2D measurements		
LV end-diastolic diameter	3.5—6 cm (2.7 ± 0.4 cm/m^2)	Related to preload, with small values
LV end-diastolic area		suggesting inad-
LV end-diastolic volume	96–167 mL (67 ± 9 mL/m^2)	equate preload, and high values suggest-ing overdistension, or compensation for LV failure
RV/LV size ratio	<.5	Value 0.5–1 indicates volume overload, >1 severe

CVP and PAWP provide a pressure, which can only infer preload through its relationship to myocardial compliance, which is unpredictable in critically ill patients. The measurements provided in this section can provide an estimate of ventricular preload allowing rapid identification of hypovolemic or hypervolemic states and have been validated.[3]

Preload measurements in isolation are not sufficient to make clinical decisions on volume management, and must be taken in context. For example, a noncritically ill patient may have adequate cardiac output at relatively low preload levels, but in the face of cardiovascular dysfunction, the same level of preload may be insufficient. Preload measurements alone, except in the extremes, do not predict response to volume infusion.[4] The concept of preload responsiveness, discussed below, helps to identify patients who may respond to volume expansion even when measures of preload appear adequate.

Left Ventricular Chamber Dimensions

The *LV diameter* in the short axis view (just below the mitral valve leaflets) at the end of diastolic filling can be used as a simple measure of chamber size useful for resuscitation. The short axis view just below the mitral leaflets helps assure that the measurement is made at the center of the chamber. The TTE measurement is most commonly made from the parasternal approach, but the subcostal can be used. The TEE measurement can be made from the intragastric approach. Switching to M-mode after obtaining the 2D image allows easier identification of end-diastole (Fig. 7-11), and is also useful for simple ejection fraction measurement (see below).

If a more quantitative assessment of LV volume is desirable, *LV volume* can be estimated using single plane or biplane measurements. A good view of the entire ventricular chamber is needed, so it is not possible in all patients. A cardiac calculation capability in the ultrasound unit is required, which uses one or more of several available estimation formulas. In the apical or subcostal four-chamber view, the 2D sequence is frozen, and the LV endocardium is traced in diastole, progressing from one side of the mitral annulus to the other. For biplane measurement (and improved accuracy), this is repeated in the two-chamber view. The calculation package then calculates the volume as an ellipsoid or series of elliptical disks.

Right Ventricular Chamber Dimensions

Right ventricular function is now recognized as the Achilles heel of the circulatory system, and RV dysfunction is common in critical illness. Inflammation, pulmonary disease, and mechanical ventilation increase RV afterload, increasing dependence on systolic function and preload. RV overdistension from aggressive fluid resuscitation can dramatically impact LV function due to ventricular interdependence imposed by the confines of the pericardium.

The right ventricle has a complex shape and is not as readily imaged in its entirety as is the left ventricle. As a result, quantitative measurements

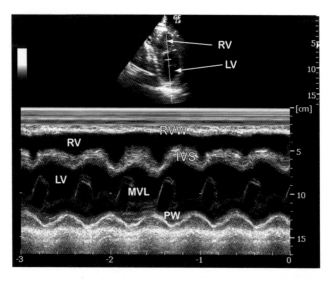

Figure 7-11. M-mode echocardiogram through the right (RV) and left (LV) ventricles. The line of interrogation is shown on the small 2D view at the top, with the resulting M-mode at the bottom. The right ventricular free wall (RVW), interventricular septum (IVS), and posterior left ventricular wall (PW) are identified, and the chamber dimensions can be measured in either systole or diastole. This view includes the leaflets of the mitral valve (MVL).

of RV size are not feasible with 2D echocardiography. RV size is assessed by its relationship to LV size, best performed in the apical or subcostal four-chamber view (Fig. 7-12). The normal value of RV/LV size is approximately 0.5, with smaller sizes suggesting inadequate preload and higher values, particularly >1, suggesting RV volume overload. In the parasternal views, the only the RV outflow tract is typically seen, but RV underfilling or volume overload can often be detected in this view.

Equally difficult to detect is volume overload, which may occur following an overly aggressive fluid resuscitation. An RV equal or larger in size than the LV in a four chamber view suggests critical RV overload that may impair both LV systolic and diastolic function. In the short axis view, flattening and shift of the interventricular septum toward the LV are also diagnostic of RV overload (see *Ventricular interdependence* below).

Inferior Vena Caval Dimension

The diameter of the inferior vena cava (IVC) near its junction with the right atrium is related to the distending pressure within the central venous system, allowing a crude estimate of preload in the spontaneously breathing patient. The IVC is imaged with the transducer directed posteriorly from

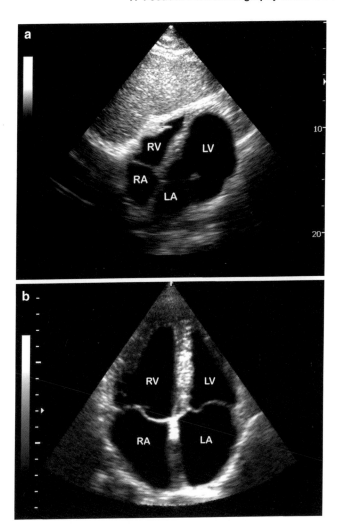

Figure 7-12. Subcostal long-axis view (**a**) showing the normal dimensions of the right ventricle (RV) in comparison to the left ventricle (LV). In this patient, the RV size is at the lower limits of normal. The apical four-chamber view in (**b**) demonstrates mild to moderate volume overload, with the size of the RV exceeding that of the LV. The right (RA) and left (LA) are seen in both views.

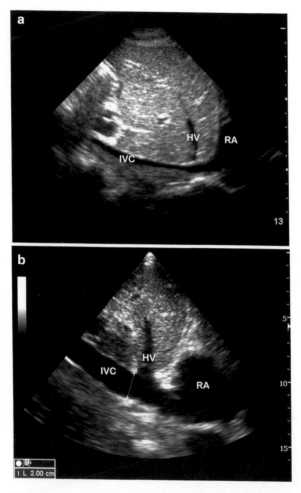

Figure 7-13. Views of the inferior vena cava (IVC) in a state of volume depletion (**a**) and with adequate intravascular volume (**b**). In (A), the IVC is nearly
collapsed, measuring about 0.3–0.4 cm. The IVC dimension in (**b**) is at the
upper limits of normal, measuring 2 cm. A hepatic vein (HV) and the right atrium
(RA) are also seen.

the subxyphoid space in the saggital plane, and the diameter measured
just below the hepatic veins about 2 cm below the caval–atrial junction
(Fig. 7-13). The transducer may need to be moved off the midline if surgical incisions or bowel gas interfere with imaging.

Normal IVC diameter is 1.5–2 cm. A diameter less than 1–1.5 cm is consistent with low preload, and can serve as an indication for volume challenge in the hemodynamically unstable patient. A full IVC (>2–2.5 cm) suggests an adequate intravascular volume. It must be recognized that this observation is most applicable in the *spontaneously breathing patient,* or in mechanically ventilated patients with low levels of PEEP and a low-level support mode. Controlled ventilation, especially with higher levels of PEEP, raises intrathoracic pressure relative to intraabdominal pressure, causing distension of the IVC even in the face of normal or even low intravascular volume. In these cases, dynamic measures of preload (i.e., assessment of preload responsiveness) or assessment of ventricular chamber sizes, are usually more helpful. However, a small IVC in a hypotensive patient on mechanical ventilation is almost always indicative of hypovolemia.

Doppler Assessment of Left Ventricular Inflow

Another approach to assessing preload is the assessment of ventricular inflow velocity, based on the observation that early (passive) filling of the ventricle is related to preload. Hypovolemia leading to diminished venous return and decreased central venous pressure is associated with a reduced early inflow velocity (E wave velocity), both absolutely and in relation to that of active filling from atrial contraction (A wave velocity), yielding a reduced *E/A* ratio (Fig. 7-14). Conversely, hypervolemia with its elevated central venous pressure results in an elevated E velocity and *E/A* ratio from the more rapid early filling.

Although *E/A* ratio can reflect volume status, it is subject to influence from two conditions affecting the myocardium. Disorders of myocardial relaxation, such as myocardial hypertrophy, myocardial ischemia, and even the aging process itself, can reduce the rate of inflow and hence the *E* wave velocity. Restrictive disorders, such as pericardial disease or pericardial effusion, can limit the filling of the ventricle following early passive filling, reducing the *A* wave velocity and thus increasing *E/A* ratio. It is important to recognize the potential contribution of these conditions, requiring evaluation of the LV on 2D as well as incorporating available clinical information. The effect of age also needs to be taken into account, since myocardial compliance decreases with advancing age. The *E/A* ratio is normally about 1.5–2 in those under the age of 50, 1–1.5 from 50 through 70, and 0.8–1 above the age of 70.

If tissue Doppler is available, additional information can be incorporated into assessment of inflow velocities. The early diastolic mitral annular velocity (*E′*) is a preload-independent index of LV relaxation, and can be used to normalize the *E* velocity for LV relaxation. This *E/E′* ratio has been shown to be well correlated to the PCWP.[5] An *E/E′* value below 8 reflects a normal PCWP, while a value above 15 is predictive of an elevated PCWP.[6] Values between 8 and 15 are variable and required further assessment. It should also perhaps be noted that one study demonstrated that in normal, healthy subjects, the *E* velocity alone was a better predictor of PCWP than was the *E/A* ratio or the *E/E′* ratio.[7]

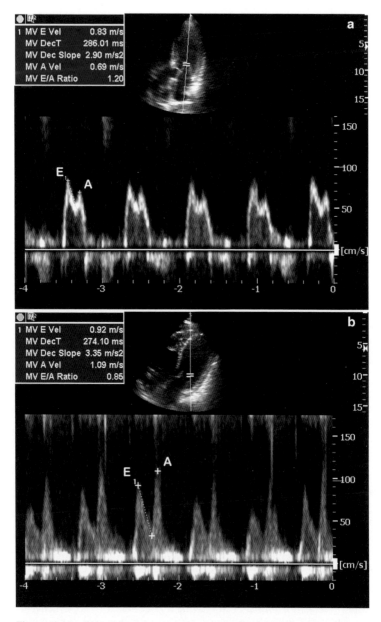

Figure 7-14. Pulsed Doppler assessment of left ventricular inflow, with the interrogation region placed in the LV at the tips of the mitral valve. The passive or early (E) and late or atrial (A) velocities can be measured. The left study (**a**) represents normal inflow velocities, with an *E/A* ratio of 1.2. The right study (**b**) demonstrates a reduced early inflow, with an *E/A* ratio of 0.85.

Preload Responsiveness

Preload or fluid responsiveness is the term used to describe an increase in cardiac performance (e.g., cardiac output) resulting from intravascular volume expansion. While the preload measurements above can help identify patients with hypovolemia, patients with a normal preload (in terms of end-diastolic volume) may still improve with a fluid challenge, and this improvement may help compensate in critical illness. The measures of preload responsiveness introduced in this section can help identify the critically ill patient in whom volume expansion may be beneficial. In contrast to the static measurements of the previous section, this section describes dynamic measurements.

These measures exploit the effects of natural and mechanical ventilation on pleural and transpulmonary pressures and the resultant effect on cardiac function. In patients who are operating on the recruitable portion of the Frank-Starling ventricular performance curve, transthoracic pressure variations associated with respiration cause small variations in preload and subsequent changes in stroke volume. These preload and stroke volume changes can be measured, and used to predict response to fluid administration.

Vena Caval Dynamics

The inferior vena cava serves as a compliance chamber for venous return into the right atrium. The lower the preload, the smaller the volume in this compliance chamber, and the greater the variation in its diameter during throughout the respiratory cycle. In order for this relationship to remain valid, the patient must have a quiet respiratory pattern. The spontaneously breathing patient must be free of respiratory distress, since wide intrathoracic pressure swings during a forced breathing pattern will result in IVC size variation independent of preload. Likewise, the intubated mechanically ventilated patient must be adapted to the ventilator, in that the ventilator, and not the patient, is responsible for introducing intrathoracic pressure variation. Ventilator dysynchrony, as in respiratory distress during spontaneous breathing, induces uncorrelated changes in IVC diameter.

As described in the above section *Inferior vena caval dimension*, the IVC diameter is measured from the subxyphoid approach. Once the IVC is imaged, M-mode can be used to record and measure the ICV dimension during both inspiration and expiration (Fig. 7-15). During spontaneous breathing (or intubated patient on minimal PEEP and low pressure support settings), the variability is expressed as the *collapsibility index,* while the variability during positive pressure ventilation is expressed as the *distensibility index.* Calculation formulas and interpretations are provided in Table 7-2.[8–11]

During TEE, one can assess respiratory variation of the superior vena cava. This vessel is entirely intrathoracic, in contrast to the extrathoracic

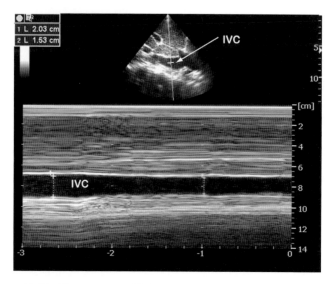

Figure 7-15. Measurement of IVC diameter with M-mode during expiration (left measurement, 2.03 cm) and inspiration (right measurement, 1.53 cm). In this patient, the collapsibility index is 0.25, within the normal range.

location of the IVC, and may be a more reliable way to assess response to fluid challenge.[11-13] The calculation and interpretation of the distensibility index for the SVC is similar to the IVC, with a different threshold value (Table 7-2).

Stroke Volume Variation

Just as respiratory variation in intrathoracic pressure results in a preload-dependent change in IVC or SVC diameter, it also results in a preload-dependent change in stroke volume. This stroke volume variation (SVV) has been exploited outside of echocardiography through the minimally invasive measurement of SVV using pulse-contour analysis. Echocardiography offers a noninvasive way to assess stroke volume, and is able to provide an assessment of SVV.

Although it is possible to assess SVV through 2D measurement of stroke volume (as described in the section on ventricular volume measurement), that approach is more difficult and error prone, and is typically performed using Doppler. Doppler measurements of aortic outflow are most commonly used, but if the apical approach is not feasible, measurement of pulmonary outflow from the parasternal view can be substituted. To perform this measurement at the aortic outflow tract, an apical five-chamber view or two-chamber view is obtained, which places aortic

Table 7-2. IVC and SVC variability indexes for fluid responsiveness.

Measurement	Calculation	Interpretation
Inferior vena cava (TTE)		
Distensibility index (mechanical ventilation)	$\dfrac{D\max_{insp} - D\min_{exp}}{D\min_{exp}}$	Value > 18% correlates with response to volume loading[8]
ΔD_{IVC} index (mechanical ventilation)	$\dfrac{D\max_{insp} - D\min_{exp}}{(D\max_{insp} + D\min_{exp})/2}$	Value > 12% correlates with response to volume loading[9]
Collapsibility index (spontaneous breathing[a])	$\dfrac{D\max_{exp} - D\min_{insp}}{D\max_{exp}}$	Value >50% correlates with low central venous pressure[10]
Superior vena cava (TEE)		
Collapsibility index (spontaneous breathing[a])	$\dfrac{D\max_{exp} - D\min_{insp}}{D\max_{exp}}$	Value >36% correlates with low central venous pressure[11]

[a] Similar values may be expected from intubated patients breathing quietly on low-level PEEP and pressure-support ventilation.

ejection along the axis of the ultrasound beam. Pulsed Doppler is used to interrogate the velocity in the aortic outflow tract at the level of the aortic valve (the narrowest point). If this view is not obtainable, an alternative is the pulmonary outflow tract, which can be viewed with the parasternal short-axis approach tilted toward the base of the heart.

The calculation of stroke volume is based on Doppler principles of velocity measurement. Integrating velocity over time yields distance, thus performing an integration of ejection velocity during a single stroke volume yields the ejection (or stroke) distance. This measurement, the velocity–time integral (VTI), is easily calculated as the area under the velocity curve during ejection using the calculation tools on the beside ultrasound machine (Fig. 7-16). The product of VTI and the cross-sectional area (CSA) through which the blood is ejected gives the stroke volume. The CSA is calculated by measuring the aortic outflow diameter in 2D and calculating its area. In practice, however, it is not necessary to complete the measurement stroke volume calculation itself, since the CSA remains constant over the respiratory cycle, simplifying the calculation of SVV using only the VTI:

$$SVV = \frac{VTI_{max} - VTI_{min}}{\left(VTI_{max} + VTI_{min}\right)/2}$$

In mechanically ventilated patients, values above about 10% predict a response to volume administration. It must be emphasized that the patient must be adapted to the mechanical ventilator, and be in a sinus rhythm or other rhythm with a stable $R–R$ interval, since variable $R–R$ interval itself results in an elevated SVV.

In the spontaneously breathing patient (with or without pressure support ventilation), the response of stroke volume to increasing preload through passive leg raising correlates with response to volume expansion.[4] For this test, baseline measurement of VTI is made in the semirecumbent position with the head of the bed elevated to 45% and the legs horizontal. The patient is then positioned with the head of the bed horizontal and the legs elevated to 45% for 90 s, and a repeat VTI measurement is made. A value greater than 12.5% predicted a response to volume loading, but with a greater specificity than sensitivity, indicating that some patients may still respond to fluid at slightly lower values (e.g., 10%).

Ventricular Performance

Evaluation of ventricular systolic function in the critically ill hemodynamically unstable patient is of substantial importance, and can identify myocardial dysfunction that can guide the application of cardiovascular agents with inotropic, vasopressor, or vasodilator actions. A goal of this

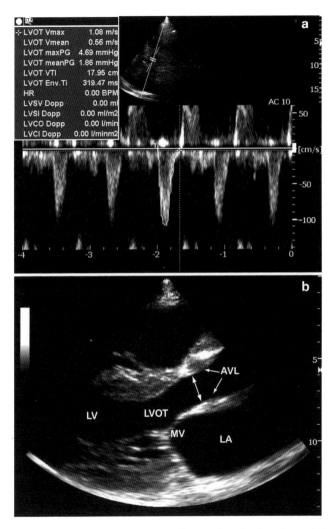

Figure 7-16. Measurement of stroke volume using the Doppler technique. The velocity profile is recorded in the aortic outflow tract (**a**), and the area of the ejection profile is traced and measured as the velocity–time integral (VTI). In this case, the VTI is about 18 cm, within the normal range. On two-dimensional echo (**b**), the diameter of the outflow tract at its narrow dimension at the base of the aortic valve is measured (*double arrow*), in this case 1.9 cm, giving a stroke volume of 51 mL. Shown for reference are the left ventricle (LV), left atrium (LA), left ventricular outflow tract (LVOT), and the aortic valve leaflets (AVL).

evaluation is evaluation of myocardial contractility. Ventricular systolic function, however, has many determinants beside contractility that need to be considered during assessment. Both preload and afterload can affect ventricular performance, and evaluation of contractility generally requires evaluation under different loading conditions. This is not feasible at the beside, so that these loading conditions must be identified and taken into consideration when trying assess contractility.

Wall Motion Abnormalities

One of the first steps in evaluating myocardial dysfunction is to identify whether dysfunction is *global* or *regional*. Global dysfunction refers to a generalized alteration in contractility that affects all portions of the ventricular myocardium nearly equally. Acute causes include global myocardial ischemia (low systemic flow), myocardial stunning from reperfusion following global ischemia, myocardial depression from sepsis and SIRS, or severe electrolyte abnormalities such as hypocalcemia. The approach to treatment involves correction of the underlying abnormality, and may require support with an inotropic or vasodilator agent.

Regional wall motion abnormalities are those which affect a portion of the left ventricular wall, most commonly associated with localized ischemia from coronary artery disease. Affected sections can be hypokinetic, akinetic, or dyskinetic. The segment(s) involved give clues to the coronary artery associated with ischemia (Fig. 7-17). Septal motion abnormalities can also result from right ventricular volume or pressure overload, and can be identified by its association with RV dilation or dysfunction.

With experience, assessment of ventricular function can be made by visual inspection of 2D images, including estimates of ejection fraction accurate to within about 10%. This visual inspection is usually all that is required during early intervention in the critically ill. Formal measurement of the indices below, however, allows for documentation for following response to therapy, especially when multiple clinicians may be involved over time. It also provides a framework from which to gain experience with visual inspection.

Fractional Shortening and Ejection Fraction

Assessment of global myocardial function includes the assessment of fractional shortening and/or ejection fraction, despite the influences of other factors described above. The fractional shortening is the degree of dimension change from diastole to systole expressed as a percentage:

$$FS = \frac{EDD - ESD}{EDD} \cdot 100\%$$

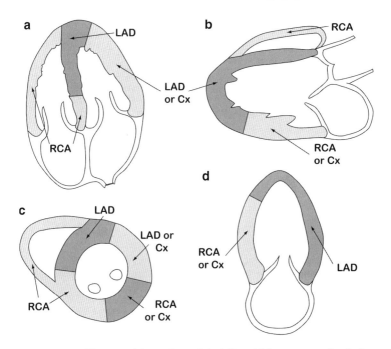

Figure 7-17. Diagram of the regions of the left ventricle corresponding to the distribution of the major epicardial coronary arteries in the apical four-chamber (**a**), parasternal long-axis (**b**), parasternal short-axis (**c**), and apical two-chamber (**d**) views. The coronary artery abbreviations are: left anterior descending (LAD), circumflex (Cx), and right coronary artery (RCA).

The dimension measurements are made from any view that allows the cross-sectional dimension of the LV to be measured. The measurement is made just below the mitral leaflet tips, and can be done in 2D mode or M-mode (Fig. 7-18). If 2D mode is used, a sequence of images is frozen and replayed to identify systole and diastole. M-mode allows more accurate assessment of cardiac cycle phase as well as measurement of chamber dimensions, in which case the axis of the beam should be perpendicular to the long axis of the heart, such as the parasternal or gastric approach. Use of a short-axis cross-sectional view allows identification of the center of the chamber, which is essential to avoid overestimation from a foreshortened view. The normal value of fractional shortening ranges from 30 to 42%, which corresponds to an ejection fraction of about 65–80% in the absence of regional wall motion abnormalities. Decreased values suggest depressed myocardial contractility, such as an acute or chronic cardiomyopathy, especially in the face of acute loading of the ventricle.

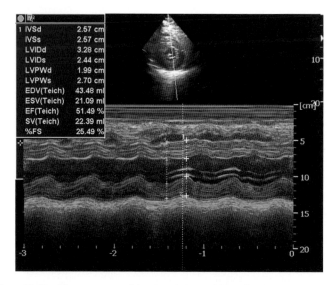

Figure 7-18. Measurement of fractional shortening and estimation of ejection fraction using M-mode echocardiography. Measurements are made of left ventricular internal diameter during diastole (left measurement) and systole (right measurement), and fractional shortening calculated, in this case 25.5%. The estimated ejection fraction by the Teicholz method in this case is 51.5%, with a stroke volume of 22.4 mL.

Higher values could result from a hyperdynamic state, either natural or catecholamine-induced, especially if associated with low preload and/or systemic vasodilatation.

In the absence of regional wall motion abnormalities, a crude estimate of ejection fraction can be made from the M-mode dimensions by assuming contraction of a spherical structure (cubic formula):

$$EF_{M\text{-}mode} = \frac{EDD^3 - ESD^3}{EDD^3} \cdot 100\%$$

More accurate measurements of ejection fraction can be made from better estimation formulas or from integration methods. The formula by Teicholz estimates ventricular volume by the empiric formula:

$$V = \frac{7}{2.4 + D} \cdot D^3$$

Substituting V for EDD^3 in the previous formula yields the Teicholz ejection fraction:

$$EF = \frac{V_{dias} - V_{sys}}{V_{dias}} \cdot 100\%$$

This calculation is usually built into bedside ultrasound machines.

Integration methods use Simpson's rule for numerically calculating the ventricular volume by the summation of the area of several disks fit to the endocardial diameter. This is achieved by tracing the outline of the ventricular chamber at the endocardial surface. The ultrasound machine can apply Simpson's technique in one plane (assuming a cylindrical cross section) or two planes (the bi-plane method, assuming an elliptical cross section). The measurements are obtained from an apical four-chamber view. The volumes at end-systole and end-diastole are computed and substituted into the EF formula above. Interpretation of ejection fraction is the same as for fractional shortening, with normal values being 55–75%. The limitation of this approach is the inability to obtain views in some patients that capture the entire endocardial surface from mitral annulus to apex.

Stroke Volume and Cardiac Output

Stroke volume can be calculated using 2D or Doppler methods. The 2D method uses the same approach for calculating end-diastolic and end-systolic volumes as described for ejection fraction in the previous section. The stroke volume is then simply calculated as the difference between these two.

Doppler methods are more commonly used for stroke volume calculation. The discussion of stroke volume variation described earlier introduced the measurement of velocity–time integral (VTI). The VTI describes the distance a column of blood ejected from the ventricle travels as a result of one systolic period. Multiplying this distance by the cross-sectional area (CSA) at the point where the image is made yields stroke volume:

$$SV = VTI \cdot CSA = VTI \cdot \frac{D^2}{4} \cdot 3.14$$

The VTI is calculated for the aortic or pulmonary valves as described above in the section on stroke volume variation (Fig. 7-16). The CSA of the aortic valve is most commonly measured from the parasternal long axis view of the aortic valve, measuring the diameter of the outflow tract at the aortic valve leaflets. The CSA is measured from the transthoracic parasternal short axis view, but in most adults, there is inadequate visualization of the pulmonary outflow tract. It is usually obtainable by TEE. The product of stroke volume and heart rate yields the cardiac output.

If the CSA cannot be obtained, the VTI alone gives a rough estimate as to whether stroke volume is normal. A normal VTI is 15–20 cm, and values below 12 indicate a significant reduction in stroke volume.

Right Ventricular Function

Quantitative measurements of RV function are not possible using the geometric formulas applicable to the left ventricle. Description of RV function is therefore qualitative, and related to LV function. RV function is best appreciated on the four chamber views, when both ventricles can be assessed simultaneously.

Afterload

Afterload represents the impedance to ejection of blood, and most commonly described as the tension generated within the myocardium during systolic ejection. The measurement of wall tension requires simultaneous measurement of echocardiographic parameters and intraventricular pressure,[14] and is therefore not suitable for the bedside. Surrogate measures are thus used, the most common being the ventricular pressure at the end of systole, measured clinically as the systemic or pulmonary systolic blood pressure (in the absence of valvular stenosis). Because of the sensitivity of the RV to increased afterload, most of the discussion will center on the right ventricle.

Right Ventricular Afterload

The right ventricle is much more afterload sensitive than is the left, and measurement of pulmonary artery pressure helps in the evaluation of RV dilatation. A dilated RV due to pulmonary hypertension describes *RV pressure overload,* whereas excessive filling leading to dilatation in the face of normal PA pressures describes *RV volume overload.* In the critically ill patient, pressure overload can result from increases in pulmonary vascular resistance associated with acute lung disease such as acute respiratory distress syndrome, and mechanical ventilation (especially high levels of support). Volume overload is most often secondary to overly aggressive fluid resuscitation, but usually has a component of pressure overload as well.

Pulmonary artery systolic pressure can be measured in most patients due to the presence of some degree of tricuspid regurgitation, especially in patients on mechanical ventilation. The peak velocity of the regurgitant jet is related to the pressure gradient across the tricuspid valve through the modified Bernoulli equation:

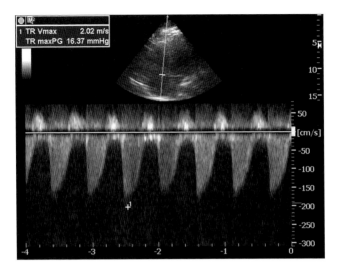

Figure 7-19. Estimation of pulmonary artery systolic pressure using continuous Doppler measurement of tricuspid regurgitant velocity. The peak velocity in this case is 2.02 m/s, yielding a systolic pressure gradient across the valve of 16.4 mmHg, from which systolic pressure can be estimated by adding to this value the known or estimated central venous pressure.

$$\Delta P = 4 \cdot V^2.$$

P is in mmHg when V is measured in m s^{-1}. Applied to the tricuspid regurgitant jet, the pressure represents PA–RA pressure, so adding in the known or estimated RA pressure gives the estimate of PA systolic pressure. The measurement is made from the apical view in most cases, using color Doppler to locate the regurgitant jet and define the best plane for its measurement. Continuous wave Doppler is applied, with the beam targeting the jet. The Doppler signal is then frozen and the peak velocity is measured (Fig. 7-19). With the calculation package, the pressure gradient is automatically displayed. The identification of elevated PA pressure then can direct appropriate treatment, such as volume reduction or use of vasodilators, such as inhaled nitric oxide, depending on the underlying cause. With echocardiography, the response to vasodilators can also be determined by repeated measurements following initiation of therapy.

Ventricular Interdependence

The right and left ventricles share the pericardial space, and acute dilatation of the right ventricle can impair left ventricular function. This interdependence can be appreciated with 2D echocardiography, and is identified by enlargement of the right ventricle and flattening of the interventricular septum, or even displacement into the left ventricular chamber (Fig. 7-20). Two consequences are impairment of left ventricular filling, and altered contraction due to the geometric distortion, leading to both

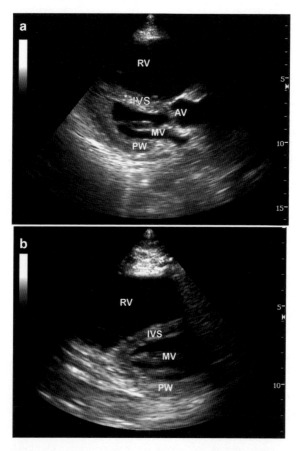

Figure 7-20. Examples of ventricular interdependence in which right ventricular volume overload has led to impairment of left ventricular systolic and diastolic function. The parasternal long axis view (**a**) demonstrates a greatly enlarged right ventricle (RV) causing flattening of the interventricular septum (IVS) and reduction in left ventricular volume. A similar finding is noted in the short axis view (**b**). Shown for reference are the mitral valve (MV), aortic valve (AV), and left ventricular posterior wall (PW).

diastolic and systolic LV dysfunction. These patients usually manifest as hemodynamic deterioration, and this condition is usually unrecognized without echocardiography. Without recognition, the usual treatment involves further fluid administration, which compounds the problem. Management involves reduction of PA pressure through pulmonary vaso-dilatation, and may require rapid volume reduction.

Cardiac Arrest and Resuscitation

Resuscitation from cardiac arrest is typically performed with limited information about underlying cardiac function, relying only on elec-trocardiographic rhythms and external pulse checks to infer the state of cardiac function. The ECG is helpful during ventricular fibrillation, but if organized electrical activity is present, peripheral assessment is very unreliable. Pulseless electrical activity, for example, can be due to overwhelming myocardial failure that is difficult to treat, but reversible causes amenable to treatment, such as cardiac tamponade, hypovolemia, cardiogenic shock, or pulmonary embolism, cannot be reliably diagnosed without echocardiography. Ultrasound can be used to identify noncardiac causes of arrest such as tension pneumothorax. It can also identify the presence of cardiac contraction that may not be detectable as a pulse, in which inotropic and/or vasopressor support may be indicated, and con-tinued unsynchronized cardiac compression may be detrimental. Given the information afforded from this modality, focused echocardiography during cardiac arrest resuscitation can provide important information.[15]

CPR is most successful if it is uninterrupted, posing a challenge for the echocardiographer to be able to image with limited or no interrup-tion of chest compression. The subcostal approach can be used to image during compressions, but may be technically inadequate and a helpful image is often not obtainable. Thus chest compressions may need to be interrupted, but an experienced echocardiographer can obtain a great deal of information in a brief period of time. Prolonged interruption of chest compressions should not be allowed to result from attempts at image acquisition. It is best if coordinated with scheduled interruptions for other reasons, such as rhythm identification.

Evaluation of wall motion provides important clues. The absence of any wall motion confirms cardiac standstill and can help decision mak-ing for continued resuscitation or discontinuation of efforts. Wall motion with adequate contractility indicates the presence of circulation and usu-ally coincides with the ability to palpate a carotid pulse. A poorly contracting ventricle indicates myocardial depression or stunning and suggests the need for an inotrope or inopressor. Very poor contractility may indicate the need to continue external compression. If the ventricle is found to be adequately contractile but underfilled, hypovolemia is present and dic-tates the need for rapid fluid infusion. The presence of a pericardial effu-sion with compression of the ventricle suggests tamponade and the need for emergent pericardiocentesis. The presence of right ventricular overload should lead one to consider the possibility of pulmonary embolism as the etiology of circulatory collapse.

■ STRUCTURAL ASSESSMENT

While the focus of this chapter has been on function assessment and hemodynamics, circulatory failure can result from structural abnormalities that may require other approaches to treatment. Most of the conditions discussed below can be identified on 2D and M-mode imaging, with color Doppler imaging providing important additional information on some cases. The goal of this section is not to provide a comprehensive review of the echocardiographic exam, but rather to focus on conditions that may cause acute instability in the ICU that should be recognizable on the focused exam.

Pericardial Effusion and Tamponade

Two-dimensional echocardiography by the transthoracic approach allows rapid identification of pericardial fluid or other space-occupying problems (e.g., postoperative hematoma) (Fig. 7-21). The size of an effusion capable of causing tamponade depends on multiple factors, including

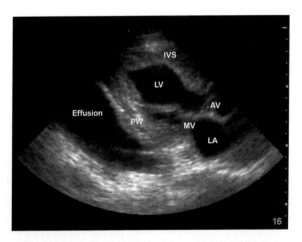

Figure 7-21. Parasternal long axis view of a large pericardial effusion. The effusion is seen posterior to the heart and extends around the apex (not visible in this image). Shown for reference are the left ventricle (LV), interventricular septum (IVS), aortic (AV) and mitral (MV) valves, and the left atrium (LA).

rapidity of development. Chronic effusions can be large without evidence of tamponade, while acute effusions or hemopericardium can induce tamponade with a much smaller volume.

Imaging is best performed from multiple windows, since pleural effusions can be confused with pericardial fluid. The parasternal approach can identify fluid around the base of the heart, acknowledging that the descending thoracic aorta can be mistaken for posterior fluid. Apical views provide imaging of fluid at the apex of the heart. The subcostal view provides imaging of fluid adjacent to the right ventricle and can be helpful for locating an approach for pericardiocentesis.

The diagnosis of pericardial tamponade remains primarily a clinical diagnosis, but several echocardiographic signs can be helpful. Collapse of the right atrium during atrial systole (late ventricular diastole) and of the right ventricle during ventricular diastole carry good sensitivity and specificity for tamponade (Fig. 7-22). Paradoxical changes in right ventricular volume, leading to the finding of pulsus paradoxus, may be identified. In contrast to the normal situation, tamponade can result in an increase in RV volume during inspiration while spontaneously breathing, and a decrease during exhalation. Finally, the elevated right atrial pressure associated with tamponade can be identified as a markedly distended inferior vena cava associated with pericardial fluid in the absence of RV dilatation.

Valvular Regurgitation

Acute valvular abnormalities leading to cardiogenic shock can be identified by a number of echocardiographic techniques, but the application of color Doppler can allow identification of life-threatening conditions. Severe acute regurgitation of the aortic or mitral valves can be identified with color Doppler as large volume regurgitant jets. Care must be taken to evaluate the anatomic extent (volume) of regurgitation into the cavity and not just the velocity, since small regurgitant jets that are not the cause of hemodynamic instability can have high velocity jets. Association with volume overload into the regurgitant chamber provides secondary information. Guidelines for evaluation of valvular regurgitation are available in standard textbooks on echocardiography.

Intracardiac Shunts

Intracardiac shunts can lead to acute hemodynamic deterioration or to persistent hypoxemia if associated with right-to-left flow. With acute lung disease, especially when requiring mechanical ventilation, a functional right-to-left shunt can develop through a patent foramen ovale in up to 25% of individuals. In most of these cases, the shunt is clinically insignificant, and these patients do not have hemodynamic instability. The development of an acute ventricular septal defect following myocardial

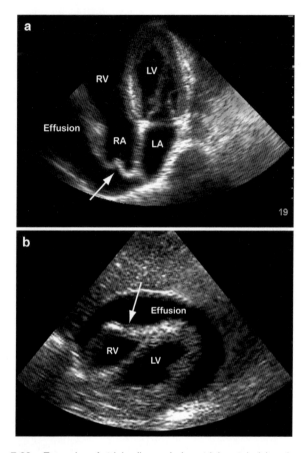

Figure 7-22. Examples of atrial collapse during atrial systole (**a**) and ventricular collapse during ventricular diastole (**b**), suggesting the possible presence of cardiac tamponade.

infarction produces life-threatening hemodynamic instability, and early identification is necessary. This defect can be identified with high sensitivity by color Doppler as a flow disturbance crossing the ventricular septum associated with dilatation of the right ventricle.

The identification of more subtle right-to-left atrial shunts can be performed with an echo contrast study. Peripheral or central venous injection of echo contrast (microbubbles in agitated saline) produces bright images on 2D echo, and bubbles crossing to the left atrium are readily identified.

■ GLOSSARY

2D real-time imaging   see B-mode imaging.

Acoustic impedance   a measure of the resistance of tissue to the propagation of ultrasound. It is largely dependent on the density of the tissue and the speed of sound propagation through the tissue.

Apical window   Insonation window located at the apex of the heart, approachable from the transthoracic and transesophageal modalities.

B-mode imaging   two dimensional imaging based on scanning over an area and mapping intensity in two dimensions. By repeating the imaging at a sufficiently fast scan rate, a real-time image can be obtained.

Color flow Doppler imaging   A form of imaging in which Doppler velocity signals are measured over an area, converted to a color map, and overlaid onto the corresponding 2D image.

Compression waves   refers to the longitudinal waves associated with sound traveling through a medium. Longitudinal waves consist of alternating pressure deviations.

Continuous wave Doppler   A form of Doppler interrogation in which a continuous ultrasound is transmitted, with continuous receiving of the reflected waves and calculation of velocity. This mode is sensitive to velocities all along the beam, and thus is useful for finding the maximum velocity only but not where it is located.

Insonation window   A location on the surface of the body or in the esophagus/stomach that is free of interfering structures, allowing acquisition of an image.

M-mode imaging   an imaging mode consisting of a one-dimensional view recorded against time.

Parasternal window   Transthoracic insonation window located to the left of the sternum, about the fourth intercostal space.

Pulse repetition frequency   In pulsed Doppler or B-mode imaging, represents the rate at which the transducer is pulsed. Imaging of deeper structures requires more time for the ultrasound signal to be reflected from the deep structures, requiring a lower PRF, and less information that can be recorded.

Pulsed wave Doppler   A form of Doppler interrogation in which a pulse of ultrasound is transmitted, with the signal received during a specified time window corresponding to a known depth. This mode allows recording of velocities at a particular intracardiac location.

Reflection   A mechanism of ultrasound signal loss that occurs when a wave is reflected away from a tissue interface of differing acoustic impedances.

Scan area   The anatomic area that can be imaged at one time. For linear transducers, the scan area is a square below the transducer. For phased-array sector transducers such as that used in echocardiography, the scan area is pie-shaped, with the narrow angle directly under the transducer.

Subcostal window   Transthoracic insonation window located in the epigastrum below the xyphoid process.

■ REFERENCES

1. Slama M, Maizel J. Echocardiographic measurement of ventricular function. *Curr Opin Crit Care*. 2006;12(3):241–248.
2. Rivers E, Nguyen B, Havstad S, et al. Early goal-directed therapy in the treatment of severe sepsis and septic shock. *N Engl J Med*. 2001;345(19):1368–1377.
3. Schiller NB, Shah PM, Crawford M, et al. Recommendations for quantitation of the left ventricle by two-dimensional echocardiography. American Society of Echocardiography Committee on Standards, Subcommittee on Quantitation of Two-Dimensional Echocardiograms. *J Am Soc Echocardiogr*. 1989;2(5):358–367.
4. Lamia B, Ochagavia A, Monnet X, Chemla D, Richard C, Teboul JL. Echocardiographic prediction of volume responsiveness in critically ill patients with spontaneously breathing activity. *Intensive Care Med*. 2007;33(7):1125–1132.
5. Nagueh SF, Middleton KJ, Kopelen HA, Zoghbi WA, Quinones MA. Doppler tissue imaging: a noninvasive technique for evaluation of left ventricular relaxation and estimation of filling pressures. *J Am Coll Cardiol*. 1997;30(6):1527–1533.
6. Ommen SR, Nishimura RA, Appleton CP, et al. Clinical utility of Doppler echocardiography and tissue Doppler imaging in the estimation of left ventricular filling pressures: A comparative simultaneous Doppler-catheterization study. *Circulation*. 2000;102(15):1788–1794.
7. Firstenberg MS, Levine BD, Garcia MJ, et al. Relationship of echocardiographic indices to pulmonary capillary wedge pressures in healthy volunteers. *J Am Coll Cardiol*. 2000;36(5):1664–1669.
8. Barbier C, Loubieres Y, Schmit C, et al. Respiratory changes in inferior vena cava diameter are helpful in predicting fluid responsiveness in ventilated septic patients. *Intensive Care Med*. 2004;30(9):1740–1746.
9. Feissel M, Michard F, Faller JP, Teboul JL. The respiratory variation in inferior vena cava diameter as a guide to fluid therapy. *Intensive Care Med*. 2004;30(9):1834–1837.
10. Kircher BJ, Himelman RB, Schiller NB. Noninvasive estimation of right atrial pressure from the inspiratory collapse of the inferior vena cava. *Am J Cardiol*. 1990;66(4):493–496.
11. Vieillard-Baron A, Chergui K, Rabiller A, et al. Superior vena caval collapsibility as a gauge of volume status in ventilated septic patients. *Intensive Care Med*. 2004;30(9):1734–1739.
12. Vieillard-Baron A, Augarde R, Prin S, Page B, Beauchet A, Jardin F. Influence of superior vena caval zone condition on cyclic changes in right ventricular outflow during respiratory support. *Anesthesiology*. 2001;95(5):1083–1088.
13. Charron C, Caille V, Jardin F, Vieillard-Baron A. Echocardiographic measurement of fluid responsiveness. *Curr Opin Crit Care*. 2006;12(3):249–254.

14. Ratshin RA, Rackley CE, Russell RO Jr. Determination of left ventricular preload and afterload by quantitative echocardiography in man. *Circ Res*. 1974;34(5):711–718.
15. Breitkreutz R, Walcher F, Seeger FH. Focused echocardiographic evaluation in resuscitation management: concept of an advanced life support-conformed algorithm. *Crit Care Med*. 2007;35(5 suppl):S150–S161.

8

Procedures in Critical Care: Dialysis and Apheresis

Matthew J. Diamond and Harold M. Szerlip

■ INTRODUCTION

Acute renal injury in the intensive care unit (ICU) is associated with significant excess mortality. A rise in the serum creatinine of 0.3 mg/dl is associated with worse outcomes in critically ill patients.[1,2] Using the consensus definition of acute renal injury, the so-called RIFLE criteria[3,4] (Fig. 8-1), the odds ratio for death increases from approximately 2.5 in those patients classified as having renal *R*isk to 5 for renal *I*njury and finally to 10 for those with *F*ailure.[5] Even after adjusting for other comorbidities, renal injury in the ICU is an independent risk factor for death[6–8] and the need for acute dialytic therapy in the ICU is associated with 50–60% mortality.[9,10]

Various extracorporeal therapies are available to treat patients in the ICU. Hemodialysis and hemofiltration can be used to remove urea and

H.M. Szerlip (✉)
Department of Hypertension and Transplant Medicine, Section of Nephrology, Medical College of Georgia, Augusta, Georgia, USA
e-mail: hszerlip@mail.mcg.edu

H.L. Frankel and B.P. deBoisblanc (eds.), *Bedside Procedures for the Intensivist*,
DOI 10.1007/978-0-387-79830-1_8,
© Springer Science+Business Media, LLC 2010

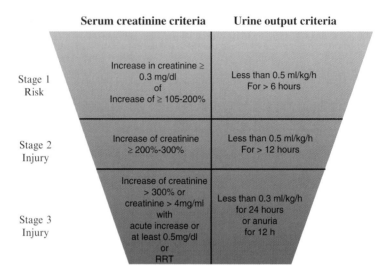

	Serum creatinine criteria	Urine output criteria
Stage 1 Risk	Increase in creatinine ≥ 0.3 mg/dl of Increase of ≥ 105-200%	Less than 0.5 ml/kg/h For > 6 hours
Stage 2 Injury	Increase of creatinine ≥ 200%-300%	Less than 0.5 ml/kg/h For > 12 hours
Stage 3 Injury	Increase of creatinine > 300% or creatinine > 4mg/ml with acute increase or at least 0.5mg/dl or RRT	Less than 0.3 ml/kg/h for 24 hours or anuria for 12 h

Figure 8-1. Modified RIFLE criteria for classification of acute kidney injury. Classification can be based on a serum creatinine or urine output.

creatinine, normalize acid-base and electrolyte abnormalities, remove fluid, and clear certain drugs and toxins from the body. Hemoperfusion, although infrequently utilized, is a therapy available to remove drugs that are highly protein bound or lipid soluble. Finally, plasmapheresis can be beneficial to treat certain antibody-mediated diseases, remove high molecular weight proteins or to replenish missing plasma factors.

■ WHEN TO INITIATE RENAL SUPPORT AND WHAT MODE OF THERAPY TO USE

Dialysis, unfortunately, only provides support and does not replace the many functions of the kidney; exactly when to start dialysis remains controversial. It is clear that when the kidneys can no longer effectively facilitate clearance of uremic toxins, maintain electrolyte balance or rid the body of excess volume, dialysis is indicated. Waiting, for these complications, however, is counterintuitive. Although there are no randomized trials explicitly comparing "early" to "late" initiation, review of the existing literature suggests that starting dialysis early appears to be associated with a better outcome than starting late.[11,12] Our own preference is to begin dialysis in a patient who after receiving adequate volume resuscitation either still has urine output less than 0.25 cc/kg/h for 24 h or is anuric for 12 h.

In a nonoliguric patient who has a rising creatinine, we suggest initiating dialysis if the patient is hemodynamically unstable or has another organ system dysfunction.

The type of dialysis provided depends on the equipment available and the comfort the nephrologists/intensivists have with the technique. Although veno-venous therapies have become the treatment of choice in most ICUs, peritoneal dialysis may be beneficial in units that are not capable of providing hemodialysis.

■ PERITONEAL DIALYSIS

Peritoneal dialysis (PD) involves the instillation and subsequent drainage of dialysate into and out of the peritoneal cavity using a percutaneously placed catheter. The peritoneal membrane serves as a semipermeable membrane allowing small molecular solutes such as electrolytes, urea, and creatinine to diffuse from the peritoneal capillaries into the dialysate down their concentration gradients. The ultrafiltration of water is accomplished by increasing the osmolality of the dialysate, usually by changing the concentration of glucose. A theoretical concern with PD is that infusion of fluid into the peritoneum may cause abdominal compartment syndrome, compromising ventilation and venous return. This form of therapy has fallen out of favor because it is difficult to achieve adequate clearance. In a recent multinational study evaluating renal failure in the ICU, <2% of patients received PD.[10] A small study, comparing hemofiltration to PD in patients with falciparum malaria found a markedly worse outcome in the PD group.[13] Another more recent study, although also under-powered study, compared high volume PD to daily hemodialysis and found no difference in metabolic control, recovery of renal function or mortality between the two modalities.[14]

■ BLOOD SIDE THERAPIES

The clearance of nitrogenous waste as well as the normalization of electrolytes can be accomplished by hemodialysis, hemofiltration, or a combination of both. There are no studies comparing the outcomes among these different forms of therapy. Therefore, as with many practices in the ICU, which one should be utilized is dependent on the comfort of the nephrologist/intensivist with the technique.

Each of these therapies is delivered by placement of a large-bore double-lumen catheter into a central vein. Blood is mechanically pumped from the proximal port of the catheter, through a semipermeable membrane consisting of thousands of hollow fibers (artificial kidney), and back to the patient through the distal port (Fig. 8-2).

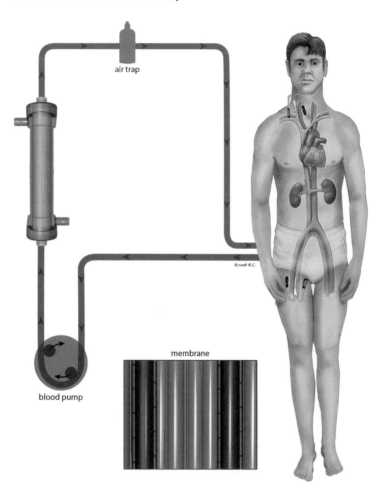

Figure 8-2. Dialysis circuit. Vascular access is obtained by placement of a large-bore double-lumen catheter into the superior vena cava from the internal jugular vein or the inferior vena cava from the femoral vein. A blood pump moves the blood from the "arterial" circuit through a membrane consisting of thousands of porous semipermeable hollow fibers. After exiting the membrane the blood passes through an air trap and is returned to the body via the "venous" limb of the catheter.

Hemodialysis

In hemodialysis, blood flows through the inside of the hollow fibers and a dialysate of the appropriate composition flows on the outside in a counter-current fashion. Small- and medium-sized solutes (<1,000 Da) diffuse across a semipermeable membrane driven by the concentration gradient established by dialysate flowing around the membranes. (Fig. 8-3, top) This modality clears solutes by diffusion. The diffusive clearance is dependent on multiple factors, including the characteristics of the semipermeable membrane, the size of the solute and the trans-membrane concentration gradient. The variables that can be controlled are the size and composition of the membrane, blood flow (up to 500 ml/min), dialysate flow (up to 800 ml/min), and treatment time. Dialysis can be provided as short (3–5 h) intermittent therapy (IHD), Continuous Veno-Venous HemoDialysis (CVVHD) (18–24 h), or hybrid therapy (8–12 h) also known as Slow Extended Dialysis (SLED)

Hemofiltration

In contrast to hemodialysis, hemofiltration does not use a dialysate. Clearance is obtained convectively by increasing the hydrostatic pressure within the blood compartment of the dialyzer. The trans-membrane pressure drives an ultrafiltrate through a porous membrane (Fig. 8-3, bottom). The composition of the ultrafiltrate depends on the sieving coefficient of the membrane for that solute, i.e., the higher the molecular weight, the lower the clearance. Electrolytes, urea, and creatinine have a sieving coefficient of 1 meaning that the concentration in the plasma and the ultrafiltrate are identical. Hemofiltration can remove solutes as high as 30,000 Da. In order to avoid intravascular volume depletion and maintain normal electrolyte composition, replacement fluid with a similar electrolyte composition as plasma is infused either pre- or postfilter. There are several commercially available sterile replacement fluids. Clearance can be increased by using a membrane filter with a higher ultrafiltration coefficient (larger pore size) or by applying a greater trans-membrane pressure. Hemofiltration is usually provided daily for 18–24 h (i.e., Continuous Veno-Venous Hemofiltration, CVVH).

Hemodiafiltration

In this technique, clearance is accomplished by both diffusion and convection. Similar to hemofiltration, hemodiafiltration is usually provided as continuous daily therapy (Continuous Veno-Venous HemoDiaFiltration, CVVHDF).

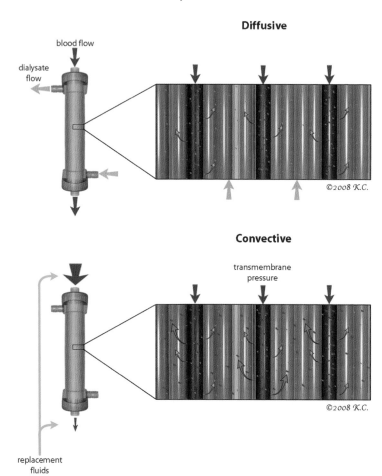

Figure 8-3. In diffusive clearance (*top*), solutes cross a semipermeable membrane down their concentration gradient. In convective clearance (*bottom*), the trans-membrane pressure drives an ultrafiltrate though a porous membrane. The size of the pores and the trans-membrane pressure determines the amount and composition of ultrafiltrate.

■ CONTINUOUS VERSUS INTERMITTENT THERAPIES

In 1977, Kramer et al introduced the concept of continuous hemofiltration for renal support in hemodynamically unstable patients in the ICU.[15,16] As originally described, access catheters were placed in both the femoral artery and femoral vein and one connected to each end of a hemofilter. The patient's blood pressure served as the driving force to move blood through the filter and back into the venous circulation. Trans-membrane pressure was varied by raising or lowering the height of the filter relative to the patient's phlebostatic axis. Because the driving pressure varied with blood pressure, this arteriovenous technique was eventually replaced by veno-venous therapy utilizing a blood pump and a double-lumen catheter placed in the central venous system. By spreading the removal of volume and solute over a 24-h period, it was hypothesized that effective dialytic therapy could be accomplished without compromising blood pressure in hemodynamically tenuous patients. This technique has gained rapid acceptance in many ICUs and has replaced intermittent hemodialysis as the treatment of choice. Advocates of continuous renal replacement therapy (CRRT) believe that it is safer and provides a mortality benefit over IHD. There are several volumetrically controlled machines available that are relatively easy to use and provide multiple clearance modalities.

Several recent studies, however, have challenged the concept that CRRT has advantages over IHD.[17–19] Not only do these studies show a lack of mortality benefit, they also demonstrate that IHD can be safely performed in critically ill patients. In fact, one retrospective study[17] comparing CRRT to IHD showed worse outcomes in the group receiving CRRT even after risk adjustment. The authors speculated that removal of soluble vitamins and small molecular weight proteins, the need for continuous anticoagulation, and poorly established dosing guidelines for antibiotics may have been responsible for the observed differences. It should be emphasized that none of these studies were adequately powered to definitively answer the question. Until such a large, randomized trial is done, the choice of continuous or intermittent therapy will remain dependent on the comfort of the practitioners.

We prefer continuous or hybrid (SLED) therapy in patients who are extremely catabolic or who are receiving large volumes of fluids. In these patients it is unlikely that a 4-h intermittent treatment could effectively remove adequate solute or volume. Other factors that might favor CRRT include vasopressor-dependent shock and the presence of cerebral edema. The latter, because of animal studies and case reports, suggest that cerebral perfusion can be better maintained during CRRT. When using IHD in a critically ill patient, hemodynamic stability can be more easily maintained by cooling the dialysate to 350°C to induce peripheral vasoconstriction; setting the dialysate sodium equal to or slightly higher than the patient's, thus minimizing solute flux; and using the smallest possible filter to minimize the amount of blood in the extracorporeal circuit.

■ INTENSIVE VERSUS CONVENTIONAL THERAPIES

Because normal kidneys function on a continuous basis, most nephrologists/intensivists have advocated instituting intensive renal support in critical ill patients in a dose that attempts to normalize renal chemistries.

Such an approach had been supported by studies showing both that IHD performed six times per week improved survival compared to three times per week[20] and that in CVVH an ultrafiltration rate of 35 ml/kg/h was superior to an ultrafiltration rate of 20 ml/kg/h.[21] A recently completed large multicentered trial, however, failed to show any benefit of intensive therapy.[9] In view of the lack of a clearly defined survival benefit to intensive therapy, it has become difficult to justify the added cost of this approach.

■ DIALYSIS ACCESS

Peritoneal Access

Temporary peritoneal catheters are easily placed into the abdominal cavity. Blind percutaneous insertion should be avoided in patients with previous abdominal surgery. Catheters are usually inserted through the Linea Alba between the right and left rectus muscles approximately 4–5 cm below the umbilicus. To avoid accidental puncture of the bladder a Foley catheter should be inserted. Pre-procedural ultrasound at the intended puncture site can add an additional margin of safety.

1. Full barrier protection is recommended. The area below the umbilicus is prepped in a sterile manner and infiltrated with 1–2% lidocaine down to the serosal peritoneal membrane.
2. Using a 14-gauge needle the peritoneum is entered. The peritoneal tubing set is attached to the needle and 1–2 L of peritoneal dialysate is infused to distend the abdomen.
3. If using a Cook Medical acute dialysis catheter the tubing is removed and a guide-wire inserted through the needle aimed at the right or left pelvic gutter. The needle is removed and using a scalpel a small incision is made over the wire to enlarge the puncture site and facilitate the insertion of the catheter. The catheter is placed over the wire; using a twisting motion while maintaining control of the proximal aspect of the wire, the catheter is inserted into the peritoneum and the wire removed. The catheter is secured to the skin.
4. If using the Trocath® peritoneal catheter (Braun Medical), the needle is removed and the puncture site enlarged with a scalpel. A stylet is inserted into the catheter and the peritoneum is again punctured. The peritoneum is entered when a sudden drop in resistance is felt. The stylet is withdrawn 3–4 cm and the curved tip of the catheter is directed toward the right or left pelvic gutter. Without moving the stylet the catheter is advanced. When in position the stylet is removed and the catheter secured to the skin.

Venous Access

Temporary hemodialysis catheters are placed in the central venous circulation in the same manner as other central venous access devices (see Chap. 5) Because it is necessary for these double-lumen catheters to support blood flows up to 400 ml/min, they are somewhat larger in diameter than standard triple-lumen central venous catheters and require larger dilators for proper insertion. There are a number of brands of duel-lumen catheters available that are made of several different materials and with varying luminal shapes. Which catheter to use depends on the user's preference. All catheters have a distal "venous" port and a more proximal "arterial" port to limit recirculation of blood.

Unlike conventional central venous catheters it is recommended that temporary dialysis catheters be placed using the internal jugular or femoral vein. The subclavian vein is seldom used for placement of hemodialysis catheter because of the high incidence of subclavian vein stenosis, which limits the use of the distal veins for future chronic hemodialysis access. In addition, because of the larger bore of these catheters it is preferable to have an easily compressible site in case of bleeding. To allow for high blood flows and to prevent recirculation, internal jugular catheters should be positioned in the right atrium; if using the femoral approach, the catheter tip should be in the inferior vena cava, preferentially above the renal veins. To allow for proper positioning acute hemodialysis catheters come in a variety of lengths: 15–24 cm.

Current guidelines suggest that due to the risk of catheter-related infection, acute hemodialysis catheters be used for no more than one week. To reduce the risk of infection, in those patients requiring dialysis for more than a week, tunneled catheters with subcutaneous cuffs should be placed. These catheters are softer; requiring a pull away sheath for insertion. They are inserted in a similar manner to cuffless catheters except for creation of a subcutaneous tunnel. Unfortunately, it is often not possible to identify which patients will recover renal function within 7 days.

■ DIALYSIS PRESCRIPTION

Table 8-1 outlines dialysis prescriptions for several modalities.

Peritoneal Dialysis

1. *Frequency*: Continuous
2. *Dose*: Two liters of dialysate infused over 10 min with a dwell time of 40–50 min and a drain time 20 min (36–40 L/day). This can be done manually or by using an automated machine.

Table 8-1. Dialysis prescriptions for various modalities.

Mode	Frequency	Duration	Clearance	Blood Flow	Dialysate Flow	Hemofiltration Rate	Replacement Fluid
IHD	3×/week	3–5 h	Kt/V > 1.2	300–400 ml/min	500–800 ml/min	N/A	N/A
CVVH	Daily	21–24 h	Effluent rate 20–35 ml/kg/min	100–300 ml/min	N/A	20–35 ml/kg/h	20–35 ml/kg/h
CVVHD	Daily	21–24 h	Effluent rate 20–35 ml/kg/h	100–300 ml/min	20–35 ml/kg/h	N/A	N/A
CVVHDF	Daily	21–24 h	Effluent rate 20–35 ml/kg/h	100–300 ml/min	10–17.5 ml/kg/h	10–17.5 ml/kg/h	10–17.5 ml/kg/h
SLED	3×/week	8–12 h	Kt/V > 1.2	100–300 ml/min	300 ml/min	N/A	N/A
PD	Daily	24 h	100–300 ml/min	N/A	100–300 ml/min	N/A	N/A

3. *Dialysate*: There are several different commercial solutions available.
4. *Dialysate composition*: PD solutions are potassium free. Potassium needs to be added to the bags depending on the patient's potassium. Commonly available solutions use lactate as the base.
5. *Ultrafiltration*: Volume is removed by increasing the glucose concentration and thus the osmolality of the dialysate (1.5–2.5–4.25%). The higher the glucose concentration the greater the ultrafiltration volume.

Intermittent Hemodialysis

1. *Frequency*: Three times a week. Additional treatments may be necessary for extremely catabolic patients. More intensive therapy is not routinely recommended.
2. *Dose*: The effectiveness of hemodialysis is expressed by the dimensionless term, Kt/V. Where K is the dialysis membrane's clearance of urea (L/h), t is treatment time, and V is volume of distribution of urea. Kt/V can be calculated by using the following formula, which is also available on most medical calculators found on handheld computers:

$$Kt/V = -\ln\left(R - 0.008 \times t\right) + \left(4 - \left(3.5\right)R\right) \times 0.55\left(\text{UF}/V\right.$$

$\quad R \;=\; 1 - (\text{postprocedure BUN/preprocedure BUN})$
$\quad \text{UF} =\; \text{ultrafiltration volume}$
$\quad V \;=\;$ Volume of distribution of urea. Although there are several different nomograms to estimate volume, because none have been validated in critically ill patients a gross estimate of total body water can be used:
$\quad\quad =\; \text{wt (kg)} \times 0.6 \text{ for males}$
$\quad\quad =\; \text{wt (kg)} \times 0.55 \text{ for females}$

This formula corrects for nitrogenous waste generation during the dialysis treatment and accounts for postdialysis volume reduction. The Kt/V should exceed 1.3 for effective dialysis treatment. Clearance of urea is dependent on blood flow and treatment time. In most patients achieving a $Kt/V = 1.2$–1.3 will require 3–5 h of treatment depending on blood flow. Because it is often not possible to predict actual clearance, it is important that the clinician measure Kt/V at least once a week.
3. *Dialysate composition*: Hemodialysis can be used to manipulate nearly any electrolyte measured on a basic chemistry panel by adjusting the composition of the dialysate solution (Table 8-2).
4. *Dialysate flow rate (Qd)*: In IHD, dialysate is generated on line using an electrolyte concentrate that is proportionately mixed with water that has been passed though a carbon filter to remove chloramines and treated by reverse osmosis to reduce electrolytes. It is further

Table 8-2. Electrolyte concentrations for intermittent hemodialysis.

Electrolyte	Available Concentration (meq/1)	Standard Concentration (meq/1)
Na	125–145	135–145
K	0–4	2–3
HCO$_3$	25–40	30–35
Ca	2.5–3.5	2.5 –3.5
Mg	0.75–1	0.75–1

filtered through a micropore membrane to remove any bacterial con-taminates. As opposed to the use of sterile pre-packaged dialysate used in CRRT, this inexpensive generation of dialysate enables the use of higher dialysate flows. The Qd is kept greater than the blood flow (500–800 ml/min) to maximize clearance.

5. *Blood flow rate (Qb)*: In the ICU setting, Qb is dependent on dialysis access. Despite using large-bore catheters placed in the central circu-lation, thrombus formation; fibrin sheaths; or occlusion of the ports by the vessel wall often limits flow. The maximum blood flow rates vary among catheters, but generally reach 400 ml/min before perfor-mance declines and flow mechanics are compromised. Because in IHD blood flow determines urea clearance, flows between 300–400 ml/min are desirable. Increasing blood flow will increase pressure within the extracorporeal circuit causing expansion of the tubing and dialyzer with a resultant increase in the volume of blood in the circuit. Although this is minimized with hollow fiber dialyzers, in hemodynamically unstable patients this may, nevertheless, compro-mise blood pressure.

6. *Membranes*: Dialysis membranes are made of various substances including cellulose, substituted cellulose, and several different bio-synthetic materials. Synthetic dialyzers activate complement to a lesser degree than cellulose membranes and are considered to be more biocompatible. These have become the membrane of choice in the ICU. In addition, membranes can have different surface areas and varying pore sizes. The larger the surface area the greater the clearance of urea but also the greater the volume of blood in the extracorporeal circuit. It is therefore best to use a smaller membrane (1.0–1.4 m^2) in patients who require vasopressors. Most nephrolo-gists will use leakier high flux membranes to improve clearance of middle-sized molecules, although the benefits of this are unproven.

7. *Ultrafiltration rate (UF)*: The pressure gradient across the membrane will drive an ultrafiltrate of plasma out of the blood compartment. The amount of ultrafiltrate is dependent on the pressure gradient and the ultrafiltration coefficient of the membrane. Membranes with a large pore size (high flux membranes) produce more ultrafiltrate per any given pressure. Modern volumetric machines allow precise

ultrafiltration rates and can remove several liters per hour if desired. UF can be adjusted to meet the volume needs of the patient and maintain euvolemia. Given the patient's cardiovascular and hemodynamic status, effective UF may be difficult to achieve without incurring further hypotension or increasing vasopressor support. The rate should be adjusted accordingly.

Continuous Renal Replacement Therapy

1. *Frequency*: CRRT is delivered on a daily basis until the patient can tolerate more conventional forms of renal replacement therapy. Treatment is usually ordered daily for 24 h. Because critically ill patients often require off-unit studies, it is not unusual for therapy to be truncated.
2. *Dose*: The advantage of CRRT is the ability to deliver renal replacement therapy over a 24-h period. Because of the continuous nature of the therapy Kt/V is usually not calculated. In CVVH, the clearance is dependent on the volume of hemofiltration; while in CVVHD because blood flow is greater than dialysis flow the clearance is dependent on dialysis flow. Whether using hemodialysis, hemofiltration or a combination of the two the volume of the effluent determines the clearance of urea. Effluent flow of 20–35 ml/kg ideal body weight/h is standard. In a 70 kg that could be accomplished with a dialysate flow of 1.4–2.5 L/h, an equivalent hemofiltration rate (with replacement fluid) or a combination (e.g., 1.25 L/h of both). As previously discussed, a recent large randomized control trial found no mortality benefit comparing 20 ml/kg/h to 35 ml/kg/h.[19]
3. *Electrolyte management*: As with IHD, in CRRT electrolytes can be manipulated by varying their concentration in the dialysate or replacement fluid. There are several commercial sterile dialysis solutions with varying electrolyte concentrations on the market; or dialysate can be custom made by the hospital pharmacy. Normocarb HF ® (Dialysis Solutions Inc.) and Prismasol® (Gambro) are FDA approved to be used as replacement fluid; sterile replacement fluid can also be made by pharmacy. Because none of these solutions contain phosphorus, levels of phosphorus need to be monitored and replacement given if low.
4. *Blood flow rate (Qb)*: Blood flow for CRRT is set at 150–300 ml/min.
5. *Dialysate flow rate (Qd)*: 1–3 L/h (see dose above) using commercially available solutions or custom solutions made by pharmacy.
6. *Ultrafiltration rate (UF)*: 1–3 L/h (see dose above).
7. *Replacement fluids*: With hemofiltration, the ultrafiltrate is replaced with an electrolyte solution similar to plasma so that the net fluid removal is zero. Replacement fluid can be infused pre- or postdialyzer. There are two FDA-approved hemofiltration solutions available or one can be custom made by the hospital pharmacy.

8. *Machines/membranes*: There are presently four different dedicated CRRT machines on the market. They all have integrative systems that volumetrically control the rate of ultrafiltration and replacement fluid. Some come with pre-assembled tubing and filter modules for ease of use. This limits the choice of filter and requires replacement of the entire module if the system clots. We recommend using a system that allows the physician to choose the filter.

Slow Extended Dialysis

SLED is a hybrid technique similar to IHD but with lower blood and dialysate flows and extended running time. It utilizes a Fresenius hemodialysis machine that has been modified to allow for lower dialysate flows than used for conventional HD. Because of the online generation of dialysate, dialysis flow can be kept greater than or equal to blood flow thus providing a greater urea clearance than CRRT.

1. *Frequency*: Can be done on a daily basis or three per week. There are no data that support a benefit of one frequency over the other.
2. *Dose*: Similar to IHD, *Kt/V* should be calculated. To achieve a *Kt/V* of >1.3 usually requires between 8 and 12 h of therapy. In hemodynamically unstable patients who are volume overloaded the time can be extended to enable volume removal over a longer period.
3. *Blood flow*: 150–300 ml/h
4. *Dialysis flow*: 200–300 ml/h

Slow Continuous Ultrafiltration

In volume-overloaded patients with preserved or only minimally impaired renal function pure ultrafiltration can be performed for volume removal. Slow Continuous Ultrafiltration (SCUF) is similar to hemofiltration but without the use of replacement fluid. SCUF allows for the continuous removal of volume and is ideal for patients with congestive heart failure or other volume overloaded patients who cannot adequately be diuresed using pharmacologic agents.

1. *Blood flow*: 100–300 ml/h
2. *Ultrafiltration rate*: 100–300 ml/h

■ ANTICOAGULATION

As blood flows through the extracorporeal circuit it encounters a multitude of different surfaces and flow dynamics. As would be expected, these nonbiological surfaces activate the clotting cascade resulting in thrombus formation within the dialyzer and tubing. This compromises blood flow and limits clearance, requiring replacement of the dialyzer and sometimes the entire extracorporeal circuit. The risk of clot formation increases with treatment time, thus patients on IHD are less likely to clot the circuit than patients on continuous therapy.

In patients who have an underlying coagulopathy, are actively bleeding, or who have a high risk of bleeding, several nonpharmacologic strategies can be used to prevent thrombosis of the circuit, including higher blood flow rates through the dialyzer and intermittent saline flushes to flush out microthrombi. Despite these measures, when no pharmacologic anticoagulation is used clotting within the dialysis circuit occurs in 10–20% of patients who are on continuous therapy. Therefore, pharmacologic anticoagulation is an important part of RRT especially for patients on continuous therapy. Anticoagulation is usually accomplished by the use of unfractionated heparin or trisodium citrate. We recommend that an institution use one or the other technique to avoid confusion.

Unfractionated Heparin

Heparin changes the conformation of antithrombin, leading to rapid inactivation of multiple coagulation factors, particularly Factor Xa. This effectively halts the coagulation cascade at multiple points, preventing thrombus formation.

In renal replacement therapy, heparin is often prescribed empirically, without monitoring the magnitude of anticoagulation. In patients with a relative increased risk of bleeding, it is appropriate to monitor coagulation levels to ensure a proper level of anticoagulation if these tests are readily available.

There are several general protocols for heparin administration during renal replacement therapy. The three general methods discussed are regular, "tight," and heparin in the prime only. It needs to be stressed that the doses noted are only an approximation. More accurate dosing requires monitoring. In patients with suspected or documented heparin induced thrombocytopenia heparin should not be used at all.

Anticoagulation Protocols

1. *Regular heparin*: In patients without a risk of bleeding heparin can be given as an initial bolus 2,000 units infused prefilter followed by a continuous infusion of approximately 1,000 units an hour. The goal is to keep the activated clotting time (ACT) approximately 80% above baseline.
2. *Tight heparin*: A more conservative strategy is used in patients who are considered at higher risk for bleeding. An initial bolus of 500–750 units followed by 500 units/h. The goal is to keep the activated clotting time approximately 40% above baseline.
3. *Heparin in prime*: In patients who are at high risk the circuit should be flushed with 5,000 units of heparin in a liter of 0.9% saline.

Because of heparin's propensity to bind to positively charged surfaces this will coat the inside of the circuit and decrease clotting. The circuit is flushed with 0.9% saline to remove any unbound heparin. This method has been shown to significantly decrease clotting within the extracorporeal circuit without increasing risk of bleeding.[22]

4. *Citrate anticoagulation*: Heparin can be avoided and bleeding risk markedly reduced by using a citrate solution to prevent thrombosis within the dialyzer circuit. Citrate chelates calcium, preventing activation of key elements of the coagulation cascade. Calcium gluconate is then infused either in the venous return line or through another central venous catheter to maintain normal levels of ionized calcium and avoid hypocalcemia. It is important to closely monitor both the ionized calcium in the extracorporeal circuit to ensure that the citrate infusion is correctly titrated and the systemic ionized calcium to adjust the calcium infusion and prevent hypocalcemia. The use of citrate, a base equivalent, requires not only reduction in the HCO_3 concentration of the dialysate but also the use of calcium free dialysate. Several protocols have been published outlining citrate administration during renal replacement therapy.[23,24] The clinician is advised to choose a single protocol and then modify it to fit the needs of the ICU.

■ COMPLICATIONS OF RENAL SUPPORT

1. Secondary to access placement
   (a) Retroperitoneal hematoma
   (b) Arteriovenous fistula formation
   (c) Pneumothorax
   (d) Hemothorax
   (e) Line infection
   (f) Bowel perforation (PD catheter)
2. Air embolism
3. Bleeding from over anticoagulation
4. Bleeding from line disconnection
5. Disequilibrium syndrome secondary to rapid solute removal
6. Hypotension
7. Hypophosphatemia
8. Hypokalemia

■ USE OF HEMODIALYSIS AND HEMOPERFUSION IN POISONING

Drug overdoses and poisonings are two indications for emergent renal replacement therapy in the ICUs.[25] Dialysis or hemoperfusion should be seen as an important, but adjunctive, therapy when treating acute drug

Table 8-3. Drug removal by hemodialysis or hemoperfusion[25]

Drug	Volume of Distribution	Molecular Weight	Water Solubility	Protein Binding (%)	Method of Removal
Ethylene glycol	0.6	62	Yes	0	Hemodialysis
Isopropyl alcohol	0.6	60	Yes	0	Hemodialysis
Methanol	0.7	32	Yes	0	Hemodialysis
Lithium	0.7	7	Yes	0	Hemodialysis
Salicylate	0.2	138	Yes	50	Hemodialysis
Valproic acid	0.13–0.22	144	Yes	90	Hemoperfusion/Hemodialysis
Theophyline	0.5	180	Yes	56	Hemoperfusion/Hemodialysis
Carbamazepine	1.4	236	No	74	Hemoperfusion
Disopyramide	0.6	340	No	10–70	Hemoperfusion
Phenobarbitol	0.5	232	No	24	Hemoperfusion
Phenytoin	0.5	252	No	90	Hemoperfusion

intoxications or frank poisonings. Conservative, supportive measures should be taken first and foremost: protecting and maintaining a patent airway, cardiovascular support, early gastric lavage (when appropriate and safe) with activated charcoal, and appropriate alkalinization or acidification of the urine.

Hemodialysis, peritoneal dialysis, and hemoperfusion can all be used to increase the removal of drugs and toxins from the body. The treatment modality is based primarily on the substance to be removed (Table 8-3). The efficacy of these methods for drug/toxin removal will depend on the substances' molecular size, water solubility, degree of protein/lipid binding, volume of distribution (V_D), and rate of transfer from the intracellular to the extracellular compartment.

The V_D is critical in determining the ability of renal therapies to remove a substance. The V_D can range from 0.06 L/kg for drugs confined to the intravascular space (heparin) to far greater than total body weight for drugs that are bound to tissue proteins and lipids (e.g., glutethimide 3 L/kg). Obviously, a drug with a large V_D will have only a small proportion of its total body drug burden within the intravascular space. Thus, hemodialysis or hemoperfusion will remove only a small fraction of drug for any given treatment.

Indications for Using Hemodialysis/Hemoperfusion for Drug/Toxin Removal

1. Decompensation despite intensive supportive therapy
2. Severe intoxication with depression of midbrain function
3. Impairment of normal drug excretion function due to hepatic, renal, or cardiac dysfunction

4. Intoxication with agents with metabolic effects
5. Intoxication with agents with delayed effects
6. Intoxication with agents that are extractable via RRT at a rate exceeding that of endogenous renal or hepatic function

Hemodialysis

IHD will remove small-to-medium molecular weight water-soluble particles (e.g., methanol, ethylene glycol, lithium, salicylates). The equipment and setup is similar to conventional dialysis. Blood flow should be maximized (400 ml/min) and a large surface area membrane used. Although the ultrafiltration coefficient of the dialysis membrane is not important for small molecules, more porous high flux membranes are necessary for larger molecular weight drugs such as Vancomycin. Although there are no supporting data, continuous therapy should be considered to remove lipid-soluble drugs with a large V_D.

Hemoperfusion

In hemoperfusion blood is pumped through a cartridge packed with polymer coated charcoal, which can either replace the hemodialysis membrane or be connected in series with the dialysis membrane. Drugs that are highly protein bound or lipid soluble are better removed by hemoperfusion than by hemodialysis. Bound drugs will preferentially bind to the activated carbon. The polymer coating prevents direct contact of the blood with the activated carbon particles but will allow small- to moderate-sized molecular weight drugs/toxins diffuse through. Thrombocytopenia occasionally occurs with charcoal hemoperfusion.

Hemoperfusion is ideal for removal of such drugs as dilantin, barbiturates, and glutethimide. Blood flow should be maximized (400 ml/min). The duration of treatment is usually 4–6 h. If necessary, time can be extended but because these cartridges become saturated they need to be replaced every 4 h. The only hemoperfusion cartridge available in the USA is the Adsorba ® (Gambro). These cartridges are expensive and have a short shelf life. For these reasons few hospitals stock them. For cost purposes, it is best for several area hospitals to form a consortium and share hemoperfusion cartridges.

PD is far less efficient than HD or HP, but can be a valuable tool when institution of hemodialysis cannot be done quickly, as in children.

■ PLASMAPHERESIS IN THE ICU

Therapeutic plasmapheresis (TPE) removes the patient's plasma which is then replaced with either fresh frozen plasma or albumin (Table 8-4).[25] TPE removes large molecular weight proteins/lipid and drugs that are highly protein bound.[26,27] TPE is ideal for the treatment of antibody-mediated

Table 8-4. Diseases treated by therapeutic plasmapheresis with the level of evidence grade.

Disease	Level of Evidence
Guillain–Barre Syndrome (acute inflammatory demyelinating polyneuropathy)	I
Chronic inflammatory demyelinating polyneuropathy	I
Anti-glomerular basement membrane disease (Goodpasture's syndrome)	I
Myasthenia gravis	I
Cryoglobulinemia	I
Thrombotic thrombocytopenic purpura	I
Paraproteinemic polyneuropathies	I
Thrombotic microangiopathy, hemolytic-uremic syndrome, and transplant-associated microangiopathy	II
Hyperviscosity syndrome in monoclonal gammopathies	II
Lambert–Eaton myasthenic syndrome	II
ANCA-associated rapidly progressive glomerulonephritis	II
Myeloma with acute renal failure	II
Mushroom poisoning	II
Paraneoplastic Neurologic Syndromes	II
Focal Segmental Glomerulosclerosis	II
Familial Hypercholesterolemia	II

Level I evidence is supported by randomized studies.
Level II evidence implies case series or anecdotal reports.

diseases. In addition, components deficient in the native plasma can be replenished, such as the von Willebrand factor cleaving protease, ADAMTS13, associated with thrombotic thrombocytopenic purpura.

TPE can be performed using either membrane plasma separators (MPS) or centrifugation. Plasma separators are similar to a dialysis membrane except that the pore size is much greater allowing for filtration of particles of much larger molecular weight. In centrifugation the various components of blood are separated in a spinning chamber based on their densities. Erythrocytes being the densest accumulate on the outside of the spinning chamber, whereas plasma, the least dense, accumulates on the inside of the chamber.

The benefit of MPS is that most standard hemodialysis machines are capable of using this methodology and therefore the purchase of expensive equipment is unnecessary. Centrifugation, however, allows for the separation and collection of the individual cellular element and is thus more versatile than membrane separation.

■ PLASMAPHERESIS PRESCRIPTION

1. *Vascular access*: With continuous modalities, a large-bore double-lumen catheter is mandated to allow for appropriate blood flow velocities. A temporary hemodialysis catheter can be used for this

modality, and is placed in the same manner and position as previously described.

2. *Calculation of patient's plasma volume*: Several formulae exist that can be used to calculate a patient's exact plasma volume; most of these are weight-based. Two formulae that can be used to estimate plasma volume are as follows:

$$(\text{wt in kg})(0.065)(1 - \text{Hct}) = \text{estimated plasma volume (PV)}$$

$$(65 - 100\,\text{mL})(\text{wt in Kg}) = \text{estimated plasma volume}$$

3. *Volume of exchange*: Most treatment prescriptions require 1–1.5 PV exchanges per treatment. Caution should be used in patients with impaired renal function, as excessive volume replacement could result in pulmonary edema, compounding an already critical situation.

4. *Treatment duration*: Based upon blood flow rates, which dictate plasma exchange velocity. Optimal blood flow rates are around 100–150 ml/min, which correlates to a plasma removal rate of 30–50 ml/min.

5. *Treatment schedule*: Varies depending on what is being treated, but in the critical care setting, one exchange should occur daily until symptoms improve; then treatment can be tapered to every other day or several times a week, depending on the underlying cause.

6. *Anticoagulation*: Heparin, Citrate.

■ REFERENCES

1. Chertow GM, Burdick E, Honour M, Bonventre JV, Bates DW. Acute kidney injury, mortality, length of stay, and costs in hospitalized patients. *J Am Soc Nephrol*. 2005;16(11):3365–3370.
2. Lassnigg A, Schmidlin D, Mouhieddine M, et al. Minimal changes of serum creatinine predict prognosis in patients after cardiothoracic surgery: a prospective cohort study. *J Am Soc Nephrol*. 2004;15(6):1597–1605.
3. Bellomo R, Ronco C, Kellum JA, et al. Acute renal failure—definition, outcome measures, animal models, fluid therapy and information technology needs: the Second International Consensus Conference of the Acute Dialysis Quality Initiative (ADQI) Group. *Crit Care*. 2004;8(4):R204–R212.
4. Mehta RL et al. Acute Kidney Injury Network: report of an initiative to improve outcomes in acute kidney injury. *Crit Care*. 2007;11(2):R31.
5. Uchino S et al. An assessment of the RIFLE criteria for acute renal failure in hospitalized patients. *Crit Care Med*. 2006;34(7):1913–1917.
6. Barrantes F et al. Acute kidney injury criteria predict outcomes of critically ill patients. *Crit Care Med*. 2008;36(5):1397–1403.

7. Ricci Z, Cruz D, Ronco C. The RIFLE criteria and mortality in acute kidney injury: a systematic review. *Kidney Int*. 2008;73(5):538–546.

8. Bagshaw SM et al. A multi-centre evaluation of the RIFLE criteria for early acute kidney injury in critically ill patients. *Nephrol Dial Transplant*. 2008;23(4):1203–1210.

9. Palevsky PM et al. Intensity of renal support in critically ill patients with acute kidney injury. *N Engl J Med*. 2008;359(1):7–20.

10. Uchino S et al. Acute renal failure in critically ill patients: a multinational, multicenter study. *Jama*. 2005;294(7):813–818.

11. Liu KD et al. Timing of initiation of dialysis in critically ill patients with acute kidney injury. *Clin J Am Soc Nephrol*. 2006;1(5):915–919.

12. Seabra VF et al. Timing of renal replacement therapy initiation in acute renal failure: a meta-analysis. *Am J Kidney Dis*. 2008;52(2):272–284.

13. Phu NH et al. Hemofiltration and peritoneal dialysis in infection-associated acute renal failure in Vietnam. *N Engl J Med*. 2002;347(12):895–902.

14. Gabriel DP, Caramori JT, Martim LC, Barretti P, Balbi AL. High volume peritoneal dialysis vs daily hemodialysis: a randomized, controlled trial in patients with acute kidney injury. *Kidney Int Suppl*. 2008;108:S87–S93.

15. Kramer P et al. Elimination of cardiac glycosides through hemofiltration. *J Dial*. 1977;1(7):689–695.

16. Kramer P et al. Continuous arteriovenous haemofiltration. A new kidney replacement therapy. *Proc Eur Dial Transplant Assoc*. 1981;18: 743–749.

17. Cho KC et al. Survival by dialysis modality in critically ill patients with acute kidney injury. *J Am Soc Nephrol*. 2006;17(11):3132–3138.

18. Uehlinger DE et al. Comparison of continuous and intermittent renal replacement therapy for acute renal failure. *Nephrol Dial Transplant*. 2005;20(8):1630–1637.

19. Vinsonneau C et al. Continuous venovenous haemodiafiltration versus intermittent haemodialysis for acute renal failure in patients with multiple-organ dysfunction syndrome: a multicentre randomised trial. *Lancet*. 2006;368(9533):379–385.

20. Schiffl H, Lang SM, Fischer R. Daily hemodialysis and the outcome of acute renal failure. *N Engl J Med*. 2002;346(5):305–310.

21. Ronco C et al. Effects of different doses in continuous veno-venous haemofiltration on outcomes of acute renal failure: a prospective randomised trial. *Lancet*. 2000;356(9223):26–30.

22. Schwab SJ et al. Hemodialysis without anticoagulation. One-year prospective trial in hospitalized patients at risk for bleeding. *Am J Med*. 1987;83(3):405–410.

23. Tobe SW et al. A novel regional citrate anticoagulation protocol for CRRT using only commercially available solutions. *J Crit Care*. 2003;18(2):121–129.

24. Tolwani AJ et al. A practical citrate anticoagulation continuous venovenous hemodiafiltration protocol for metabolic control and high solute clearance. *Clin J Am Soc Nephrol*. 2006;1(1):79–87.

25. Goldfrank LR. *Goldfrank's toxicologic emergencies.* 7th ed. New York: McGraw-Hill Medical Pub. Division; 2002:58–68.
26. Madore F. Plasmapheresis. Technical aspects and indications. *Crit Care Clin.* 2002;18(2):375–392.
27. Rahman T, Harper L. Plasmapheresis in nephrology: an update. *Curr Opin Nephrol Hypertens.* 2006;15(6):603–609.

9

Pericardiocentesis

James Parker and Murtuza J. Ali

The use of pericardiocentesis has become increasingly common. It may be performed emergently, as in cardiac tamponade, or as part of the diagnostic workup of cryptogenic pericardial effusion. In the hands of an experienced operator with the current techniques, complication rates have been minimized.

■ HISTORY

Percutaneous pericardiocentesis was first performed in 1840 by Frank Schuh.[1] The subxiphoid approach was adopted in 1911 but because the procedure was performed "blind," it was associated with high rates of complication. The use of continuous ECG monitoring as a guiding strategy reduced complications to 15–20%.[2] With advances in ultrasound and fluoroscopy technologies, pericardiocentesis has evolved into a procedure with complication rates between 0.5 and 3.7%.[3–5]

J. Parker (✉)
Section of Cardiology, Department of Internal Medicine, Louisiana State University School of Medicine, New Orleans, LA, USA
e-mail: jpark4@lsuhsc.edu

H.L. Frankel and B.P. deBoisblanc (eds.), *Bedside Procedures for the Intensivist*,
DOI 10.1007/978-0-387-79830-1_9,
© Springer Science+Business Media, LLC 2010

■ ETIOLOGY

Most pericardial effusions are asymptomatic, idiopathic, and found incidentally. Many of the same causes of pericarditis can lead to pericardial effusions. In addition, a large number of asymptomatic healthy pregnant women have pericardial effusions. Common causes of pericardial effusion are:

- Idiopathic
- Infection (bacterial, viral, rickettsial, fungal, or parasitic)
- Neoplasm
- Early and late post-MI (Dressler), rupture of a ventricular aneurysm, or dissecting aortic aneurysm
- Drugs (procainamide, hydralazine, minoxidil, Coumadin, thrombolytics, isoniazid, cyclosporine)
- Autoimmune disorders (lupus, rheumatoid arthritis, scleroderma, polyarteritis nodosa, sarcoidosis, and myasthenia gravis, mixed connective tissue disorder)
- Trauma (including perforation from a catheter insertion, pacemaker implantation, post-CPR or post cardiothoracic surgery)
- Hypothyroidism
- Amyloidosis
- Uremia
- Radiation
- Pneumopericardium
- Idiopathic thrombocytopenic purpura

■ DIAGNOSIS OF TAMPONADE

The suspicion of pericardial tamponade usually first arises with symptoms and signs on the physical exam:

- Beck's triad[6]:
  - Drop in arterial blood pressure
  - Elevated jugular venous pressure
  - Muffled heart sounds
- Tachycardia
- Pulsus paradoxus
- Chest pain (especially if the effusion is from an inflammatory etiology)

but the diagnosis can be aided by a number of imaging modalities. While imaging may demonstrate or confirm raised intrapericardial pressures, the diagnosis of tamponade requires the right clinical situation.

Echocardiography has been given class I recommendation by the relevant subspecialty guidelines for the diagnosis of pericardial effusion. It should be performed prior to performing a pericardiocentesis to document the location and the size of the effusion. Echocardiography can detect an effusion as small as 30 cc.[7] Small effusions collect in the posterior pericardium when a patient is supine and as the size of the effusion increases, the fluid will be seen antero-laterally and eventually circumferentially. It is important to note if the fluid appears to be free-flowing or is septated and loculated. A loculated effusion may better be drained by an open surgical approach rather than a closed percutaneous method.

Echocardiography is a critical tool in diagnosing cardiac tamponade. Echocardiographic characteristics of raised intrapericardial pressure are[8]:

- Right atrial or right ventricular wall collapse during diastole
- Reciprocal changes in left and right ventricular volumes with respiration (pulsus paradoxus and ventricular interdependence)
- Increased respiratory variation in the mitral and tricuspid valve inflow velocities
- Dilation (plethora) of the inferior vena cava and less than a 50% reduction in inferior vena caval diameter with inspiration

The presence of low voltage QRS with sinus tachycardia or electrical alternans with sinus tachycardia are additional clues to the diagnosis of tamponade.[9] The chest X-ray is very insensitive since there will likely be only minimal changes on a chest X-ray with a rapidly collecting effusion. Larger effusions maybe suggested by an increased cardiac silhouette often in a sac-like "water bottle" shape. However, it is very difficult to distinguish dilated cardiomyopathy from pericardial effusion on chest X-ray since both will show an enlarged cardiac silhouette. Occasionally, a radio-opaque band representing fluid can be seen outside of the radio-lucent epicardial fat pad.[10]

■ NONOPERATIVE MANAGEMENT

If there is no evidence of hemodynamic compromise and no need for diagnostic fluid sampling, a pericardial effusion can be managed conservatively. Treatment is focused on management of the underlying cause of the effusion, e.g., dialysis in a patient with uremic pericarditis.

■ OPEN PERICARDIOTOMY

Surgical drainage of a pericardial effusion is preferable in recurrent or chronic large pericardial effusions, especially those that have had previous percutaneous pericardiocentesis performed. A subxiphoid pericardial window, a thoracotomy with a pleuropericardial window or a pericardiectomy may be the preferred treatment.

Large loculated pericardial effusions are difficult to adequately drain by percutaneous approach due to their complex nature. Similarly, postcardiothoracic surgical effusions often occur posteriorly and contain clotted blood, making percutaneous drainage difficult. In both of these cases, surgical evacuation is the preferred method of drainage.

■ PERICARDIOCENTESIS

Indications

Therapeutic pericardiocentesis is carried out in the setting of signs or symptoms or tamponade, whereas diagnostic pericardiocentesis is usually performed to help establish the etiolgy of large chronic effusions. Pathologic pericardial effusions may develop secondary either to increases in production of pericardial fluid (e.g., secondary to infection, trauma, surgery, radiation, malignancy, etc.) or to decreases in the drainage from the pericardium (e.g., elevated right atrial pressure). Most pericardial effusions remain clinically silent and are found incidentally on imaging studies. Although an accumulation of more than 20–30 mL of fluid in the pericardium is abnormal, a change in the cardiac silhouette on chest X-ray may not become apparent until at least 250 mL has accumulated.[11]

The rate at which fluid has deposited often is the most important determinant of whether it will cause symptoms. If fluid rapidly accumulates, the limited compliance of the pericardium will lead to elevations in pericardial pressure and impairment of cardiac filling. For this reason, cardiac tamponade is most commonly seen with problems such as hemorrhage due to trauma. In contrast, effusions that accumulate slowly may reach several liters and never become hemodynamically significant.[12]

Pericardial effusions may be classified as transudates, exudates, bloody (hemopericardium), or even air-containing (pneumopericardium). Larger effusions are more commonly neoplastic, mycobacterial, uremic, myxedematous, or due to pyogenic infections. Massive chronic effusions represent only 2–3.5% of all pathologic effusions.[13] When effusions are loculated, there is usually a history of surgery, trauma, or severe infection.

Contraindications

There are no absolute contraindications to emergent pericardiocentesis in critically ill patients with clinical evidence of tamponade. When tamponade is caused by myocardial free-wall rupture or aortic dissection that extends retrograde into the pericardium, only the minimum amount of fluid that restores intracardiac filling should be drained since removal of additional fluid can result in more rapid reaccumulation.

In more stable patients with large pericardial effusions, individual risk–benefit assessment must be used to guide the decision for pericardiocentesis. The major risk for elective pericardiocentesis is that of myocardial injury with the development of hemorrhagic pericardial tamponade. For this reason, it is best to correct any underlying coagulopathy prior to elective procedures.

Procedure

It has become a common practice to perform cardiac pericardiocentesis in the cardiac catheterization lab to allow for closer monitoring of the patient's hemodynamics and provide an emergency procedure if necessary. However, this may not be an option in emergency circumstances.

- The procedure should be performed by an experienced individual.
- An echocardiogram should be obtained prior to undertaking the procedure:
  - To document the size, location, and characteristics of the effusion
  - To help guide the placement of the catheter
- Although fluoroscopy may be considered as an alternative or adjunct to echocardiography, echocardiography can be performed at bedside and avoids the exposure of the patient to contrast dye and X-rays.
- CT-guidance may be useful for patients who are poor candidates for echocardiography due to body habitus.
- If the procedure is being performed electively:
  - All anticoagulants should be held
  - A coagulation panel should be obtained prior to starting the procedure
  - (a) The INR should be <1.5
  - (b) The APTT should be <100
  - (c) If thrombolytics, anti-platelet agents, heparin or Coumadin are responsible for the effusion, the coagulopathy can be reversed with fresh frozen plasma, platelet transfusions, protamine, or vitamin K, respectively
  - The procedure should not be delayed in a patient who is hemodynamically unstable.

A 12-lead ECG should be obtained before and after pericardiocentesis. Although not required, ECG monitoring can be performed during the procedure. Items that should be included in a pericardiocentesis tray are:

- 10 cm 18- to 20-gauge cardiac needle (lumbar puncture needles have a bevel that is too long)
- Three-way stopcock
- Syringes (10, 20, and 60 mL)
- Chlorhexidine skin prep
- ECG monitor and defibrillator
- Specimen collection tubes for fluid analysis and cultures
- 25-gauge needle for local anesthetic
- 10 mL 1 % lidocaine
- Sterile gloves, mask, gown, drapes, towels, and gauze
- #11 scalpel blade
- Mosquito hemostats
- Multihole pigtail catheter

- Soft J-tipped guidewire
- 20 mL sterile isotonic sodium chloride flush solution
- Optional ECG machine and technician
- 1 Liter collection bag or bottle

ECG monitoring during pericardiocentesis can be performed by attaching an ECG lead (typically the V_1 or V_5 lead) to the needle with a sterile alligator clip and lead wire. If the needle comes in contact with the myocardium, ST segment elevation ("current of injury") will be observed.[14] Monitoring the V_1 lead from the needle is more sensitive than monitoring the same lead via surface electrodes. If this method is used, extreme care must be taken that the patient and ECG machine are well grounded. If stray electrical current passes via the lead/needle into the myocardium, fibrillation can be induced. The 2004 European Society of Cardiology has deemed this technique, when used without echocardiography, to be insufficient to safeguard against myocardial injury.[15]

Procedural Steps

1. Institute peri-procedural monitoring including continuous ECG monitoring, pulse oximetry, and noninvasive blood pressure monitoring.
2. Start a functional large bore IV line and oxygen at 2 L per nasal cannula or higher if hypoxemic.
3. Position the patient 30–45° head-up to allow the fluid to pool inferiorly.
4. Perform preprocedural echocardiography to decide the best and safest approach. A subcostal or subxiphoid approach is most commonly used; however, an apical or a parasternal approach is also an option.
5. Prepare and drape the chosen site.
6. Inject 1% lidocaine (check for allergy) with the 25-gauge needle into the needle entry site.
7. Connect the pericardiocentesis needle and a 20-mL syringe loaded with 5 mL lidocaine to the 3-way stopcock. Connect a pressure transducer to the side-port on the stopcock if pericardial pressures will be measured.
8. If used, attach a sterile ECG recording lead to the proximal metal portion of the needle.
9. Using the subcostal or subxiphoid approach (Fig. 9-1), insert the needle a few millimeters inferior and left lateral to the xiphoid process but medial to the left costal margin. Direct the needle cephalad toward the left costal margin while pressing the syringe and needle toward the patient's abdomen (at an angle of 15–20° from the abdominal wall) and slowly advance. The needle is usually directed toward the left midclavicular line but specific directional angle can be adjusted based on echocardiographic guidance.[16]

Subxiphoid approach

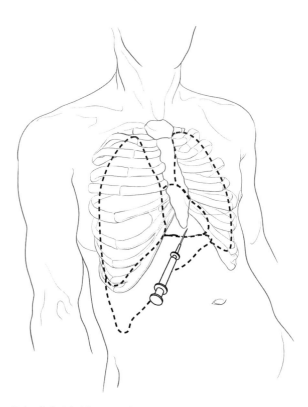

Figure 9-1. Subxiphoid approach.

10. If an apical approach (Fig. 9-2) is chosen, the needle should be inserted 1 cm lateral and one intercostal space below the apical impulse. The needle is then advanced parallel to the long axis of the left ventricle toward the aortic valve (right shoulder).[16] This approach positions the needle very close to the lingula of the left lung and can result in a pneumothorax. It is best to perform this approach only with echocardiographic guidance.

11. In the parasternal approach (Fig. 9-3), the needle insertion is made 1 cm lateral to the sternal edge in the fifth intercostal space (to avoid the internal mammary artery which lies medially and the lingula which lies laterally).[17]

Apical approach

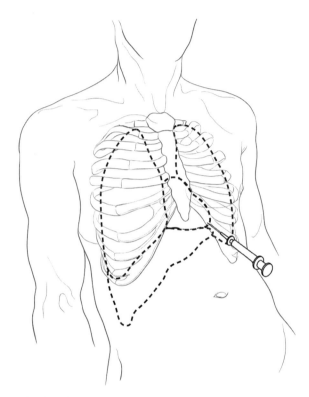

Figure 9-2. Apical approach.

12. Negative pressure should be applied by drawing back on the syringe plunger while advancing the needle. The pericardium is generally 6–8 cm below the skin in adults and 5 cm below the skin in children.[11] If the patient feels discomfort, stop the needle advancement and inject a small amount of lidocaine. Be sure to aspirate prior to lidocaine administration to ensure that the needle is not inside of a vessel or other structure. Continue to advance the needle until fluid is aspirated or ST elevation is noted on the ECG monitor. If ST elevation is noted, the needle is lodged in the myocardium and should be pulled back.

13. As the needle is advanced toward the pericardium, progress can be observed using the echocardiogram. The needle will appear as a bright

Parasternal approach

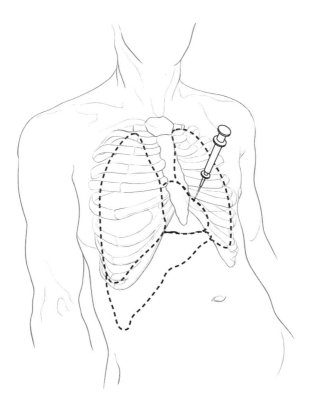

Figure 9-3. Parasternal approach.

linear structure often causing echo scatter on the image. Highly echogenic needles are commercially available. If unsure of the needle position on the echo, a slight in and out bounce or shake of the needle can be performed and the resultant shifting of tissue can be observed on the echo. Often the needle may still not be seen on the echo, even when the path of the needle is correct and the pericardium is accessed.

14. If the needle is advanced fully with no fluid being obtained or if the ECG shows ST elevation, withdraw the needle slowly while aspirating. Flush the needle with the lidocaine and reinsert the needle, advancing in a different direction.

15. Occasionally a "give" or "pop" may be felt when entering the pericardium but this is not always the case. If serous or hemorrhagic

fluid is aspirated, remove the lidocaine-filled syringe and inject a small amount of contrast material (agitated saline or radiopaque) through the needle while monitoring the echocardiogram or fluoroscopy, respectively. If the needle is positioned in the pericardial space, bubbles or radiopaque contrast will be seen filling the pericardial space on the image. If the needle tip is within the right ventricle, contrast or agitated saline will fill the cardiac chamber.

16. Once the needle is confirmed to be in the pericardial space, a soft J-tipped guidewire is passed through the needle and wrapped around the heart. The needle then removed over the guidewire. The wire should be visible on the echocardiogram. Make a 5 mm skin incision at the guidewire entry site and separate the subcutaneous tissue using the mosquito hemostats. This will allow easier passage of the catheter.

17. Insert the soft pigtail catheter over the guidewire. A pigtail catheter is used because it avoids the risk of causing trauma to the heart associated with a straight-tipped catheter. The catheter will have multiple holes at the distal end, so it must be inserted to allow all of these holes to be in the pericardial space.

18. Remove the guidewire.

19. Connect the catheter hub to the three-way stopcock connected to a 60-mL syringe and pressure transducer if pericardial pressures are to be measured. The fluid should aspirate easily via the syringe. The catheter can be flushed with 1–2 mL of saline to prevent blockage. All diagnostic laboratory samples can be drawn at this time.

20. The proximal end of the catheter should be fixed to the chest wall with suture. An initial interrupted stitch to the chest wall followed by several figure of eight loops around the catheter and closure with a surgeon's locking knot will ensure the catheter is secure.

21. Apply a clean sterile dressing over the catheter.

22. The pericardial catheter can be left in place for 24 h with continuous closed gravity-driven drainage. Negative pressure should not be applied to the catheter to assist with drainage. If the catheter is maintained for more than 24 h, risk of infection is increased greatly. However, a catheter may not be able to be removed in 24 h if fluid continues to reaccumulate rapidly. Generally, drainage should continue until the volume collected is <50 mL/day.

■ COMPLICATIONS

The incidence of major complications in experienced hands has been reported as 1.3–1.6%.[18] The greatest danger is that of laceration of a coronary artery or vein. Puncture of the left ventricle usually does not cause significant bleeding, whereas puncture of the thin-walled right ventricle or right atrium can result in tamponade.

If a cardiac chamber or coronary vessel is punctured and noted by aspiration of blood or pressure measurement or intracardiac injection of agitated saline, close monitoring of the patient's hemodynamic state must be performed. If the patient's central venous pressure increases as compared to prior to starting the procedure, cardiac tamponade must be suspected. Fluoroscopy or echocardiography can provide additional indication of acute tamponade. Emergent surgical correction is necessary in this circumstance.

Another rare complication of pericardiocentesis is acute left ventricular failure with pulmonary edema. The etiology of this complication is unknown but has been reported in association with concurrent left ventricular dysfunction. In this setting, an acute increase in venous return may cause flash pulmonary edema.[19] This has also been associated with acute right ventricular dilation.[20] Drainage of fluid in sequential steps of <1,000 mL was recommended by the 2004 ESC guidelines to help avoid these complications.[15]

Other complications of the procedure can be minor bleeding at the procedure site, ventricular or atrial ectopic beats, arrhythmias, hypotension, pneumothorax, and pulmonary edema. For serious complications, emergency surgery may be needed.

■ REFERENCES

1. Kilpatrick Z, Chapman C. On pericardiocentesis. *Am J Cardiol.* 1965;16:622.
2. Bishop LH, Estes EH, McIntosh HD. The electrocardiogram as a safeguard in pericardiocentesis. *JAMA.* 1956;162:264.
3. Duvernoy O, Borowiec J, Helmius G, Erikson U. Complications of percutaneous pericardiocentesis under fluoroscopic guidance. *Acta Radiol.* 1992;33:309.
4. Bastian A, Meissner A, Lins M, et al. Pericardiocentesis: differential aspects of a common procedure. *Intensive Care Med.* 2000;26:573.
5. Tsang T, Barnes M, Hayes S, et al. Clinical and echocardiographic characteristics of significant pericardial effusions following cardiothoracic surgery and outcomes of echo-guided pericardiocentesis for management: Mayo Clinic experience, 1979–1998. *Chest.* 1999;116:322.
6. Beck C. Two cardiac compression triads. *JAMA.* 1935;104:715.
7. Cheitlin MD, Armstrong WF, Aurigemma GP. ACC/AHA/ASE 2003 guideline for the clinical application of echocardiography; 2003.
8. Levine MJ, Lorell BH, Diver DJ, Come PC. Implications of electrocardiographically assisted diagnosis of pericardial tamponade in contemporary medical patients: detection before hemodynamic embarrassment. *J Am Coll Cardiol.* 1991;17:59.
9. Eisenberg MJ, de Romeral LM, Heidenreich PA, et al. The diagnosis of pericardial effusion and cardiac tamponade by 12-lead ECG. *Chest.* 1996;110:318.

10. Carsky E, Azimi F, Maucer R. Epicardial fat sign in the diagnosis of pericardial effusion. *JAMA*. 1980;244:2762.

11. Baue A, Blakemore W. The pericardium. *Ann Thorac Surg*. 1972;14:81.

12. Hancock E. Management of pericardial disease. *Mod Concepts Cardiovasc Dis*. 1979;48:1.

13. Soler-Soler J. Massive chronic pericardial effusion. In: Soler-Soler J, Permanyer-Miralda G, Sagrista-Sauleda J, eds. *Pericardial diseases—old dilemmas and new insights*. 6th ed. The Netherlands: Kluwer; 1990:153–165.

14. Shabetai R. *The Pericardium*. New York: Grune and Stratton; 1981:338.

15. Maisch B, Seferovic PM, Ristic AD, et al. Guidelines on the diagnosis and management of pericardial diseases executive summary; The Task force on the diagnosis and management of pericardial diseases of the European society of cardiology. *Eur Heart J*. 2004;25:587.

16. Treasure T, Cottler L. Practical procedures: how to aspirate the pericardium. *Br J Hosp Med*. 1980;24:488.

17. Brown C, Gurley H, Hutchins G, et al. Injuries associated with percutaneous placement of transthoracic pacemakers. *Ann Emerg Med*. 1985;14:223.

18. Tsang TS, Enriquez-Sarano M, Freeman WK, et al. Consecutive 1127 therapeutic echocardiographically guided pericardiocentesis: clinical profile, practice patterns and outcomes spanning 21 years. *Mayo Clin Proc*. 2002;77:429.

19. Uemura S, Kagoshima T, Hashimoto T, et al. Acute left ventricular failure with pulmonary edema following pericardiocentesis for cardiac tamponade—a case report. *Jpn Circ J*. 1995;59:55.

20. Armstrong WF, Feigenbaum H, Dillon JC. Acute right ventricular dilation and echocardiographic volume overload following pericardiocentesis for relief of cardiac tamponade. *Am Heart J*. 1984;107:1266.

10

Bedside Insertion of Vena Cava Filters in the Intensive Care Unit

A. Britton Christmas and Ronald F. Sing

The development of deep venous thrombosis (DVT) and pulmonary embolism (PE) remains a daily concern for physicians who care for critically ill patients. Diagnosing PE is challenging in the intensive care unit (ICU) because signs and symptoms are nonspecific. In greater than two-thirds of patients, acute PE occurs prior to the diagnosis of DVT. Subsequently, much emphasis on this disease process focuses on prophylaxis and prevention rather than treatment. Mechanical prophylaxis with graded compression stockings and pharmacologic anticoagulation with heparin, low molecular weight heparin, and warfarin remain the mainstays of prevention and treatment. However, there are patient populations that are at high risk for venous thromboembolism (VTE) who are candidates for the placement of vena cava filters (VCFs).[1]

R.F. Sing (✉)
Department of General Surgery, Carolinas HealthCare System,
1025 Morehead Medical Drive 275, Charlotte, NC 28204, USA
e-mail: Ron.sing@carolinashealthcare.org

H.L. Frankel and B.P. deBoisblanc (eds.), *Bedside Procedures for the Intensivist*,
DOI 10.1007/978-0-387-79830-1_10,
© Springer Science+Business Media, LLC 2010

■ HISTORY

Mechanical prophylaxis for VTE by ligation of the inferior vena cava (IVC) was introduced in the seventeenth century but it wasn't until the mid-twentieth century that suture plication of the IVC was widely practiced. In the 1960s, surgical implantation of intraluminal devices (Mobbin-Udin umbrella) via laparotomy and venotomy of the IVC became popular. Almost universally, these techniques resulted in caval occlusion accompanied by the postphlebitic syndrome and the hemodynamic consequences of decreased venous return. Not until the introduction of the Greenfield filter, with its conical design, did mechanical prevention of PE become a truly efficacious and safe treatment. As a consequence of its large (24 French) introducer, insertion of the original Greenfield filter required surgical cut down of the internal jugular vein, requiring that the procedure be performed in the operating room.

The evolution of percutaneous Seldinger techniques combined with smaller profile introducers (6–12 French) has decreased the complexity of filter insertion. Traditionally, VCFs have been inserted in either the operating suite or angiography suite. Recently percutaneous techniques have allowed the insertion of VCFs at the patient's bedside, eliminating safety issues related to the transportation of critically ill patients out of the ICU. According to previous reports, the transport of critically ill patients from the ICU to other parts of the hospital (i.e., radiology department or operating room) can result in mishaps in 5–30% of patients,[2–6] with an increase in mortality of up to 30% relating to these mishaps. Of primary concern, critically ill patients are often mechanically ventilated with endotracheal tubes that can become easily dislodged. Hemodynamic events such as hypotension, hypertension, and cardiac dysrhythmias can occur as well.[7,8] These secondary insults can worsen outcomes especially in brain-injured patients.[9]

■ CONSIDERATIONS

Performing radiologic procedures, including fluoroscopy, in the ICU is a common practice. However, concerns of radiation exposure to the ICU staff and physicians cannot be trivialized. There are three tenets of radiation safety: time, distance, and shielding. Adherence to these tenets reduces radiation risk. Staff physicians, nurses, and residents directly involved in the use of fluoroscopy must wear lead shielding while all other observers must maintain at least a 3 m distance from the X-ray source. Total fluoroscopy time for an entire procedure should be kept to <2 min. This includes advancement of the guidewire, performance of a contrast venacavogram, and insertion of the filter. The fluoroscope emits 1–2 REM/min, but collateral exposure perpendicular to the beam is only 0.5 mREM/h at 2 m. Average annual background radiation is approximately100 mREM; therefore, collateral exposure to patients and other personnel is negligible.[10] We performed a 3-month investigation of radiation exposure during approximately 1,500 radiological procedures of all types in an "open" ICU using multiple ultrasensitive dosimeters. No significant radiation exposure was observed during the study.[11]

Increased experience with portable color-flow duplex ultrasound scanning of the IVC and with intravascular ultrasound (IVUS) has led to numerous reports of ultrasound-guided IVC filter insertion in critically ill ICU patients.[12–18] Ultrasound modalities may obviate the need for fluoroscopy altogether, but are not without their limitations. For example, Rosenthal,[14] in an analysis of bedside insertion of VCF using IVUS for 94 patients, reported two filters deployed in the iliac veins. Two additional reports demonstrated failure rates of bedside duplex ultrasound of 13 and 14%, respectively,[12,13] compared to our 100% success rate using contrast or carbon dioxide venography. Furthermore, few noninterventional radiologists or nonendovascular surgeons possess adequate duplex or IVUS experience to enable them to comfortably perform this procedure. Finally, the hospital cost of disposable intravascular ultrasound probes is $600 compared to less than $150 for iodinated contrast and catheters. These findings further strengthen our belief that IVUS does not reliably identify potential IVC anomalies that can influence the risk of misplacement of VCF. To verify the position of the renal veins and recognize potential anatomic anomalies, we recommend the routine use of a preinsertion contrast cavogram rather than caval ultrasound unless the risk of contrast-induced nephropathy is high.

■ INDICATIONS FOR VCFS

General indications for the insertion of a caval filter are:

- VTE with a contraindication to anticoagulation
- Recurrence of VTE in spite of therapeutic anticoagulation in a patient with lower extremity or pelvic DVT
- High risk of recurrent VTE with poor cardiopulmonary reserve
- Large ileofemoral clot burden with >5 cm nonadherent, free-floating segment
- Planned surgical pulmonary embolectomy
- Chronic thromboembolic pulmonary hypertension with planned pulmonary thromboendarterectomy

Although supportive data are lacking, over the past decade as VCFs have become safer, easier to use, and removable, many filters have been increasingly placed prophylactically in patients at high risk for VTE – in particular, the severely injured and the bariatric surgical patient population. In actuality, all VCF are prophylactic as they do not treat DVT or PE, they only prevent PE.

Although the majority of filters are placed because of contraindications to anticoagulation, whenever possible, anticoagulation should be given after placement.

■ CONTRAINDICATIONS

Contraindications to the placement of VCFs include:

- Vena cava occlusion with an inadequate "landing zone"
- Caval diameters larger than that recommended for a specific filter (most VCFs in the United States are indicated for diameters up to 30 mm)
- Inability to advance the guidewire and/or imaging catheter (catheters and guidewires should never be forced as this may result in perforation of the vena cava or embolization of a thrombus)

■ ANATOMY

The most common insertion access point for venous cannulation is either an internal jugular or a femoral vein. However, if these sites are unavailable, several devices are also approved for insertion via a subclavian or antecubital vein. Cannulation of the vein and passage of the guidewire is performed utilizing the standard Seldinger technique that will be described below. The guidewire is advanced into the distal inferior vena cava under fluoroscopic guidance.

The anatomy of the inferior vena cava is "typical" in approximately 95% of patients. Important landmarks in the inferior vena cava are the renal veins, the iliac bifurcation, and any venous anomalies (Fig. 10-1). These anatomic landmarks are important to help determine the exact position in the IVC for deployment. Significant tilt can occur if the struts are deployed into a renal vein, which can reduce the efficacy of VCF filtration. Obviously, it is important to deploy the filter above the iliac bifurcation to ensure filtration of both legs. Finally, it is mandatory to perform a cavogram to measure the IVC diameter prior to filter insertion. This step can avoid inserting a filter that is too small in diameter to hook the caval wall resulting in migration/embolism of the filter to the heart. The filter limits are:

- 28 mm
- Titanium Greenfield
- Stainless Steel Greenfield

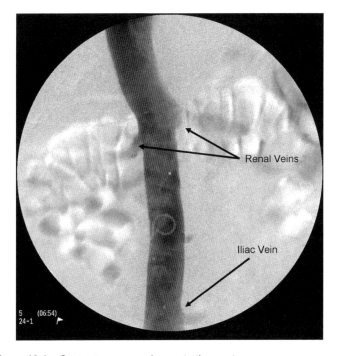

Figure 10-1. Contrast cavogram demonstrating anatomy.

- G2
- Simon Nitinol
- Vena Tech LP
- Vena Tech LGM
- 30 mm
- Gianturco Tulip
- Celect
- TrapEase
- OptEase
- 40 mm
- Bird's Nest

■ EQUIPMENT

With the exception of portable fluoroscopy (C-arm) and a contrast injector, the equipment required for bedside VCF insertion is relatively simple and readily available in the ICU[15]:

- Portable fluoroscopy (C-arm), fluoroscopy capable bed, and lead aprons
- Large sterile sheet
- Surgical cap, mask, and sterile procedure gown
- Central venous line tray
- Access needle
- 1% lidocaine
- Gauze 4×4s
- Flush valves
- No. 11 scalpel
- 500 mL saline (for flushes)
- 60-mL syringes (2)
- Portable contrast injection device
- Contrast medium
- 145-cm, 0.035-in J-tipped guidewire
- 72 in pressure tubing
- Pigtail angiography catheter
- VCF

■ SETUP, PREPARATION, AND POSITIONING

Proper preparation and positioning of the patient is imperative during the placement of VCFs as this may affect image acquisition and quality.

- Ideally, all ICU beds should be fluoroscopy-ready so a patient does not need to be transferred to a specialized stretcher or unit.
- The patient should be moved to the midline and positioned near the top of the bed. We recommend leaving the side rails in the up position for the duration of the procedure.
- The bed may need to be elevated so that the portable fluoroscopy unit C-arm can be positioned above the patient's midline.
- A bedside table should be prepared using a sterile drape so that it can be used as a sterile back table (Fig. 10-2).
- Open a sterile central venous access tray on the back table. Typical central venous access trays include much of the basic equipment necessary for VCF insertion:
- Sterile drapes
- Access needles (Seldinger)
- Lidocaine
- Flush valves
- Scalpel
- Gauze sponges
- Additional supplies opened sterilely and placed on the back table include:
- 60 ml syringes (2) for flushes

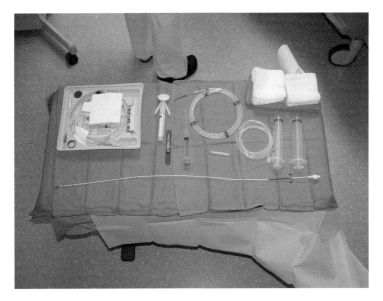

Figure 10-2. Sterile back table for supplies.

- Pressure tubing (pressure injector)
- 145-cm, 0.035-in J-tipped guidewire
- Pigtail catheter for contrast injection
- The VCF

We use either heparinized saline (2 units/mL) or normal saline to flush the catheters and prevent the development of inadvertent clots. The pigtail catheter (Pig-Cav, Cook Critical Care Inc., Bloomington, IN) used for the initial contrast injection has radio-opaque markers (28 and 30 mm) for measurement scaling to ensure that vena cava diameter is appropriate for the specified VCF (Fig. 10-3). All VCFs in the United States are approved for vena cava diameters up to 28 or 30 mm with the exception of the Bird's Nest filter (Cook Critical Care Inc., Bloomington, IN) which is approved for diameters up to 40 mm. The radio-opaque markers correct for the magnification artifact that occurs with fluoroscopy. The Cordis OptEase filter insertion apparatus includes a dilator with multiple side holes. It has 30 mm radio-opaque markers and can be employed for the preinsertion cavogram.

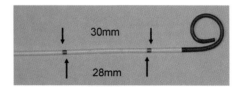

Figure 10-3. Five-French angiography catheter demonstrating premeasured radio-opaque marks to correct for fluoroscopic magnification artifact.

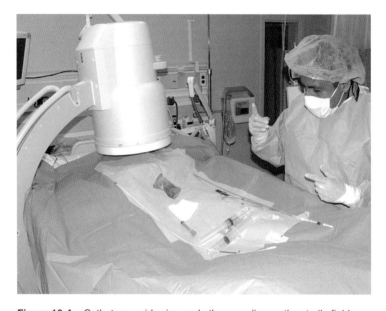

Figure 10-4. Catheters, guidewire, and other supplies on the sterile field.

■ TECHNIQUE

The insertion site should be prepared with a chlorhexidine solution and isolated with sterile drapes. We prefer a disposable, prepackaged "thyroid sheet" that will cover the entire bed regardless of whether it is used for a femoral or jugular-subclavian approach (Fig. 10-4). The side rails of the bed are left in the up position so that the overlaying sterile drape makes

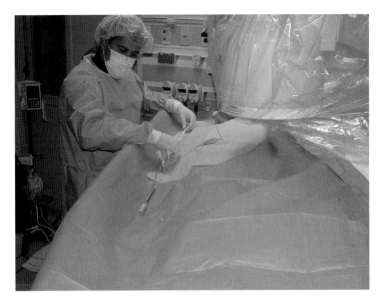

Figure 10-5. "Valley" formed by drape over side-rail in up position to keep catheters and supplies from rolling onto floor.

a "valley" between the patient and the railing where catheters, wires, and other supplies can be placed without the risk of equipment falling on the floor (Fig. 10-5). Surgeons should wear full sterile gowns and gloves, caps and face-masks with eye protection. All dilation, introduction, and imaging catheters are first flushed with heparinized saline. A portable digital-subtraction fluoroscopy unit (Philips Medical, Eindhoven, The Netherlands) is used to identify the twelfth thoracic vertebra and lumbar vertebrae. Guidewire placement, insertion of catheters, and deployment of the VCF are all fluoroscopically guided. The preferred access points are either the right internal jugular vein or the right femoral vein unless contraindicated (i.e., existing central venous catheter or injury). Using the Seldinger technique, the selected vein is cannulated and a 145-cm long, 0.035-in diameter, flexible J-tip guidewire is advanced into the vena cava (Fig. 10-6). A small stab is then made with a No. 11 scalpel to allow for the subsequent dilation and passage of imaging and/or introducer catheters. The 5-French pigtail angiography catheter is advanced into the distal inferior vena cava and positioned at approximately the

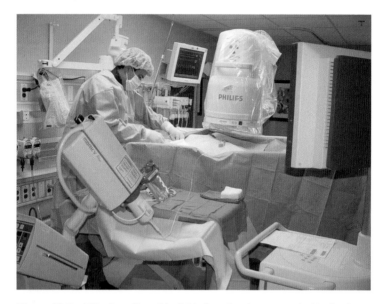

Figure 10-6. Filter insertion at bedside from jugular approach. Monitor is on the right side of the image, pressure injector is in foreground to the left.

fourth lumbar spinous interspace. A contrast venacavogram should be performed using 45 mL of intravenous, nonionic, iodinated contrast medium injected over 3 s (15 mL/s) (see Fig. 10-1). Though we prefer the use of a power injector, a hand held-injection will suffice if a power injector is not available (Fig. 10-7). Images are obtained and saved for the permanent record. Caval size, the location of the iliac bifurcation, and the location of the renal veins and any anomalies are determined. The VCF is usually deployed into the infrarenal position, and a hard copy plain film X-ray obtained. Suprarenal filters are inserted when there is a caval thrombus in the infrarenal "landing zone." Suprarenal filters are also considered in women of child-bearing age. After completion of the insertion, a cavogram of 30 mL injected over 2 s is taken to confirm the orientation and position of the VCF (Figs. 10-8 and 10-9). The introducer catheter is removed, and direct pressure to the insertion site is applied for 10 min.

In a patient with an elevated serum creatinine, carbon dioxide (CO_2) can be used as a contrast agent, since it has no hepatic or renal toxicity and is nonallergenic. Carbon dioxide imaging is performed using a hand injection system (AngioDynamics, Glen Falls, NY) with digital subtraction enhancement. This system is composed of a tubing system that has a series

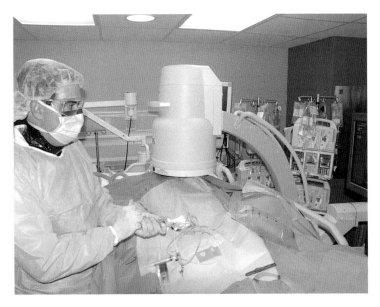

Figure 10-7. Hand injection cavogram using CO_2 gas.

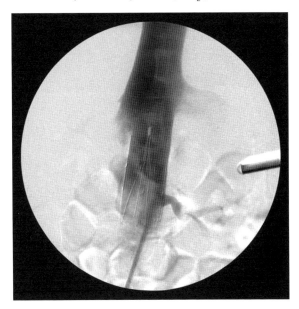

Figure 10-8. Completion cavogram showing orientation and position of Vena Tech LP filter.

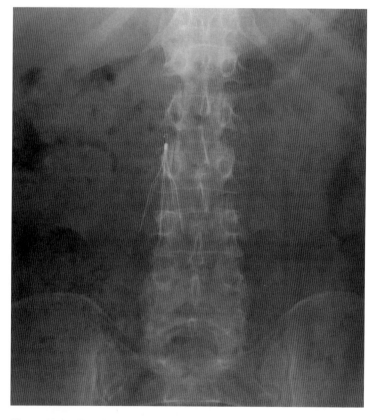

Figure 10-9. Plain film X-ray of Tulip filter.

of one-way valves to prevent the introduction of air into the system and a reservoir bag of 1,500 mL that can be filled from a tank of vascular grade CO_2 (99.99% pure) (Fig. 10-10). The pigtail catheter is positioned at the fourth and fifth lumber vertebral interspace. Injections of 60 cc are repeated with a breath hold if the first cavogram is considered to be suboptimal. There is very little cumulative effect of multiple boluses of CO_2 until several hundred milliliters are injected.[19–21] (Fig. 10-11)

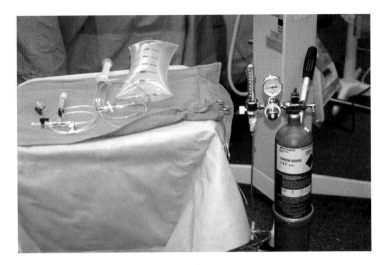

Figure 10-10. Carbon dioxide injection system showing tank of vascular grade CO_2, reservoir bag, and flush system.

■ COMPLICATIONS

Complications rate of VCFs are no different whether inserted in the radiology department, the operating room, or the ICU.[22] The procedure is performed with the same techniques and same equipment regardless of the venue. The most concerning complication of VCF insertion is caval occlusion. Although as many as 50% of patients with caval occlusion may be asymptomatic, others may have catastrophic consequences. Serious complications include acute hemodynamic collapse from decreased cardiac preload, chronic venous stasis with the development of the postphlebitic syndrome, and phlegmasia cerulean dolens with resultant limb gangrene of both lower extremities. Although additional long-term follow-up studies are needed, the incidence of caval occlusion with bedside VCF insertion has been reported to be low. The largest series of 403 patients reported <1% caval occlusion.

Although the nonionic iodinated contrast agents have significantly reduced the incidence of pain and adverse reactions, the risk of contrast nephropathy and subsequent renal failure has not diminished. This risk rises exponentially with the level of the serum creatinine.

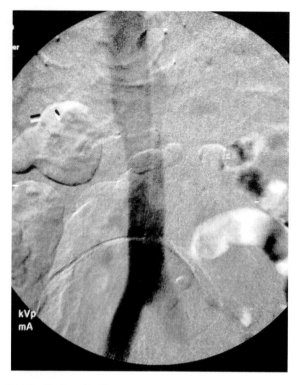

Figure 10-11. Carbon dioxide cavogram.

■ SUMMARY

The advent of percutaneously inserted devices and smaller profile filters allow this VCF placement to be safely performed in the ICU. The equipment needs for caval imaging and guidance of VCF insertion are portable and easily accessible to the bedside (Fig. 10-12). Critically ill patients in the ICU whose transport itself maybe a hazardous adventure will have the greatest benefit from VCF insertion at the bedside.

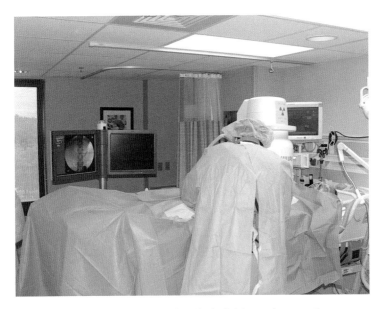

Figure 10-12. Bedside VCF insertion via the left femoral approach.

■ REFERENCES

1. Marino PL. Venous thromboembolism. In: Marino PL, ed. *The ICU Book*. 2nd ed. Philadelphia, PA: Lippincott Williams & Wilkins; 1998:106–120.
2. Ehrenwerth J, Sorbo S, Hackel A. Transport of critically ill adults. *Crit Care Med*. 1986;14:543–547.
3. Insel J, Weissman C, Kemper M, Askanazi J, Hyman AI. Cardiovascular changes during transport of critically ill and postoperative patients. *Crit Care Med*. 1986;14:539–542.
4. Taylor JO, Chulay JD, Landers CF, Hood W Jr, Abelman WH. Monitoring high-risk cardiac patients during transportation in the hospital. *Lancet*. 1970;2:1205–1208.
5. Waddell G. Movement of critically ill patients within the hospital. *Br Med J*. 1975;2:417–419.
6. Braman SS, Dunn SM, Amico CA, Millman RP. Complications of intrahospital transport in critically ill patients. *Ann Intern Med*. 1987;107:469–473.

7. Venkataraman ST, Orr RA. Intrahospital transport of critically ill patients. *Crit Care Clin.* 1992;8:525–531.

8. Van Natta TL, Morris JA, Eddy VA, et al. Elective bedside surgery in critically injured patients is safe and cost effective. *Ann Surg.* 1997;227:618–626.

9. Andrews PJD, Piper IR, Dearden NM, Miller JD. Secondary insults during intrahospital transport of head-injured patients. *Lancet.* 1990; 335:327–330.

10. Sing RF, Cicci CK, Smith CH, Messick WJ. Bedside insertion of inferior vena cava filters in the intensive care unit. *J Trauma.* 1999;47:1104–1107.

11. Mostafa G, McKeown R, Huynh TT, Heniford BT. The hazard of scattered radiation in a trauma intensive care unit. *Crit Care Med.* 2002;30:574–576.

12. Kazmers A, Groehn H, Meeker C. Duplex examination of the inferior vena cava. *Am Surg.* 2000;10:986–989.

13. Benjamin ME, Sandager GP, Cohn EJ, et al. Duplex ultrasound of inferior vena cava filters in multitrauma patients. *Am J Surg.* 1999;178:92–97.

14. Rosenthal D, Wellons ED, Levitt AB, et al. Rose of prophylactic temporary inferior vena cava filters placed at bedside under intravascular ultrasound guidance in patients with multiple trauma. *J Vasc Surg.* 2000; 40:958–964.

15. Nunn CR, Neuzil D, Naslund T, et al. Cost-effective method for bedside insertion of vena cava filters in trauma patients. *J Trauma.* 1997;43:752–758.

16. Neuzil DF, Garrard CL, Berkman RA, Pierce R, Naslund TC. Duplex-directed vena cava filter placement: report of initial experience. *Surgery.* 1998;123:470–474.

17. Sato DT, Robinson KD, Gregory RT, et al. Duplex directed caval filter insertion in multi-trauma and critically ill patients. *Ann Vasc Surg.* 1999;13: 365–371.

18. Matsumura JS, Morasch MD. Filter placement by ultrasound technique at the bedside. *Seminars in Vasc Surg.* 2000;13:199–203.

19. Schmelzer TM, Christmas AB, Jacobs DG, Heniford BT, Sing RF. Imaging of the vena cava in the intensive care unit prior to vena cava filter insertion: carbon dioxide as an alternative to iodinated contrast. *Am Surg.* 2008;74:141–145.

20. Sullivan KL, Bonn J, Shapiro MJ, Gardiner GA. Venography with carbon dioxide as a contrast agent. *Cardiovasc Intervent Radiol.* 1995;18:141–145.

21. Sing RF, Stackhouse DJ, Cicci CK, LeQuire MH. Bedside Carbon Dioxide (CO_2) preinsertion cavogram for inferior vena cava filter placement: case report. *J Trauma.* 1999;47:1140–1141.

22. Sing RF, Jacobs DG, Heniford BT. Bedside insertion of inferior vena cava filters in the intensive care unit. *J Am Col Surg.* 2001;192:570–576.

11

Percutaneous Dilational Tracheostomy

Bennett P. deBoisblanc

■ HISTORY

Tracheostomy is an ancient surgical procedure that was first described in the *Rig Veda* over 3,000 years ago.[1] Indications for tracheostomy remained unclear until the 1850s when it was advocated as a treatment for upper airway obstruction due to diphtheria.[2] However, operative mortality remained high. In 1909, Chevalier Jackson, the father of modern tracheostomy, refined the open tracheostomy technique that is still used today. During the 1940s polio epidemics, the need for improved pulmonary hygiene resulted in a resurgence of tracheostomy.[3] This period was followed by a third wave of interest in the 1960s following the birth of modern ICUs and the widespread adoption of positive pressure ventilation.

Techniques for performing tracheostomy had remained largely unchanged until 1985 when Pasquale Ciaglia described a new Seldinger-based percutaneous procedure that advanced plastic dilators over

B.P. deBoisblanc (✉)
Section of Pulmonary/Critical Care Medicine, Louisiana State University Health Sciences Center, New Orleans, LA, USA
e-mail: bdeboi@lsuhsc.edu

H.L. Frankel and B.P. deBoisblanc (eds.), *Bedside Procedures for the Intensivist*,
DOI 10.1007/978-0-387-79830-1_11,
© Springer Science+Business Media, LLC 2010

a percutaneously placed guidewire to create a tracheostoma.[4] Over the last two decades, Ciaglia percutaneous dilational tracheostomy (PDT) technique has become the preferred technique for performing tracheostomy in many ICUs. No technique is stagnant and PDT is no exception. Several modifications have improved its safety including: cannulation one or two tracheal interspaces below the cricoid cartilage, employment of videobronchoscopic guidance, adoption of a single-step dilator, and utilization of preprocedural ultrasound.

■ INDICATIONS FOR PDT

The appeal of PDT is that it is largely dilational rather than incisional and is therefore associated with less tissue devitalization. PDT has reportedly been associated with less peri-procedural bleeding, a lower risk of infectious complications, and better cosmesis. And, because it is usually performed at the bedside in the ICU, operating room scheduling and transportation of unstable patients are eliminated. Indications for tracheostomy are:

- Need for prolonged positive pressure ventilation
- Upper airway obstruction (e.g., tumor, epiglottitis, bilateral vocal cord paralysis, angioedema, sleep apnea)
- Ongoing need for bronchial hygiene

PDT could be considered as a potential alternative to open tracheostomy for all of these situations although it is most commonly performed on ICU patients requiring prolonged positive pressure ventilation. The first decision that must be made is whether to perform a tracheostomy at all or to continue with translaryngeal ventilation. Although this discussion is beyond the scope of this chapter, as a general rule, the best candidates for tracheostomy are those patients who have improved enough to benefit from the better comfort, mobility, speech, and swallowing afforded by tracheostomy but who are still dependent on positive pressure ventilation. Relative contraindications to PDT include:

- Uncorrected coagulopathy (INR > 1.5, PTT > 1.5 times the upper limit of normal, Platelets < 50,000, uremia)
- Morbid obesity (BMI > 35)
- Limited neck mobility (e.g., cervical spine injury, rheumatoid arthritis)
- Previous neck surgery that distorts anatomy
- Goiter or mass at the operative site
- High-riding innominate artery
- Requirement for PEEP > 10 or Fi02 > 60%
- Hemodynamic instability

Absolute contraindications to PDT are:

- Need for emergency airway
- Age <8 years
- Uncontrolled infection at the operative site

■ PDT TECHNIQUE

The single-dilator Ciaglia PDT technique (Blue Rhino™, Cook Medical; Ultra-Perc™, Smiths Medical) is the most widely practiced PDT technique in the USA. A long, single, curved dilator (Fig. 11-1) is used in lieu of multiple progressively larger dilators.[5,6] This improves the efficiency of the procedure. In a prospective, randomized trial of 50 trauma patients, procedural time was approximately 6 min with the single dilator technique compared to approximately 10 min with the multiple dilator technique.[7] The single dilator has additional advantages that make it attractive. Its curvature and softer consistency reduce point pressure on the posterior tracheal wall. And by not having to change dilators there is less tidal volume loss as the tracheostoma is created.

Briefly, the Ciaglia technique begins with a 2-cm skin incision and the percutaneous placement of a needle and guidewire between the first and second or second and third tracheal rings. A tracheostoma is created by the progressive advancement of a tapered plastic dilator over the guidewire until the stoma is large enough to accept a tracheostomy tube loaded on to a loading dilator. Although conceptually simple, the safe and efficient employment of this procedure requires the mastery of four

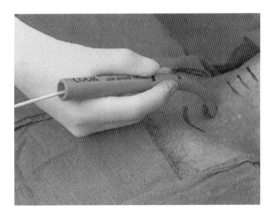

Figure 11-1. Single-step Blue Rhino™ PDT dilator (Cook Medical, Bloomington, IN).

skills which will be described in detail below: management the existing endotracheal tube, proper guidewire placement, stomal dilation, and finally tracheostomy tube placement.

Patient Selection

In the absence of contraindications, a skilled operator can safely perform PDT in any patient. However, it is best to apprentice with patients who have long thin necks and well-defined anatomy.

Monitoring

When performing any invasive procedure on a critically ill patient, be prepared for the worst-case scenario. In the case of PDT, premature loss of the endotracheal tube can have catastrophic consequences; therefore, continuous monitoring of vital signs, pulse oximetry, inhaled and exhaled tidal volumes, and airway pressures is mandatory. Continuous capnometry adds an additional margin of reassurance that the endotracheal tube is still in place. Patients are ventilated with 100% oxygen for the duration of the procedure.

Sedation

PDT is often possible with only conscious sedation and local anesthesia. However, since absolute control of the airway is critical, most operators prefer to use a deeper level of sedation and neuromuscular blockade. We use a combination of a local anesthetic, a short-acting benzodiazepine or propofol, a narcotic analgesic, and a nondepolarizing neuromuscular blocker. Paralysis is only necessary during the time that the endotracheal tube is withdrawn into the larynx. For most cases this is less than 15 min. It is important to emphasize that paralysis is not a substitute for adequate sedation, analgesia, and local anesthesia. Tachycardia and hypertension are often signs of patient discomfort but may also be early indicators of hypoxemia, hypercarbia, or other complications.

Positioning

Right-handed operators usually perform PDT standing on the right side of the bed with the patient positioned supine and close to the right edge of the mattress. In patients with normal neck mobility, rolled towels are placed under the shoulders to allow the neck to extend and open up the operative site and the tracheal interspaces. Care must be taken to make sure that the vertex is supported. Limited neck mobility, as is often seen in the aged and those with cervical spine disease, can make the procedure more difficult.

Anatomic Assessment

When the tracheostoma is properly placed between the first and second or second and third tracheal rings, it will traverse the thyroid isthmus a third of the time.[8] This rarely causes significant bleeding since PDT is dilatational below the skin. Occasionally an inferior thyroidal vein will traverse the intended operative site (Fig. 11-2), but the risk of significant bleeding with PDT is small due to the tamponading effect of the tracheostomy tube. Routine preoperative ultrasound of the base of the neck over the intended operative site (Fig. 11-3) can help identify intended landmarks and can identify large superficial and deep vessels not visible or palpable.[9–11] In one report,[11] 4 of 497 PDT procedures were associated with bleeding. The authors felt that, in each case of bleeding, ultrasound could have visualized the vessels that were ultimately determined to be the source: the inferior thyroid vein (two cases), high brachiocephalic vein (one case), and an aberrant anterior jugular communicating vein (one case). Ultrasound may be particularly useful prior to undertaking PDT in morbidly obese patients. However, randomized clinical trials from which to formulate an evidence-based recommendation are lacking and critics of routine preoperative ultrasound cite the added time and expense and the low risk of significant bleeding without its use.

Airway Management

It is imperative to maintain custody of the airway during PDT. Premature loss of the endotracheal tube, even briefly, can be lethal in a critically

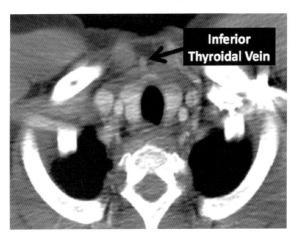

Figure 11-2. CT scan of the neck showing a large inferior thyroidal vein at the level of intended PDT.

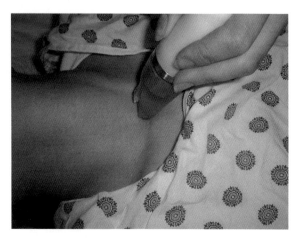

Figure 11-3. Preprocedural ultrasound of the anterior neck just cephalad to the sternal notch.

ill patient with limited cardiopulmonary reserve. The increased susceptibility of the ICU patient to adverse outcomes from airway loss is compounded by elements of the Ciaglia PDT technique that tend to promote or hide airway loss. Specifically, a patient is first paralyzed, then the neck is placed in a position that makes reintubation difficult, next the patient is hidden from view under surgical drapes while all eyes are focused on the operative site, then the endotracheal tube is withdrawn into a vulnerable position, and finally an operator tugs caudad on the trachea while the endotracheal tube is held tight to the maxilla. Reducing the potential for premature extubation and identifying premature extubation early if it does occur require a coordinated team approach.

An individual with expert airway skills should be at the head of the bed. All of the airway tools necessary to manage a difficult airway should be within reach, including a laryngoscope handle with appropriate-sized blades, an AMBU bag, a supraglottic airway (e.g., laryngeal mask), a suction apparatus, extra endotracheal tubes, a CO_2 detector, and a stiff, hollow airway exchange catheter. Once the patient has been sedated and paralyzed, a quick look with the laryngoscope will identify if a patient has a difficult airway.

Skin Incision and Blunt Dissection

The surgical field is prepped and draped and a 3×2 cm field block is created with lidocaine and epinephrine at the incision site. A 2-cm skin incision is made directly over the first and second tracheal interspaces

Table 11-1. Techniques for repositioning the endotracheal tube.

Techniques for repositioning the endotracheal tube	Safety	Accuracy	Speed
Direct laryngoscopy	++++	++++	++++
Bronchoscopic visualization	++	+++	+
Transtracheal illumination	+++	+++	++
ET cuff palpation	+	+	+
Premeasured blind withdrawal	+	+	+

(approximately halfway between the palpable cricoid cartilage and the sternal notch). Below the skin, the wound is bluntly dissected with a hemostat and an index finger down to the level of the pretracheal fascia.

To minimize risk, the endotracheal tube should not be withdrawn into the larynx until it is time to enter the trachea with the needle. Just before the needle is introduced between the first and second tracheal rings, the tip of the endotracheal tube will need to be pulled back so that its tip lies at or above the level of the cricoid cartilage. There are several methods for gauging the repositioning of the endotracheal tube prior to needle cannulation of the trachea (Table 11-1).

Withdrawing the endotracheal tube under direct laryngoscopic visualization is quick, accurate, and safe but it does not replace the need to use videobronchoscopy to guide the needle and guidewire placement as described below.[1,12,13] When using direct laryngoscopy, the endotracheal tube should be withdrawn until the superior edge of its cuff is visible between the true vocal cords. In an adult patient, this will usually place the tip of the endotracheal tube at the level of the cricoid cartilage. Because of its conical shape, the endolarynx is a location where inflation of the cuff will not secure the position of the endotracheal tube regardless of how much air is instilled. In fact, overinflating the cuff within the larynx will actually force the cuff further cephalad and out of the larynx. Therefore, one assistant should always have custody of the endotracheal tube and manually hold it in position during the entire case. Placing a hollow endotracheal tube exchanger through the endotracheal tube before repositioning it can add a significant margin of safety.[14]

Video Bronchoscopy

Video bronchoscopy can be used in lieu of direct laryngoscopy to reposition the endotracheal tube. The video bronchoscope is inserted into the endotracheal tube until just the tip of the tube is visible at the periphery of the image. Gripping both the scope and the tube as one unit, the endotracheal tube cuff is then deflated and the tube slowly withdrawn while visualizing the endotracheal anatomy. At the same time, the operator deforms the anterior tracheal wall with a hemostat at the point where the tracheostoma will be created. When "tenting" of the anterior tracheal wall by the hemostat can be seen (Fig. 11-4) or when the corrugated appearance

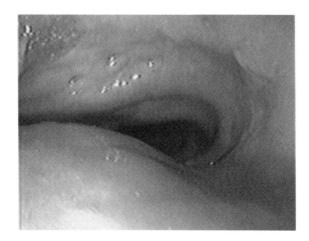

Figure 11-4. Tenting of the anterior tracheal wall by the hemostat to verify that the site of needle puncture will be below the tip of the endotracheal tube.

of the tracheal rings transitions to the smooth conical appearance of the endolarynx, the tube is held in place and the cuff gently reinflated.

Finally, two methods of repositioning the endotracheal tube, palpating the trachea while rapidly inflating and deflating the cuff and premeasured withdrawal, are not reliable and should not be relied on as the only means of confirming endotracheal tube position. Alternative methods of maintaining the airway during PDT, for example, use of a laryngeal mask airway (LMA) and use a microlaryngeal tube, have their advocates but have not gained popularity in the United States.[15,16]

Once the endotracheal tube is in the proper position, the video bronchoscope is used to position the tip of the needle prior to actual entry of the needle into the trachea. This is accomplished by gently deforming the anterior tracheal wall with the needle tip, as was done with the hemostat, while observing for tenting of the anterior tracheal mucosa. The operator adjusts the position of the needle tip so that it enters the trachea between the 11 and 1 o'clock positions below the cricoid cartilage, in between two tracheal rings, (preferably between the first and second or second and third), and away from the posterior tracheal wall. The J-tipped guidewire can then be advanced through the needle toward the carina and the needle withdrawn.

A "guiding catheter" is placed over the guidewire to stiffen it and reduce pressure on the posterior tracheal wall. A single-step beveled plastic dilator is then placed over the guiding catheter and guidewire and advanced in steps to create a tracheostoma of adequate size. The best technique for passing the dilator is to rest the hypothenar eminence of

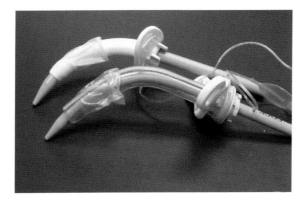

Figure 11-5. A standard and a bariatric tracheostomy tube loaded onto appropriate-sized, beveled plastic obturators. The obturator–tracheostomy tube combination is then placed onto the guiding catheter and guidewire combination and advanced through the tracheostoma into the trachea as one unit.

the dominant hand on the sternum and grip the dilator firmly like a pencil. A rocking motion in a posterior and caudad direction is used while visualizing the video image to reduce posterior wall pressure. Difficulty in advancing the dilator is most often due to an inadequate skin incision or blunt dissection. If excessive resistance is encountered and the skin is dimpling inward, extend the incision and repeat the blunt dissection. The tracheostoma must be slightly overdilated and the dilator left in place for a minute or two to overcome tissue memory.

The single-step dilator is removed from the guiding catheter and guidewire. A specialty tracheostomy tube is then loaded onto an appropriately sized, beveled plastic obturator (Fig. 11-5). This combination is then placed onto the guiding catheter and guidewire combination and advanced into the trachea as one unit. The obturator, guiding catheter, and guidewire are removed and the tracheostomy tube tip location is confirmed by briefly placing the video bronchoscope through the tracheostomy tube. The bronchoscope is then removed, the inner cannula of the tracheostomy tube is inserted, and positive pressure ventilation is begun through the tracheostomy tube. The wings of the tracheostomy tube flange should be sutured snugly and then tied in place.

■ SPECIAL SITUATIONS

Performing PDT in morbidly obese patients (BMI > 30 kg/m^2) can be difficult. Direct laryngoscopy is more challenging, surface landmarks may be obscured, and extra-long custom tracheostomy tubes (Fig. 11-5) may be necessary. In a small series, PDT was successfully performed in 13 consecutive obese patients with a BMI > 27 kg/m². [17] Peri-procedural complications were limited to temporary paratracheal tube placement in one patient and a cuff leak in another.

The lack of cervical spine clearance and inability to extend the neck are relative contraindications for PDT. In a series of 28 patients who underwent PDT without cervical spine clearance, 13 patients had known cervical spine fractures (6 stabilized with a halo or operative fixation and 7 stabilized with a cervical collar). [18] The PDT success rate was 96% while complications occurred in only 7%. There were no cases of aggravated spinal cord injury and there were no procedure-related deaths. In another series, 16 patients with anterior cervical fusions following spinal cord injury were randomized to surgical tracheostomy or ultrasound-guided PDT (Griggs dilational forceps technique). [19] Neither group experienced major perioperative complications and outcomes were similar for the two procedures.

■ PERI-PROCEDURAL COMPLICATIONS

Performing PDT in a patient with a small endotracheal tube (e.g., <7.5 mm internal diameter) while using an adult-sized fiber optic bronchoscope (5–6 mm outside diameter) can reduce minute ventilation and cause hypercapnia. [20] Equally worrisome is the potential for dynamic hyperinflation if expiration is incomplete due to high expiratory airways resistance. If vigilance is not maintained, barotrauma or hemodynamic embarrassment may occur. Videobronchoscopic visualization is critical only during the needle/guidewire introduction and dilator passage. It is therefore possible to use an intermittent bronchoscopic technique that withdraws the scope into the swivel adapter and readvances it into position every few breaths. If episodes of desaturation, excessive loss of tidal volume, or hemodynamic instability occur at a time when secretions or blood obscure the video image, then we use direct laryngoscopy to confirm endotracheal tube position.

Posterior wall tears that occur during PDT can rapidly lead to tension pneumothorax in a patient on positive pressure ventilation. [21] Rising peak airway pressures, oxyhemoglobin desaturation, hemodynamic instability, or the rapid development of subcutaneous emphysema or pneumomediasinum are clues to the diagnosis. Emergent tube thoracostomy can be life saving if a pneumothorax develops in a patient on positive pressure ventilation. Advancing the endotracheal tube to a level below the tear may control the air leak. Management of posterior wall tears ranges from observation in stable patients to operative repair.

Most peri-procedural bleeding originates from the skin edge. Completing the PDT and placing a snug fitting tracheostomy tube into the stoma can tamponade this type of bleeding. If skin edge oozing continues, sutures can be placed above and below the tracheostomy tube to snug up the fit even more. Rarely we have had to use hemostatic foam packed into the stoma along side of the tracheostomy tube.

In the event that the tracheostomy tube becomes dislodged before the patient is liberated from positive pressure ventilation, it is safer to reintubate orally even if the tracheostoma is mature. The tracheostomy tube can then be electively replaced.

■ POSTOPERATIVE CARE

There are no convincing data to support the use of prophylactic antibiotics for PDT. The incidence of stomatitis is only about 5%,[22] even though the trachea is often heavily colonized with pathogenic bacteria by the time that a tracheostomy is performed. The stoma should be cleaned daily with a prep solution, for example, chlorhexidene, and covered with clean dry gauze. If mild stomatitis does develop, it can often be managed with the use of topical antibiotics alone. There are no controlled data to support the practice of routine tracheostomy tube changes and we prefer to change a tube only if it malfunctions or if a smaller or uncuffed tube is needed for speech. Retaining sutures can be removed when the stoma is mature, usually around 7–10 days.

■ CONCLUSIONS

PDT is a bedside procedure that can be performed in the ICU with very low morbidity. Practitioners of PDT should also be skilled in basic ultrasound techniques, advanced airway management, videobronchoscopy,

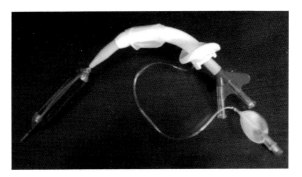

Figure 11-6. New balloon PDT device (Blue Dolphin™, Cook, Bloomington, IN).

tube thoracostomy, and mechanical ventilation. Established techniques are being constantly refined and new techniques such as balloon-facilitated PDT (Fig. 11-6) are coming on to the market. As techniques evolve, practitioners will need to continually update skill sets. Independence to perform PDT should be accrued through a process that includes didactic training, simulation, apprenticeship, peer review, and continuing medical education.

■ REFERENCES

1. Frost EAM. Tracing the tracheostomy. *Ann Otol Rhinol Laryngol.* 1976;85:618–624.
2. Salmon LFW. Tracheostomy. *Proc R Soc Med.* 1975;68:347–356.
3. Galloway TC. Tracheotomy in bulbar poliomyelitis. *J Am Med Assoc.* 1943;123:1096–1097.
4. Ciaglia P, Firsching R, Syniec C. Elective percutaneous dilatational tracheostomy; a new simple bedside procedure; preliminary report. *Chest.* 1985;87:715–719.
5. Byhahn C et al. [Ciaglia blue rhino: a modified technique for percutaneous dilatation tracheostomy. Technique and early clinical results]. *Anaesthesist.* 2000;49(3):202–206.
6. Byhahn C et al. Percutaneous tracheostomy: CIaglia Blue Rhino versus the basic Ciaglia technique of percutaneous dilational tracheostomy. *Anesth Analg.* 2000;91:882–886.
7. Johnson JL et al. Percutaneous dilational tracheostomy: a comparison of single- versus multiple-dilator techniques. *Crit Care Med.* 2001;29(6):1251–1254.
8. Dexter TJ. A cadaver study appraising accuracy of blind placement of percutaneous tracheostomy. [comment]. *Anaesthesia.* 1995;50(10):863–864.
9. Hatfield A, Bodenham A. Portable ultrasonic scanning of the anterior neck before percutaneous dilatational tracheostomy. *Anaesthesia.* 1999;54(7):660–663.
10. Sustic A et al. Ultrasonographically guided percutaneous dilatational tracheostomy after anterior cervical spine fixation. *Acta Anaesthesiol Scand.* 1999;43(10):1078–1080.
11. Muhammad JK et al. Percutaneous dilatational tracheostomy under ultrasound guidance. *Br J Oral Maxillofac Surg.* 1999;37(4):309–311.
12. Hill SA. An unusual complication of percutaneous tracheostomy. *Anaesthesia.* 1995;50(5):469–470.
13. Masterson GR, Smurthwaite GJ. A complication of percutaneous tracheostomy. *Anaesthesia.* 1994;49:452–453.
14. Deblieux P et al. Facilitation of percutaneous dilational tracheostomy by use of a perforated endotracheal tube exchanger. [comment]. *Chest.* 1995;108(2):572–574.

15. Ambesh SP et al. Laryngeal mask airway vs endotracheal tube to facilitate bedside percutaneous tracheostomy in critically ill patients: a prospective comparative study. *J Postgrad Med*. 2002;48(1):11–15.

16. Fisher L et al. Percutaneous dilational tracheostomy: a safer technique of airway management using a microlaryngeal tube. *Anaesthesia*. 2002;57(3):253–255.

17. Mansharamani NG et al. Safety of bedside percutaneous dilatational tracheostomy in obese patients in the ICU. *Chest*. 2000;117(5):1426–1429.

18. Mayberry JC et al. Cervical spine clearance and neck extension during percutaneous tracheostomy in trauma patients. *Crit Care Med*. 2000;28(10):3436–3440.

19. Sustic A et al. Surgical tracheostomy versus percutaneous dilational tracheostomy in patients with anterior cervical spine fixation: preliminary report. *Spine*. 2002;27(17):1942–1945. discussion 1945.

20. Reilly PM et al. Hypercarbia during tracheostomy: a comparison of percutaneous endoscopic, percutaneous Doppler, and standard surgical tracheostomy. *Intensive Care Med*. 1997;23(8):859–864.

21. Trottier SJ et al. Posterior tracheal wall perforation during percutaneous dilational tracheostomy: an investigation into its mechanism and prevention. *Chest*. 1999;115(5):1383–1389.

22. Higgins KM, Punthakee X. Meta-analysis ccomparison of open versus percutaneous tracheostomy. *Laryngoscope*. 2007;117:447–454.

12

Open Tracheostomy

Adam M. Shiroff and John P. Pryor

■ INTRODUCTION

Open tracheostomy has been performed, in its modern definition, since the early 1900s.[1] Since its first use, the indications for tracheostomy have varied widely, from inflammatory disease and malignancy to airway protection and ventilatory support. Tracheostomy is one of the most common procedures that the intensive care unit (ICU) patient population will undergo. Bedside open tracheostomy (BOT) has become an attractive option for critically ill patients; it obviates the need for transport to the operating room, has been shown to decrease costs, and can be done safely.[2,3]

■ INDICATIONS

Indications for tracheostomy in the critically ill are debated. When considering a tracheostomy, consider the complications of endotracheal intubation and the specific advantages tracheostomy has over endotracheal intubation.

J.P. Pryor (✉)
Department of Surgery, Division of Traumatology and Surgical Critical Care,
University of Pennsylvania School of Medicine and University of Pennsylvania
Medical Center, 2 Dulles, 3400 Spruce Street, Philadelphia, PA 19104, USA
e-mail: Pryorj@uphs.upenn.edu

H.L. Frankel and B.P. deBoisblanc (eds.), *Bedside Procedures for the Intensivist*,
DOI 10.1007/978-0-387-79830-1_12,
© Springer Science+Business Media, LLC 2010

Prolonged intubation has multiple potential problems such as laryngeal edema, pressure injury to the trachea, and subsequent stenosis. Thus patients who are not expected to be liberated from the ventilator for 3–7 days should be considered for tracheostomy.[4]

There are several advantages of tracheostomy over endotracheal intubation. Critically ill patients will frequently have difficulty in managing their secretions. Access for frequent suctioning is an established benefit to tracheostomy. Once a patient has undergone tracheostomy, the need for sedation and analgesia is decreased, nursing care is easier, the patient is more comfortable and may potentially phonate and enjoy oral nutrition.[5] Tracheostomy confers a significant reduction in airway resistance that translates to a shorter time to wean from the ventilator.[6] Tracheostomy may also decrease the likelihood of ventilator-associated pneumonia.[7]

■ TIMING

The timing of tracheostomy has been a subject of much debate in the literature. Some of the difficulty is that there is no unified definition of what is an "early" or a "late" tracheostomy. There is still no clear consensus on the optimal time to perform the procedure. Once meeting an indication for tracheostomy, each patient should be assessed individually for risks vs. benefits of the procedure. It has been shown that early tracheostomy reduces the length of stay in the ICU and hospital and reduces morbidity and mortality.[8–10]

■ OPEN VS. PERCUTANEOUS

Although the debate between BOT and bedside percutaneous dilatational tracheostomy (PDT) is beyond the scope of this chapter it deserves mention. It has been shown that both BOT and PDT can be performed safely by experienced practitioners.[11] It has been shown that there is no significant outcome benefit to one technique over the other, but PDT may offer some cost savings.[2]

■ ANATOMY

The trachea lies in the midline of the neck. The importance of a thorough knowledge of the anatomy in this region cannot be overemphasized. Surface anatomy varies depending on patient body habitus and position and may provide little to no information. Careful palpation of the thyroid cartilage and cricoid cartilage along with the supra-sternal notch will help guide the operating surgeon. From superficial to deep at the level of the second to third tracheal rings in the midline of the neck the surgeon will encounter several structures in consecutive order:

1. Skin and subcutaneous tissue
2. Platysma muscle
3. Junction of the strap muscles in the midline
4. Isthmus of the thyroid gland
5. Pretracheal fascia
6. Trachea

It is important to note the direct posterior location of the esophagus. Trauma to the posterior wall of the trachea can lead to communication with the esophagus and fistula formation. The key to safe dissection and placement of the tracheostomy tube is knowledge of the surrounding structures and maintenance of a midline position throughout the procedure.

■ ICU ROOM SETUP

The ICU patient room is not an operating room. However, it can easily function as one with some careful planning and the proper equipment. Lighting is often suboptimal for surgical procedures in the ICU. Portable OR-style overhead lights are available but they are cumbersome and expensive. Headlamps are an excellent option for focused lighting. OR-caliber electrocautery is used and must fit in the room along with a bedside table or Mayo stand capable of holding the necessary instruments within comfortable reach of the operating surgeon and the assistant. The ICU bed is typically larger than an OR table and this can present several issues. First, the bed must be able to be pulled away from the wall so that the respiratory therapist can be positioned to manipulate the endotracheal tube (ETT) and allow room for endotracheal intubation should the airway need to be secured from above. The width of the bed can make operating uncomfortable when the patient is in the middle of the bed; this can be remedied by either moving the patient toward the side of the surgeon or, on rare occasion, switching the ICU bed for a hospital gurney which is more closely matched to an OR table in terms of width. The position of the surgeon should not compromise the ability to safely manipulate the airway.

■ EQUIPMENT

Bedside tracheostomy requires the same essential instrumentation as in the operating room. When choosing instruments for a bedside procedure tray one must have the essential tools without excessive, rarely used items that will clutter the instrument tray. In addition to the electrocautery base unit and adequate overhead lighting or a headlamp, the surgical instruments and number needed for the procedure are:

- Scalpels #11 and #15
- Electrocautery pencil and grounding pad

- 12 F Frazer suction
- Yankaur suction
- Sterile suction tubing
- Adson forceps × 2
- DeBakey forceps × 2
- Trousseau–Jackson tracheal dilator
- Tracheal hook, sharp
- Weitlaner retractor
- Senn retractor × 2
- Green thyroid retractor × 2
- Army-Navy retractor × 2
- Metzenbaum curved scissors
- Curved blunt scissors
- Needle holder × 2
- Allis clamp × 2
- Hemostat, curved × 4
- Towel clamps × 4
- 10-cc syringe, slip tip × 2
- Needle 19 gauge, 1.5 in
- Needle 22 gauge, 1.5 in
- Gauze sponges × 10
- 2–0 Silk ties
- 3–0 Silk ties
- 2–0 polypropylene suture x 2

■ TYPES OF TRACHEOSTOMY TUBES

There are a variety of tracheostomy tubes available. The numbering of the tubes (i.e., #8) conveys the internal diameter in millimeters. Based on the body habitus of the patient, there are tracheostomy tubes that are longer in the anterior–posterior dimension as well as the superior–inferior dimension. There are tubes that require air to fill the cuff (Shiley) as well as tubes that are largely filled with foam (Bivona). The size and type of tracheostomy tube used is a clinical decision made by the operating surgeon in concert with the critical care team, keeping in mind the needs of the patient from a respiratory and pulmonary toilet standpoint.

■ ANESTHESIA

A well-sedated and motionless patient is optimal for bedside tracheostomy. A combination of narcotic analgesia, an amnestic agent, and a muscle relaxant provide the needed anesthesia for this procedure. These drugs are readily available in the ICU and critical care nurses are comfortable with their administration. For example, fentanyl, versed, and cisatracurium in doses appropriate for the patient's hemodynamic status will yield excellent results. Note that the surgeon should confirm adequate sedation prior to the administration of the muscle relaxant and an increase in heart rate and blood pressure during the procedure should prompt supplementation with additional narcotic and amnestic agents. Local anesthesia at the site of incision will prevent some of the postoperative discomfort and is recommended. It is important to have a distinct anesthesia or airway team at the head of the bed. This team can consist of an intensivist, an anesthesiologist, or an experienced respiratory therapist, but comfort with the bedside procedure and experience in orotracheal intubation is a must.

■ TECHNIQUE

After consent is reviewed and all appropriate patient identifying standards are met the procedure can begin.

1. A roll is placed behind the shoulders of the supine patient extending the neck if the cervical spine is without injury. If the cervical spine can not be extended, spine precautions must be maintained using bolsters taped along the sides of the patient's head. The respiratory therapist is at the head of the bed; the patient should be sedated (fentanyl and midazolam) and given muscle relaxation (cisatracurium) by the ICU nurse.
2. The neck is then prepped and draped in the usual sterile fashion. A U-drape is used with the limbs toward the head of the bed to facilitate the transition of the ventilator tubing from ETT to tracheostomy.
3. The function of the electrocautery (pencil and grounding pad) and the positioning of the operating surgeons headlamp are confirmed. The balloon of the tracheostomy tube is checked.
4. 1% lidocaine with epinephrine is injected along the proposed incision line.
5. A 4–6 cm horizontal incision is made approximately two finger breaths above the sternal notch.
6. Dissection is carried through subcutaneous fat and platysma muscle using electrocautery. Care is taken not to injure the two anterior jugular veins. If encountered, they are tied with 3–0 silk suture and divided to avoid injury during retraction and troublesome bleeding.
7. A self retaining retractor is placed to keep the wound open.
8. An incision vertically through midline junction of the strap muscles brings the surgeon onto pretracheal fascia; the strap muscles are retracted laterally.
9. An Army-Navy retractor is placed in the inferior aspect of the wound.
10. If thyroid isthmus is encountered, careful dissection of the inferior

aspect in the pretracheal plain to allow cephalad retraction is completed.

11. If the thyroid gland cannot be mobilized, the isthmus is dissected off the trachea, clamped, divided, and oversewn with nonabsorbable suture (silk).

12. Green retractors at 10 and 2 o'clock are useful to elevate the thyroid and stabilize the trachea.

13. The second and third rings of the trachea are identified.

14. The ETT needs to be freed from attachments (tape to the patient's face, the NG tube, etc.) This is typically done by the respiratory therapist, who is ready to manipulate the ETT. The balloon of the ETT is then deflated

15. A horizontal incision is made in the space between the second and third tracheal rings and a small T-incision is made vertically down through the third tracheal ring.

16. The tracheal spreader is used to enlarge the opening and to visualize the ETT being withdrawn slowly. Suction is useful at this time; there are often pulmonary secretions that can obstruct the view of the ETT.

17. Once the ETT is just cephalad of the tracheotomy, the tracheal spreader is removed and with care the tracheostomy tube is placed. If the angle of the trachea is steep such that further elevation of the trachea would allow a more direct entrance into the airway, a tracheal hook is placed under the cricoid cartilage. This will allow additional control of the trachea. Too much tension or counter-tension, however, can lead to tearing of the hook from the trachea and loss of control of the airway.

18. End tidal carbon dioxide monitoring or color capnography must be used to confirm placement of the tube in the airway, as well as breath sounds and the return of tidal volume on the ventilator.

19. Only after placement is confirmed should the retractors and/or hook be removed from the incision and the ETT then can be withdrawn from the upper airway.

20. The lateral aspects of the incision may require a single interrupted stitch each to decrease the size of the wound.

21. The tracheostomy tube is then secured with permanent monofilament suture at the four corners of the flange. A soft Velcro or cotton trach-tie is used for further securing the tracheostomy tube around the patient's neck.

■ COMPLICATIONS

The complications of tracheostomy are well described and significant complications are rare.[12] Early complications are most often technical in nature. Bleeding, pneumothorax, pneumomediastinum, subcutaneous emphysema, decannulation, and obstruction can largely be prevented by meticulous operative technique and attention to detail. Late complications include tracheal stenosis, tracheo-innominate fistula (TIF), and tracheo-esophageal fistula.[13,14] Another complication is early decannulation. In the event that the tracheostomy tube becomes dislodged, the appropriate maneuver is to re-intubate in an orotracheal manner. Attempts at replacing a tracheostomy tube in relatively recent tracheostomy tract can lead to significant delay in re-establishing an acceptable airway. Although rare, TIF does occur and if not managed immediately is rapidly fatal. Often there is a sentinel bleed that terminates on its own and requires evaluation. In the actively bleeding TIF, there are several maneuvers that can temporize the situation and these depend on if the bleeding is into the airway; rapid bronchoscopy can help make this diagnosis if it is in question. If the trachea is contaminated with blood, the tracheostomy balloon should be maximally inflated. If this controls bleeding, the patient should then go for immediate surgical exploration. In the event that bleeding continues pressure should be applied to the stoma site, or the tracheostomy itself can be displaced anteriorly, compressing the overlying vessel against the sternum as the patient is transported to the OR. Bleeding into the airway proper is an even more life-threatening situation and if the initial overinflation of the cuff does not control bleeding the patient should be orotracheally intubated and the tracheostomy removed. Once removed, digital compression of the bleeding source is done through the stoma site. It is important to ensure that the ETT cuff is distal to the bleeding site to provide oxygenation and ventilation. The patient must then go emergently to the operating room for a median sternotomy and control of the bleeding vessel.[15]

■ REFERENCES

1. Jackson C. Tracheostomy. *Laryngoscope.* 1909;19:285–290.
2. Bacchetta MD, Girardi LN, Southard EJ, et al. Comparison of open versus percutaneous dilatational tracheostomy in the cardiothoracic surgical patient: outcomes and financial analysis. *Ann Thorac Surg.* 2005;79:1879–1885.
3. Terra RM, Fernandez A, Bammann RH, et al. Open bedside tracheostomy: routine procedure for patients under prolonged mechanical ventilation. *Clinics.* 2007;62(4):427–432.
4. MacIntyre NR, Cook DJ, Ely EW Jr, et al. Evidence-based guidelines for weaning and discontinuing ventilatory support: a collective task force facilitated by the American College of Chest Physicians; the American Association for Respiratory Care; and the American College of Critical Care Medicine. *Chest.* 2001;120(6 Suppl):375S–395S.
5. Niesezkowska A, Combes A, Luyt CE, et al. Impact of tracheostomy on sedative administration, sedation level, and comfort of mechanically ventilated intensive care unit patients. *Crit Care Med.* 2004;33:2527–2533.

6. Diehl JL, El Atrous S, Touchard D, et al. Changes in work of breathing induced by tracheotomy in ventilator-dependent patients. *Am J Respir Crit Care Med*. 1999;159:383–388.

7. Nseir S, Di Polmeo C, Jozefowicz E, et al. Relationship between tracheotomy and ventilator-associated pneumonia: a case control study. *Eur Respir J*. 2007;30(2):314–320.

8. Rumback MJ, Newton M, Truncale T, et al. A prospective, randomized, study comparing early percutaneous dilational tracheotomy to prolonged translaryngeal intubation (delayed tracheotomy) in critically ill medical patients. *Crit Care Med*. 2004;32:1689–1694.

9. Moller MG, Slaikeu JD, Bonelli P, et al. Early tracheostomy versus late tracheostomy in the surgical intensive care unit. *Am J Surg*. 2005;189:293–296.

10. Flaatten H, Gjerde S, Heimdal JH, et al. The effect of tracheostomy on outcome in intensive care unit patients. *Acta Anaethesiol Scand*. 2006;50:92–98.

11. Silvester W, Goldsmith D, Uchino S, et al. Percutaneous versus surgical tracheostomy: a randomized controlled study with long-term follow-up. *Crit Care Med*. 2006;34:2145–2152.

12. Goldenberg D, Ari EG, Golz A, et al. Tracheotomy complications: a retrospective study of 1130 cases. *Otolaryngol Head Neck Surg*. 2000;123(4):495–500.

13. De Leyn P, Bedert L, Delcroix M, et al. Tracheotomy: clinical review and guidelines. *Eur J Cardiothorac Surg*. 2007;32(3):412–421.

14. Epstein SK. Late complications of tracheostomy. *Respir Care*. 2005;50(4):542–549.

15. Grant CA, Dempsey G, Harrison J, Jones T. Tracheo-innominate artery fistula after percutaneous tracheostomy: three case reports and a clinical review. *Br J Anaesth*. 2006;96(1):127–131.

13

Transbronchial Biopsy in the Intensive Care Unit

Erik E. Folch, Chirag Choudhary, Sonali Vadi, and Atul C. Mehta

■ INTRODUCTION

Since its introduction in 1968, the fiberoptic bronchoscope has had a remarkable impact in the diagnosis and management of patients with respiratory maladies.[1] The physicians entrusted with the care of critically ill patients are often faced with an array of chest roentgenographic abnormalities for which flexible bronchoscopy (FB) can be a valuable diagnostic tool.

The etiologies of radiographic abnormalities on chest imaging of intensive care unit (ICU) patients are multivariate. Empiric therapy is frequently initiated on the basis of clinical suspicion with uncertain accuracy. This can lead to inappropriate treatment in some patients with the ensuing risk of possible adverse events, including the emergence of antibiotic resistance, while potentially reversible causes may go unrecognized. In critically ill patients, use of FB and its diagnostic capabilities can help guide therapy.

A.C. Mehta (✉)
Sheikh Khalifa Medical City managed by Cleveland Clinic, Abu Dhabi, UAE
e-mail: mehtaa1@ccf.org

H.L. Frankel and B.P. deBoisblanc (eds.), *Bedside Procedures for the Intensivist*,
DOI 10.1007/978-0-387-79830-1_13,
© Springer Science+Business Media, LLC 2010

Often, broncho-alveolar lavage (BAL) performed via FB is insufficient when used alone for the diagnosis of tissue invasion or histologic assessment of parenchymal involvement.[2]

The diagnostic yield of open lung biopsy has been reported to be 46–100% with an alteration in treatment in approximately 73% of patients.[3] However, the procedure is associated with a high incidence of desaturation, need for thoracotomy tubes, peri-operative bleeding, and in some cases bronchopleural fistula. The postoperative course can further be complicated by pleural space and skin infections and occasionally death. In addition to concerns about morbidity of open lung biopsy, no study has shown an improvement in the survival of mechanically ventilated patients with this technique.[4,5] For these reasons, FB with transbronchial lung biopsy (TBLB) remains a viable option to obtain lung tissue under the circumstances faced by critical care physicians.

■ INDICATIONS FOR FB

The flexible bronchoscope allows physicians in the ICU the ability to visualize the airways and perform a variety of procedures in order to obtain samples for histologic and microbiologic studies. These modalities include BAL, TBLB, endobronchial biopsy (EBBx), bronchial brushings, transbronchial needle aspiration (TBNA), and a special double lumen specimen brush for quantitative cultures. FB can also be used to remove foreign bodies, diagnose and control hemoptysis, and perform other advanced interventional bronchoscopic procedures.[6]

Diagnostic and therapeutic indications for FB in the ICU are:

- Diagnostic
  - Diffuse or focal lung infiltrates (e.g., lung mass, ventilator-associated pneumonia)
  - Evaluation of persistent or recurrent pneumonia
  - Position of:
    (a) Endotracheal tube
    (b) Double lumen endotracheal tube
  - Evaluation of:
    (a) Airway trauma
    (b) Acute inhalational injury
    (c) Broncho-pleural fistula
    (d) Foreign body aspiration
  - Diagnosis of acute lung rejection in allogenic lung transplant recipients

- Therapeutic
  - Airway management
    (a) Difficult intubation [7]
    (b) Double-lumen endotracheal tube placement [7]

(c) Placement of Combitube™ by endotracheal tube [8]
- Atelectasis due to mucus plugs despite conservative treatment [9]
- Removal of excessive airway secretions
- Adjunct to percutaneous dilatational tracheostomy [10]
- Management of massive hemoptysis [11]
- Removal of aspirated material
- Foreign-body removal [12]
- Closure of bronchopleural fistula [13]
- Management of central obstructive airway lesions [6]

Compared to BAL alone, TBLB via FB increases the yield for a wide array of lung diseases affecting patients in the ICU, but it carries risks above and beyond those of bronchoscopy alone. This is especially true in patients who are on mechanical ventilation since this group of patients is usually poorly tolerant of complications. Absolute contraindications to bronchoscopy or transbronchial biopsies in the ICU:

- Lack of informed consent[14]
- Uncooperative patient
- Serious uncorrected electrolyte abnormalities
- Inability to maintain patent airway
- Inability to ventilate or oxygenate during the procedure[14]
- Inadequate facilities[14]
- Hemodynamic instability
- Malignant arrhythmias[15,16]
- Antiplatelet medications (Clopidogrel)[17–19]
- Inexperienced operator[14]

Relative contraindications are:

- Elevated intracranial pressure[20,21]
- Impending respiratory failure
- Laryngeal edema
- Coagulopathy[22,23]
- Uremia[22,24]
- Pulmonary hypertension
- Lung abscess
- Use of high positive end-expiratory pressure (PEEP)
- Pregnancy[25]
- Cardiac ischemia[16,26,27]

Most procedural complications of bronchoscopy and TBLB occur in patients with known risk factors for adverse outcome. Recognition of potential risk factors for complications of bronchoscopy and TBLB is important prior to beginning these procedures. Some risk factors, such as coagulopathy, may be reversible while others, such as immunocompromised state, alert the operator to be prepared for potential adverse events.

Risk factors for TBLB associated complications in critically ill patients include:

- Coagulopathy
- Medications
- Renal insufficiency
- Immunocompromised state
- Unstable cardiovascular disease
- Recent acute myocardial infarction (<48 h)
- Hemodynamic instability
- Arrhythmias
- Increased intracranial pressure
- Reactive airway disease
- Hypoxia ($PaO_2 < 60$ mmHg or $FiO_2 > 0.7$)
- PEEP > 10 cm H_2O
- Auto-PEEP > 15 cm H_2O

■ COAGULOPATHY

Based on a retrospective review of bleeding complications, a platelet count $<50 \times 10^9/l$, an international normalized ratio (INR) >1.5, or activated partial thromboplastin time >2.0 times the control are contraindications to TBLB.[22]

TBLB should not be attempted during clopidogrel therapy. Instead, clopidogrel should be discontinued 5–7 days before TBLB if TBLB is deemed necessary. A prospective cohort study of clopidogrel was stopped prematurely due to excessive bleeding rates in those treated with the drug.[18] Bleeding occurred in 89% of patients on clopidogrel vs. 3.4% of the control group. None of the patients in either group had laboratory evidence of coagulopathy. Aspirin may be an acceptable substitute to clopidogrel since the risk of severe bleeding with aspirin alone has been reported to be 0.9%[17] as compared to 100% bleeding risk in patients on both drugs.[19]

Oral anticoagulants (warfarin) should be withheld at least 3 days prior to FB for TBLB or the effects of anticoagulation should be reversed with low-dose vitamin K. Low molecular weight heparin (LMWH) should be withheld the evening before and on the morning of the procedure. In patients who require continuous anticoagulation, unfractionated heparin (UFH) can be commenced on withholding the LMWH. UFH should then be discontinued 4–6 h prior to the planned procedure. In a retrospective review on the safety of BAL and TBLB in mechanically ventilated patients, no association between use of LMWH used for venous thromboembolism prophylaxis and the occurrence of bleeding was noted.[23] Additional guidelines on the use of anticoagulants during the peri-operative period exist.[28]

These guidelines can be extrapolated for bronchoscopy in view of the invasiveness of the procedure and risk of bleeding.

Azotemia (BUN > 30 mg/dl) has been associated with an incidence of bleeding of 4–45% following TBLB.[22,24,29] However, clinically significant bleeding was observed in only 6% of the patients and bleeding usually resolved with FB tamponade or epinephrine instillation.

Interventions undertaken to try to prevent excessive bleeding in uremic patients have included:

- Preprocedural hemodialysis
- Use of Desmopressin 0.3–0.4 mcg/kg subcutaneous or intravenously 30 min prior to TBLB[30]
- Platelet transfusions
- Preprocedural administration of cryoprecipitate, or administration of conjugated estrogen 0.6 mg/kg IV over 30–40 min[29,31]

Intravenous desmopressin has been recommended as the first line therapy to prevent bleeding in this group of patients. While, studies reporting dialysis for prevention or management of bleeding in uremic patients have shown inconsistent effects of dialysis on coagulation parameters and platelet function,[30] hemodialysis when used in combination with other treatments does appear to be beneficial. Cryoprecipitate administered within 30 min of the procedure has an effect that lasts for 4–12 h.

Although FB with TBLB is associated with a higher diagnostic yield (81%) in immuno-compromised patients with pulmonary infiltrates than in nonimmunocompromised patients,[32] the immunosuppressed host is at greater risk for a bleeding complication.[33] The reported incidence of bleeding in this population varies from 15 to 29%.[22,34] Interestingly, the results from a prospective, cohort study did not reveal any correlation between immunosuppressive medication use after transplantation and the propensity to bleed.[17]

■ UNSTABLE CARDIOVASCULAR DISEASE

Reported cardiovascular effects of FB have included a rise in mean arterial pressure (MAP), stroke volume, and pulmonary artery pressure; a fall in arterial oxygen saturation; tachydysrhythmias and bundle branch blocks; and myocardial ischemia.[35,36] Although major complications are uncommon in patients who are undergoing FB with a history of recent myocardial infarction (4–6 weeks), unstable angina, or dysrhythmias,[16] risks and benefits should be carefully weighed prior to proceeding. Patients should be hemodynamically stable for at least 48 h prior to the procedure.

■ INCREASED INTRACRANIAL PRESSURE

Although FB can raise intracranial pressure in patients with head injury, it also causes a simultaneous rise in MAP, thus maintaining cerebral perfusion pressure (CPP). The rise in ICP and MAP is transient and rapidly returns to baseline postprocedure. No deterioration in neurological status or Glasgow Coma Scale was reported in two separate trials investigating FB in patients with severe head trauma.[20,21] Sedation, paralysis, analgesia, and topical anesthesia did not prevent rise in ICP in this group of patients.

■ REACTIVE AIRWAY DISEASE

FB can cause laryngospasm or bronchospasm in patients with reactive airway disease. Nebulizing bronchodilators prior to FB helps prevent bronchospasm, oxyhemoglobin desaturation, and changes in lung volumes but may not improve clinical outcomes.[37] Nevertheless, we recommend the use of a short-acting bronchodilator due to its low risk and potential benefit.

■ NECESSARY EQUIPMENT

The following pieces of equipment are necessary for an optimal FB experience:

- Protective personal equipment: gown, gloves, mask, eye shield
- Bite block to prevent damage to the bronchoscope during trans-oral insertion
- Y-adaptor to reduce the loss of delivered tidal volume
- Flexible bronchoscopes of various diameters
- Flexible forceps
- Flexible brush
- Normal saline
- Lidocaine 1 or 2% solution
- Ice-cold saline (0.9% NaCl)
- Epinephrine (1:10,000 dilution) or Norepinephrine
- Resuscitation equipment including defibrillator, Ambu-bag, laryngoscope, replacement ETT, and chest tube insertion tray.
- Anesthesia agents for moderate sedation (e.g., Midazolam, Morphine, Fentanyl, Propofol)

■ PREPROCEDURE

Informed consent for TBLB in mechanically ventilated patients varies from that in ambulatory outpatients because it carries an increased risk of bleeding and pneumothorax. The procedure and its potential complications should be explicitly explained to the patient (if awake) and/or surrogates, and an opportunity given to ask any questions prior to the procedure.[38]

The single most important factor responsible for the success of the procedure is the expertise of the bronchoscopist and assistant team. The 2007 Guidelines on Bronchoscopy Assisting[39,40] state: " … *bronchoscopy assistant should be trained in the setup and handling of equipment, collecting/preparing/labeling/handling of specimens, delivery of aerosolized medications and handling mechanical ventilation.*" The guidelines emphasize the need for vigilant monitoring of the patient's condition.

Eligible patients should be hemodynamically stable (MAP>60 mmHg) and without significant arrhythmias. Patients should be fasted for 4 h and the stomach should be emptied via the nasogastric tube to minimize the risk of aspirating tube feedings. Due to the risk of hypoxemia, mechanically ventilated patients should be placed on 100% oxygen at least 10 min before beginning. Adequate alveolar ventilation must be insured by ventilating in a volume-control mode at a respiratory rate that avoids auto-PEEP.[41–43] Set PEEP should be minimized if oxygenation permits. Pulse oximetry and capnometry should be continuously monitored. Concomitant suctioning closes the alveoli with resultant alveolar hypoventilation.[42,44]

Occurrence of pneumothorax as a result of the bronchoscopic procedure can be detected by an elevation of both peak pressure (Ppeak) and plateau pressure (Pplat), with maintained inspiratory flow rates and tidal volumes. The bronchoscopist and respiratory therapist should be aware of the peak inspiratory pressure and plateau pressure throughout the procedure.

Adequate intravenous sedation is an important element in the safe application of FB in critically ill patients. Benzodiazepines have both amnesic and anxiolytic properties. Midazolam has a fast onset and a short duration of action.[45] Propofol is an excellent sedative and induction agent that has the advantage of rapid onset of action with shorter recovery time than benzodiazepines[46], but hypotension occurs more commonly with propofol. Opioids have analgesic and antitussive properties and are important adjuncts to sedatives during FB. Fentanyl has a rapid onset of action and clearance and is associated with a low incidence of both nausea and hypotension. Due to nonlinear dose-response relationship, the dose of these drugs should be titrated to clinical effect. As a general rule, dosages of sedative and analgesics should be titrated with great care in the elderly and in patients with renal and liver disease. Specific antagonists to opiates (naloxone) and benzodiazepines (flumazenil) should be available at hand. Adequacy of sedation and ventilation ensures ease of the procedure and satisfactory oxygenation. Paralysis with neuromuscular blockers is necessary in a small percentage of patients to eliminate agitation and cough in the appropriately sedated patient.

Atropine has been routinely used prior to TBLB to prevent vasovagal episodes, bronchoconstriction, or to reduce bronchial secretions. However, neither a clinical benefit nor any increase in the frequency of complications could be demonstrated in two double-blind, placebo controlled studies.[47,48] Therefore, we do not recommend the use of atropine prior to the procedure.

Facilities for resuscitation and difficult airway management should be at hand. Health care professionals involved should be mandatorily trained as per AHA cardio-pulmonary resuscitation. Thoracostomy tube set or a pig-tail catheter with an expertise in its placement should be on site prior to the procedure of TBLB to manage inadvertent complication of pneumothorax.

Infection, a dreaded complication post-FB, especially in critically ill patients, has a reported incidence of 6.5%.[49] Use of prophylactic antibiotics in high-risk patients such as those with a history of infective endocarditis, prosthetic heart valves, hemophilia, malnutrition, immunocompromised status, or insulin-dependent diabetes who will undergo FB or TBLB have been described.[50] Prophylactic antibiotics should be administered to asplenic patients, patients with artificial valves or those with history of endocarditis prior to any intervention in the respiratory tract.

■ PROCEDURE

Guidelines for the hand hygiene and the use of personal protective equipment (gown, gloves, mask, and eye shield) should be followed.[50]

Even when performing FB via an oral ETT, a bite-block (Fig. 13-1) should be inserted to prevent the patient crushing the fiberoptic broncho-scope. Even adequately sedated patients can experience an unprovoked seizure. This is mandatory, even in a patient receiving muscle relaxants, to prevent both destruction of the instrument and respiratory embarrass-ment due to jamming of the scope within the ETT (Fig. 13-2).

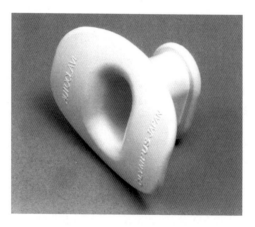

Figure 13-1. Bite block.

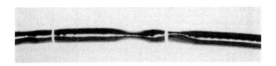

Figure 13-2. Damage to flexible bronchoscope as a result of patient biting during examination.

Transbronchial lung biopsies are usually performed through the working channel of the scope. The procedure is performed by inserting the scope either through the ETT or tracheostomy tube in a mechanically ventilated patient. In a nonventilated patient, the bronchoscope can be inserted via the trans-nasal or trans-oral route. The bronchoscope will allow direct visualization of the airways and can then be directed to the area of interest as suggested by the chest imaging.

Patients with a tenuous respiratory status prior to bronchoscopy may require intubation and mechanical ventilation immediately after the procedure is performed. In such cases, it is preferred to electively intubate the patient prior to the procedure to avoid emergent airway management issues and associated risks. In mechanically ventilated patients, a swivel adaptor with a rubber diaphragm is attached to the proximal end of the ETT through which the bronchoscope is inserted (Fig. 13-3). This helps in preventing loss of delivered respiratory volumes and PEEP during the course of the procedure.[42,51] Alternatively, the bronchoscopist may decide to use a laryngeal-mask airway (LMA) (Fig. 13-4).[52]

In rare cases, the bronchoscopist is faced with situations in which patients require noninvasive positive pressure ventilation (NIPPV) and a bronchoscopy is indicated. The options available in this case include elective intubation for the procedure, or the use of a Patil-Syracuse mask to minimize air-leak during the procedure, while continuing to use NIPPV[7,53,54] (Figs. 13-5 and 13-6).

The elucidative study by Lindholm et al. demonstrates the significance of a larger ETT while performing FB.[42] This study demonstrated that the fiberoptic bronchoscope can occupy the entire cross-sectional area of the airway in an intubated patient. A 5.7 mm outer diameter (OD) scope obstructs 40% of the total cross-section of a 9 mm internal diameter ETT, 51% of an 8 mm ETT, and 66% of a 7 mm tube. ETTs with an inner diameter (ID) of <8.0 mm hinder expiratory airflow causing auto-PEEP. Intratracheal pressures during spontaneous breathing varied from −5 to +3.5 cm H_2O, whereas in ventilated patients they varied from −10 to +9 cm H_2O. Smaller ID ETTs can also reduce tidal volume delivery. On average, using a 5.9 mm OD scope, tidal volume decreased by 12% with 8.5 mm ID ETT, by 30% with 8.0 mm ID, and by 87% with 7.5 mm ID. A good rule of thumb is that the ID of the ETT should be at least 2.0 mm greater than the ID of the fiberoptic bronchoscope.[43]

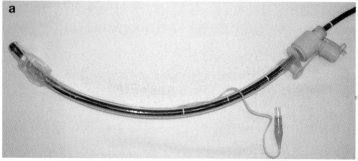

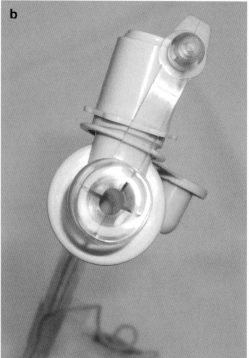

Figure 13-3. Disposable swivel adaptor used for flexible bronchoscopy during mechanical ventilation. Note the cuts made in the plastic diaphragm to prevent excessive traction on the bronchoscope.

The tracheostomy tubes are stiffer and hinder easy maneuverability during FB. The increased fixed curvature of a tracheostomy tube also offers resistance to scope passage. In addition, tracheostomy tubes with

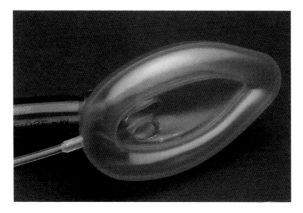

Figure 13-4. Laryngeal-mask airway (LMA) may be used as an alternative to endotracheal intubation when a difficult airway is encountered or when a subglottic obstruction is suspected.[52]

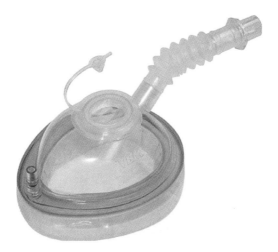

Figure 13-5. Silicone endoscopy mask (VBN Medical).

an inner cannula often have a narrower lumen than single lumen tubes of the same external diameter. Replacing the tracheostomy tube with a more flexible ETT through the stoma can facilitate scope passage and prevent damage to the instrument (Figs. 13-7 and 13-8).

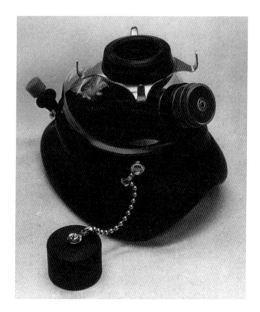

Figure 13-6. Patil-Syracuse mask for bronchoscopic procedures while receiving NIPPV.

Diagnostic yield from TBLB has varied from 76 to 92%, while the complication rates have varied from 3.4 to 8.6%.[55–58] The number of biopsies required is dictated by the clinical presentation. A study of 530 TBB for diffuse lung disease demonstrated a yield of 38% with 1–3 biopsies, versus 69% yield with 6–10 biopsies.[59] In the case of sarcoidosis, the overall diagnostic yield is estimated to be 73–80%. However, in stage I sarcoidosis, as many as 10 TBB are needed, while in stage II and III the diagnostic yield is 95% with 4 TBB.[60–62]

Fluoroscopic guidance for TBLB has been advocated but is usually not available while performing the procedure in the ICU. Although one study observed a reduction in the incidence of barotrauma with fluoroscopically guided TBLB,[2] other studies comparing fluoroscopy to no fluoroscopy have not shown major differences in complication rates between the two. Neither was the diagnostic yield for diffuse infiltrates improved with fluoroscopy.[63] However, the diagnostic yield for focal infiltrates does appear to be improved with fluoroscopy use. A routine postprocedure chest X-ray is not needed when TBLB is performed under fluoroscopy guidance as the patients can be screened postprocedure.[64]

Topical anesthesia can be obtained with lidocaine 1–2%. Lidocaine has a quick onset of action but short duration of action. It can be used as

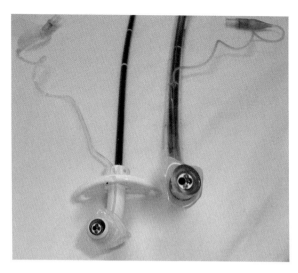

Figure 13-7. Comparison of adult bronchoscope in endotracheal tube (#8.5 F) and tracheostomy tube (#6) requiring the use of pediatric bronchoscope. Stiffness of the tracheostomy tube increases the resistance, and the probability of getting stuck.

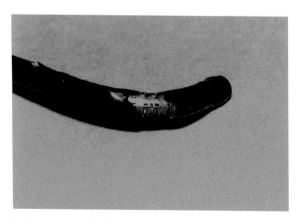

Figure 13-8. Damaged flexible bronchoscope after difficult passage through a tracheostomy tube.

a local spray or can be nebulized or instilled via the working channel of the bronchoscope during the procedure. Recommended maximal dose is 4–5 mg/kg ideal body weight or 300 mg per procedure.[65,66] Patients with liver disease are particularly prone to the adverse effects of lidocaine. These include arrhythmias, seizures, cardiorespiratory arrest, and death. Local anesthetic agents have antimicrobial properties and their use may yield false-negative culture results on BAL and bronchial washings but quantitative culture may aid proper interpretation of the results.[67,68] Use of BAL dilutes the concentration of the lidocaine in the airway.

With the patient in supine position, and the ETT in place, the "time-out" or verification of the patient's identity and the planned procedure is performed.

The following steps illustrate the appropriate sequence of performing FB and TBLB:

1. Disconnect the ventilator from the ET tube for the placement of the "Y" adaptor with immediate reconnection to the ventilator. Place the bite-block to protect the bronchoscope.
2. Instill an aliquot of 2 cc of 1–2% lidocaine in the ETT.
3. After application of lubricant gel at the distal tip of the flexible bronchoscope, it is inserted into the ETT through the "Y" adapter.
4. Visually corroborate the adequate placement of the ETT in relation to the carina (ending at 2–3 cm from the carina).
5. Instill topical lidocaine into the trachea, both mainstem bronchi and the subsegmental bronchus of interest. This will allow a complete airway exam while minimizing coughing.
6. Complete the airway exam by examining each segmental bronchus, and advancing the bronchoscope as far as possible without causing excessive mucosal injury. If the differential diagnosis includes infection, a BAL is performed prior to the airway exam in order to minimize contamination of the suction channel. For the same reason, we recommend avoiding the use of suction prior to performing the BAL.
7. Advance the bronchoscope into the preselected area to be sampled. Assume a "wedge position", which is defined as the position where the bronchoscope cannot be advanced further while the distal lumen is still visible. This would serve as a seal in the case of bleeding localizing it to the involved segment.
8. The biopsy forceps are then inserted into the working channel of the bronchoscope. The forceps can be safely passed until the premarked length of the forceps reaches the proximal port of the working channel. From this point, the forceps are gently advanced until resistance is met indicating a location near the visceral pleura.
9. After approximating the visceral pleura, the forceps are pulled back 2–3 cm and opened during inspiration or while delivering tidal volume. They are then slowly advanced forward anchoring

them onto the bifurcation of a respiratory bronchiole. The forceps are closed during exhalation allowing more alveoli to fall into the cusps of the forceps. The forceps are then withdrawn with a sharp snapping motion and the sequence repeated until the adequate number of biopsy specimens is obtained.

10. After the adequate number of biopsies have been obtained from a particular subsegment, the bronchoscope is kept "wedged" in that position for approximately 4 min allowing clot formation and in turn tamponade the bleeding site.

11. After ensuring adequate hemostasis in one area, other areas of the lung can be biopsied in a similar manner if necessary.

■ SUMMARY

FB is a valuable tool in both the diagnosis and treatment of a variety of respiratory conditions encountered in the ICU. With appropriate patient selection and preparation and technical expertise, BAL and TBLB can have a high diagnostic yield and a low complication rate.

■ REFERENCES

1. Sackner MA. Bronchofiberscopy. *Am Rev Respir Dis*. 1975;111(1):62–88.
2. Papin TA, Grum CM, Weg JG. Transbronchial biopsy during mechanical ventilation. *Chest*. 1986;89(2):168–170.
3. Kao KC, Tsai YH, Wu YK, et al. Open lung biopsy in early-stage acute respiratory distress syndrome. *Crit Care*. 2006;10(4):R106.
4. Meduri GU, Chinn AJ, Leeper KV, et al. Corticosteroid rescue treatment of progressive fibroproliferation in late ARDS. Patterns of response and predictors of outcome. *Chest*. 1994;105(5):1516–1527.
5. Potter D, Pass HI, Brower S, et al. Prospective randomized study of open lung biopsy versus empirical antibiotic therapy for acute pneumonitis in nonneutropenic cancer patients. *Ann Thorac Surg*. 1985;40(5):422–428.
6. Folch E, Mehta AC. Airway interventions in the tracheobronchial tree. *Semin Respir Crit Care Med*. 2008;29(4):441–452.
7. Ovassapian A. *Fiberoptic Airway Endoscopy in Anesthesia and Critical Care*, vol. xix. New York: Raven Press; 1990:172.
8. Gaitini LA, Vaida SJ, Somri M, Fradis M, Ben-David B. Fiberoptic-guided airway exchange of the esophageal-tracheal combitube in spontaneously breathing versus mechanically ventilated patients. *Anesth Analg*. 1999;88(1):193–196.
9. Milledge JS. Therapeutic fibreoptic bronchoscopy in intensive care. *Br Med J*. 1976;2(6049):1427–1429.

10. Grundling M, Pavlovic D, Kuhn SO, Feyerherd F. Is the method of modified percutaneous tracheostomy without bronchoscopic guidance really simple and safe? *Chest*. 2005;128(5):3774–3775.
11. Dweik RA, Stoller JK. Role of bronchoscopy in massive hemoptysis. *Clin Chest Med*. 1999;20(1):89–105.
12. Limper AH, Prakash UB. Tracheobronchial foreign bodies in adults. *Ann Intern Med*. 1990;112(8):604–609.
13. Lois M, Noppen M. Bronchopleural fistulas: an overview of the problem with special focus on endoscopic management. *Chest*. 2005;128(6):3955–3965.
14. American Thoracic Society. Medical Section of the American Lung Association. Guidelines for fiberoptic bronchoscopy in adults. *Am Rev Respir Dis*. 1987;136(4):1066.
15. Katz AS, Michelson EL, Stawicki J, Holford FD. Cardiac arrhythmias. Frequency during fiberoptic bronchoscopy and correlation with hypoxemia. *Arch Intern Med*. 1981;141(5):603–606.
16. Dweik RA, Mehta AC, Meeker DP, Arroliga AC. Analysis of the safety of bronchoscopy after recent acute myocardial infarction. *Chest*. 1996;110(3):825–828.
17. Diette GB, Wiener CM, White P Jr. The higher risk of bleeding in lung transplant recipients from bronchoscopy is independent of traditional bleeding risks: results of a prospective cohort study. *Chest*. 1999;115(2):397–402.
18. Ernst A, Eberhardt R, Wahidi M, Becker HD, Herth FJ. Effect of routine clopidogrel use on bleeding complications after transbronchial biopsy in humans. *Chest*. 2006;129(3):734–737.
19. Herth FJ, Becker HD, Ernst A. Aspirin does not increase bleeding complications after transbronchial biopsy. *Chest*. 2002;122(4):1461–1464.
20. Peerless JR, Snow N, Likavec MJ, Pinchak AC, Malangoni MA. The effect of fiberoptic bronchoscopy on cerebral hemodynamics in patients with severe head injury. *Chest*. 1995;108(4):962–965.
21. Kerwin AJ, Croce MA, Timmons SD, Maxwell RA, Malhotra AK, Fabian TC. Effects of fiberoptic bronchoscopy on intracranial pressure in patients with brain injury: a prospective clinical study. *J Trauma*. 2000;48(5):878–882; discussion 882–873.
22. Zavala DC. Pulmonary hemorrhage in fiberoptic transbronchial biopsy. *Chest*. 1976;70(5):584–588.
23. Bulpa PA, Dive AM, Mertens L, et al. Combined bronchoalveolar lavage and transbronchial lung biopsy: safety and yield in ventilated patients. *Eur Respir J*. 2003;21(3):489–494.
24. O'Brien JD, Ettinger NA, Shevlin D, Kollef MH. Safety and yield of transbronchial biopsy in mechanically ventilated patients. *Crit Care Med*. 1997;25(3):440–446.
25. Bahhady IJ, Ernst A. Risks of and recommendations for flexible bronchoscopy in pregnancy: a review. *Chest*. 2004;126(6):1974–1981.

26. Matot I, Kramer MR, Glantz L, Drenger B, Cotev S. Myocardial ischemia in sedated patients undergoing fiberoptic bronchoscopy. *Chest.* 1997;112(6):1454–1458.

27. Dunagan DP, Burke HL, Aquino SL, Chin R Jr, Adair NE, Haponik EF. Fiberoptic bronchoscopy in coronary care unit patients: indications, safety, and clinical implications. *Chest.* 1998;114(6):1660–1667.

28. Douketis JD, Berger PB, Dunn AS, et al. The perioperative management of antithrombotic therapy: American College of chest physicians evidence-based clinical practice guidelines (8th Edition). *Chest.* 2008;133(6 suppl):299S–339S.

29. Mehta NLMD, Harkin TJMD, Rom WNMD, Graap WET, Addrizzo-Harris DJMD. Should renal insufficiency be a relative contraindication to bronchoscopic biopsy? *J Bronchol.* 2005;12(2):81–83.

30. Hedges SJ, Dehoney SB, Hooper JS, Amanzadeh J, Busti AJ. Evidence-based treatment recommendations for uremic bleeding. *Nat Clin Pract.* 2007;3(3):138–153.

31. Livio M, Mannucci PM, Vigano G, et al. Conjugated estrogens for the management of bleeding associated with renal failure. *N Engl J Med.* 1986;315(12):731–735.

32. Jain P, Sandur S, Meli Y, Arroliga AC, Stoller JK, Mehta AC. Role of flexible bronchoscopy in immunocompromised patients with lung infiltrates. *Chest.* 2004;125(2):712–722.

33. Cordasco EM Jr, Mehta AC, Ahmad M. Bronchoscopically induced bleeding. A summary of nine years' Cleveland clinic experience and review of the literature. *Chest.* 1991;100(4):1141–1147.

34. Hanson RR, Zavala DC, Rhodes ML, Keim LW, Smith JD. Transbronchial biopsy via flexible fiberoptic bronchoscope; results in 164 patients. *Am Rev Respir Dis.* 1976;114(1):67–72.

35. Bein T, Pfeifer M, Keyl C, Metz C, Taeger K. Right ventricular function and plasma atrial natriuretic peptide levels during fiberbronchoscopic alveolar lavage in critically ill, mechanically ventilated patients. *Chest.* 1995;108(4):1030–1035.

36. Davies L, Mister R, Spence DP, Calverley PM, Earis JE, Pearson MG. Cardiovascular consequences of fibreoptic bronchoscopy. *Eur Respir J.* 1997;10(3):695–698.

37. Stolz D, Pollak V, Chhajed PN, Gysin C, Pflimlin E, Tamm M. A randomized, placebo-controlled trial of bronchodilators for bronchoscopy in patients with COPD. *Chest.* 2007;131(3):765–772.

38. Schweickert W, Hall J. Informed consent in the intensive care unit: ensuring understanding in a complex environment. *Curr Opin Crit Care.* 2005;11(6):624–628.

39. AARC clinical practice guideline. Fiberoptic bronchoscopy assisting. American Association for Respiratory Care. *Respir Care.* 1993;38(11):1173–1178.

40. American Association for Respiratory Care (AARC). Bronchoscopy assisting – 2007 revision and update. *Respir Care.* 2007;52(1):74–80.

41. Meduri GU, Chastre J. The standardization of bronchoscopic techniques for ventilator-associated pneumonia. *Chest*. 1992;102(5 Suppl 1):557S–564S.
42. Lindholm CE, Ollman B, Snyder JV, Millen EG, Grenvik A. Cardiorespiratory effects of flexible fiberoptic bronchoscopy in critically ill patients. *Chest*. 1978;74(4):362–368.
43. Lawson RW, Peters JI, Shelledy DC. Effects of fiberoptic bronchoscopy during mechanical ventilation in a lung model. *Chest*. 2000;118(3):824–831.
44. McArthur CD. AARC clinical practice guideline. Capnography/capnometry during mechanical ventilation – 2003 revision and update. *Respir Care*. 2003;48(5):534–539.
45. Williams TJ, Nicoulet I, Coleman E, McAlaney C. Safety and patient acceptability of intravenous midazolam for fibre optic bronchoscopy. *Respir Med*. 1994;88(4):305–307.
46. Clarkson K, Power CK, O'Connell F, Pathmakanthan S, Burke CM. A comparative evaluation of propofol and midazolam as sedative agents in fiberoptic bronchoscopy. *Chest*. 1993;104(4):1029–1031.
47. Cowl CT, Prakash UB, Kruger BR. The role of anticholinergics in bronchoscopy. A randomized clinical trial. *Chest*. 2000;118(1):188–192.
48. Williams T, Brooks T, Ward C. The role of atropine premedication in fiberoptic bronchoscopy using intravenous midazolam sedation. *Chest*. 1998;113(5):1394–1398.
49. Yigla M, Oren I, Bentur L, et al. Incidence of bacteraemia following fibreoptic bronchoscopy. *Eur Respir J*. 1999;14(4):789–791.
50. Mehta AC, Prakash UB, Garland R, et al. American College of Chest Physicians and American Association for Bronchology [corrected] consensus statement: prevention of flexible bronchoscopy-associated infection. *Chest*. 2005;128(3):1742–1755.
51. Reichert WW, Hall WJ, Hyde RW. A simple disposable device for performing fiberoptic bronchoscopy on patients requiring continuous artificial ventilation. *Am Rev Respir Dis*. 1974;109(3):394–396.
52. Benumof JL. Management of the difficult adult airway. With special emphasis on awake tracheal intubation. *Anesthesiology*. 1991;75(6):1087–1110.
53. Antonelli M, Conti G, Riccioni L, Meduri GU. Noninvasive positive-pressure ventilation via face mask during bronchoscopy with BAL in high-risk hypoxemic patients. *Chest*. 1996;110(3):724–728.
54. McGrath G, Das-Gupta M, Clarke G. Bronchoscopy via continuous positive airway pressure for patients with respiratory failure. *Chest*. 2001;119(2):670–671.
55. Anders GT, Johnson JE, Bush BA, Matthews JI. Transbronchial biopsy without fluoroscopy. A seven-year perspective. *Chest*. 1988;94(3):557–560.
56. de Fenoyl O, Capron F, Lebeau B, Rochemaure J. Transbronchial biopsy without fluoroscopy: a five year experience in outpatients. *Thorax*. 1989;44(11):956–959.

57. Milligan SA, Luce JM, Golden J, Stulbarg M, Hopewell PC. Transbronchial biopsy without fluoroscopy in patients with diffuse roentgenographic infiltrates and the acquired immunodeficiency syndrome. *Am Rev Respir Dis*. 1988;137(2):486–488.

58. Puar HS, Young RC Jr, Armstrong EM. Bronchial and transbronchial lung biopsy without fluoroscopy in sarcoidosis. *Chest*. 1985;87(3):303–306.

59. Descombes E, Gardiol D, Leuenberger P. Transbronchial lung biopsy: an analysis of 530 cases with reference to the number of samples. *Monaldi Arch Chest Dis*. 1997;52(4):324–329.

60. Statement on sarcoidosis. Joint Statement of the American Thoracic Society (ATS), the European Respiratory Society (ERS) and the World Association of Sarcoidosis and Other Granulomatous Disorders (WASOG) adopted by the ATS Board of Directors and by the ERS Executive Committee, February 1999. *Am J Respir Crit Care Med*. 1999;160(2):736–755

61. Armstrong JR, Radke JR, Kvale PA, Eichenhorn MS, Popovich J Jr. Endoscopic findings in sarcoidosis. Characteristics and correlations with radiographic staging and bronchial mucosal biopsy yield. *Ann Otol Rhinol Laryngol*. 1981;90(4 Pt 1):339–343.

62. Roethe RA, Fuller PB, Byrd RB, Hafermann DR. Transbronchoscopic lung biopsy in sarcoidosis. Optimal number and sites for diagnosis. *Chest*. 1980;77(3):400–402.

63. Killeen D, Chin R, Conforti J. Bronchoscopic myths and legends. *Clin Pulm Med*. 2005;12(1):53–55.

64. Frazier WD, Pope TL Jr, Findley LJ. Pneumothorax following transbronchial biopsy. Low diagnostic yield with routine chest roentgenograms. *Chest*. 1990;97(3):539–540.

65. Fulkerson WJ. Current concepts. Fiberoptic bronchoscopy. *N Engl J Med*. 1984;311(8):511–515.

66. Dellinger RP, Bandi V. Fiberoptic bronchoscopy in the intensive care unit. *Crit Care Clin*. 1992;8(4):755–772.

67. Shelley MP, Wilson P, Norman J. Sedation for fibreoptic bronchoscopy. *Thorax*. 1989;44(10):769–775.

68. Wimberley N, Willey S, Sullivan N, Bartlett JG. Antibacterial properties of lidocaine. *Chest*. 1979;76(1):37–40.

14

Percutaneous Endoscopic Gastrostomy

Jennifer Lang and Shahid Shafi

■ INTRODUCTION

Malnutrition is a common problem in patients in the intensive care unit (ICU). Enteral nutrition has been shown to be superior to improve morbidity and mortality rates compared to parenteral nutrition.[1] Enteral feeding prevents gut atrophy and bacterial translocation, thereby reducing infectious complications, such as pneumonias and intra-abdominal abscesses.[1] Traditionally, long-term enteral access for nutrition was provided via surgically placed feeding gastrostomy or feeding jejunostomy tubes. Percutaneous endoscopic gastrostomy (PEG) tube placement, as described by Gauder and Ponsky in 1980, is now the method of long-term enteral access for nutrition.[2]

S. Shafi (✉)
Department of Surgery, Baylor Health Care System, Grapevine, TX, USA
e-mail: Shahid.shafi@utsouthwestern.edu

H.L. Frankel and B.P. deBoisblanc (eds.), *Bedside Procedures for the Intensivist*,
DOI 10.1007/978-0-387-79830-1_14,
© Springer Science+Business Media, LLC 2010

Surgical placement of feeding tubes is associated with a higher risk of morbidity and mortality compared to percutaneous placement, especially in higher risk older patients with significant comorbidities. Major complication rates of surgical feeding tube placement have been reported around 20%, compared to 5% for percutaneous.[3–6] Similarly, mortality risk is also increased with surgical placement at about 4%, compared to less than 1% for percutaneous placement.[5] Percutaneous placement also obviates the need for an operating room or a laparotomy, decreases time for placement, decreases cost, and is associated with a shorter recovery time.[6]

Nasogastric tubes (NGTs) are another option for enteral feeding when the anticipated duration of use is relatively short (days to a few weeks). However, NGTs are poorly tolerated by patients, often get obstructed, and are associated with aspiration, irritations, ulcerations, and bleeding.[3,7] In a randomized controlled trial of PEG vs. fine bore NGT, tube failures, defined as inability to position, displacement, blockage, self-removal, or refusal to continue with tube, occurred in 95% of the NGT patients compared to none in the PEG patients.[7] PEG tubes were also superior in amount of nutrition delivery (55% of goal in the NGT vs. 93% in the PEG group) with significantly higher associated weight gain (0.6 kg vs. 1.4 kg).[7]

■ INDICATIONS AND CONTRAINDICATIONS

The primary indication for PEG placement is the inability to orally feed a patient with an intact gastrointestinal tract that can be used for nutrition. Common indications are[3,4,6,8]:

- Neurological disorders, such as head injuries, strokes, neuromuscular disorders, severe dementia
- Oropharyngeal dysfunction
- Esophageal motility disorders
- Wasting/failure to thrive
- Decompression of bowel

Absolute contraindications are[3,9]:

- Coagulopathy
- Interposed organs
- Carcinomatosis
- Severe ascites
- Peritonitis
- Anorexia nervosa
- Severe psychosis
- Inability to perform endoscopy

Relative contraindications are:

- Failure to transilluminate
- Mild to moderate ascites

- Ventriculoperitoneal shunt
- Peritoneal dialysis

■ PREOPERATIVE PREPARATION

- Informed consent
- NPO for 8 h
- Personnel
- Nurse to monitor patient and assist with supplies
- Endoscopist (physician's assistant, trained RN, MD)
- Surgeon
- Equipment
- Endoscope with viewers
- Commercially available kits for PEG placement
- Supplies
- Clorhexidine prep
- 2% Lidocaine with epinephrine
- 10 cc syringe with 25 gauge and 18 gauge needles
- #11 Blade scalpel
- 2-0 Nylon suture
- Sterile dressing
- A single dose of a preoperative antibiotic[3,10,11]
- Sedation
- Monitoring devices

■ DESCRIPTION OF PROCEDURES

Pull Method

The patient is placed in supine position, and the abdomen is prepped with a topical antiseptic. Orogastric endoscopy is performed and the stomach is inspected for any abnormalities. The stomach is then insufflated to transilluminate the abdominal wall in the left upper quadrant. The surgeon, standing on the left side of the bed, marks the insertion site by palpating the transilluminated abdominal wall while the endoscopist visually confirms the indentation of the stomach wall. The target area is anesthetized with 2% lidocaine with epinephrine and a small stab incision is made. We advocate using the safe tract method to prevent injuring another hollow organ, such as the colon. An 18 g needle attached to the syringe is inserted through the stab wound with continuous aspiration while visualizing the needle entry into the stomach through the endoscope. If air is aspirated prior to endoscopic visualizing of the tip of your needle in the stomach, it is likely that another hollow organ has been punctured unintentionally. In that case, the procedure should be aborted and converted into an open procedure in the operating room. Upon successful insertion of the needle in the stomach confirmed by endoscopic visualization, a guide wire is threaded into the stomach. The guide wire is grasped with a snare passed through the endoscope, and the needle is removed. The endoscope and guide wire are removed out of the mouth, and the snare is released. In this position, the guide wire enters through the abdominal wall into the stomach, through the esophagus and out of the mouth. The gastrostomy tube is then secured to the guide wire outside the mouth. The tube is then advanced into the stomach through the mouth by gently pulling the guide wire from the skin incision. The endoscope is placed again to confirm the placement of the internal bumper of the gastrostomy tube flat against the stomach wall with no bleeding. An external bumper is placed on the gastrostomy tube to secure the stomach to the abdominal wall. The external bumper should be snug but not too tight, allowing for about 360° turn and 3–5 mm of free movement[9,12] (Fig. 14-1).

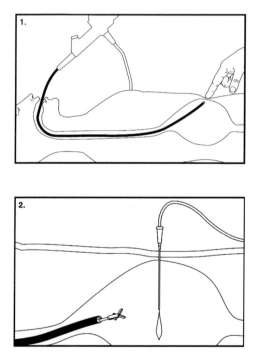

Figure 14-1. Pull method. Permission for use granted by Cook Medical Incorporated, Bloomington, Indiana.

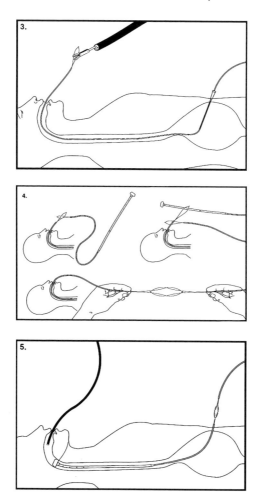

Figure 14-1. (continued)

■ PUSH METHOD

The push method is done exactly the same way as the pull with one exception. Once the guidewire has been passed through the oral cavity, the gastrostomy tube is threaded over the wire through the oral cavity and the esophagus and then pushed into the stomach and out the skin incision (Fig. 14-2).

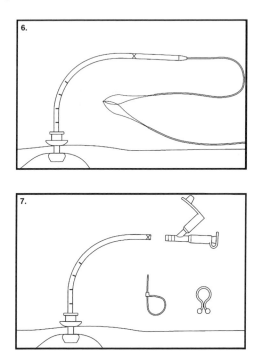

Figure 14-1. (continued)

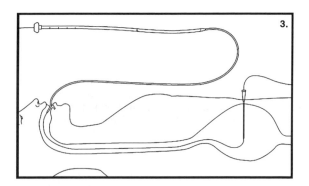

Figure 14-2. Push method. Permission for use granted by Cook Medical Incorporated, Bloomington, Indiana.

Introducer/Serial Dilating Method (Russell Technique)

The stomach is accessed with a needle similar to the pull technique, and a guidewire is placed into the stomach. A skin incision is made along that guide wire approximately one centimeter in length, bluntly splitting the muscle and fascia of the abdominal wall while leaving the peritoneum intact. A peel away introducer kit (such as the 16F Desilets-Hoffman Sheath Set®) is used in this procedure. The entire unit, containing the dilator and the sheath are passed over the guide wire. Once the dilator and sheath are visualized in the stomach, the guide wire and the dilator are removed, leaving the sheath in place. A gastrostomy tube is then passed through the peel-away sheath into the stomach. The balloon near the end of the tube is inflated with approximately 5 cc of water to secure the tube. The sheath is pulled away, and the catheter is pulled back to allow opposition of the balloon to the abdominal wall. The catheter is then sutured to the skin using nylon sutures. A sterile dressing is placed[13] (Fig. 14-3).

■ SLiC METHOD

The SLiC technique uses a modification of the introducer/peel away sheath described above, and requires a 7–8 mm AutoSuture Mini Step cannula, a 20 French Malecot catheter, and a 10–13 French metal stylet. After localizing the stomach with a needle, an incision is made in the abdominal wall. The cannula with its blunt trocar is thrust into the gastric lumen in one swift motion, with the insufflation valve in the off position. The blunt trocar is withdrawn leaving the cannula in place. The Malecot tube, with the stylet in place, is then inserted into the stomach through the cannula. The stylet and the cannula are removed over the Malecot tube. Position of the Malecot tube in the stomach is confirmed endoscopically, and the tube is sutured to the skin[14] (Fig. 14-4).

■ POSTPROCEDURE MANAGEMENT

1. Fixation to abdominal wall: PEG tube fixation devices should not be secured too tightly as it causes pressure necrosis of the abdominal wall. The tube should have about 5 mm of free movement.
2. Site care: The dressing should be changed daily to keep the site clean and dry until healing has occurred, which usually takes about 1 week. Afterwards, the dressing changes may be every 2–3 days depending on patient requirements.
3. Tube care: After each feeding (or daily if using continuous feeding), the tube should be flushed with 40 cc of water to prevent occlusions.[3]
4. Feeding through the tube: Traditionally, feedings are withheld for 24 h after tube placement. Feedings are then started with water or half

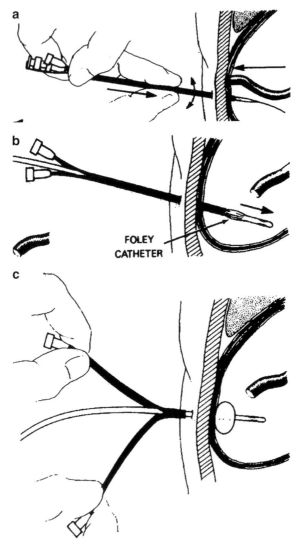

Figure 14-3. Introducer technique. From Russell et al.[13]; used with permission.

strength formulas for the first 24 h, and advanced as tolerated. Several studies have attempted alternative methods. In a randomized control trial of feeding at 3 h postprocedure vs. 24-h, both starting with full

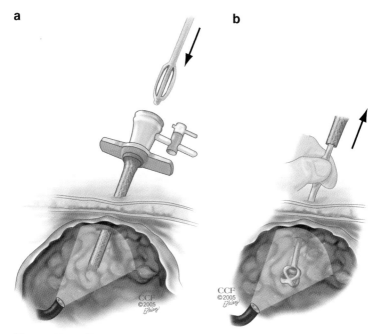

Figure 14-4. SLiC method. Courtesy of the Cleveland Clinic; used with permission.

strength feeds at 30 cc per hour for 24 h, there was no significant difference between the two approaches.[15] Another prospective randomized trial started feeding at 1 h postprocedure vs. 24 h and found no significant difference.[16] We recommend beginning tube feeds immediately after the procedure with full strength feeds, and advancing to the goal rate over the next 24 h. However, these decisions should be based on individual patient considerations.

■ COMPLICATIONS

PEG tube placement is a very safe procedure with complication rates of 1–4% for major complications and 10–30% for minor complications.[3,8,17] Complications are[3,5,6,8,9,16,18]:

- Aspiration during endoscopy
- Colon injury
- Hemorrhage (abdominal wall)

- Esophageal perforation
- Gastric leak
- Gastro-colo-cutaneous fistula
- Small bowel injury
- Buried bumper syndrome
- Incisional site herniation
- Migrating Foley balloon causing obstruction
- Bowel/gastric volvulus around PEG tube
- Tumor implants at stoma
- Peristomal pain
- Wound infection
- Peristomal leakage
- Ileus
- Obstruction of tube
- Dislodgement of tube

The presence of pneumoperitoneum after the procedure is not considered a complication as it is a relatively common finding on chest radiographs following PEG tube placements. A recent review found that 6.7% of patients had pneumoperitoneum on a chest X-ray performed within 24 h of PEG, which resolved in a mean of 3 days without complications.[18] A prospective study found pneumoperitoneum in 20% of patients, all of which resolved without complications, although in a few patients, the pneumoperitoneum persisted for over 72 h.[19]

■ CONCLUSION

The PEG tube is a useful tool in the ICU for providing long-term enteral nutrition. Placement requires endoscopic and bedside surgical skills. The procedure generally takes less than 30 min, and the tube can be used for feeding the patient within hours of placement. Complication rates are low, and the tubes are easy to care for with a high satisfaction rating by patients and care-givers.[8]

■ REFERENCES

1. Khaodhiar L, Blackburn G. Enteral nutrition. In: Fischer JE, ed. *Mastery of Surgery*. 5th ed. Philadelphia, PA: Wolters Kluwer Health/Lippincott Williams and Wilkins; 2006:45.
2. Gauderer MW, Ponsky JL, Izant RJ. Gastrostomy without laparotomy: a percutaneous endoscopic technique. *J Pediatr Surg*. 1980;15:872–875.
3. Loser C, Aschl G, Hebuterne X, et al. ESPEN guidelines on artificial enteral nutrition – percutaneous endoscopic gastrostomy. *Clin Nutr*. 2005;24:848–861.

4. Erdil A, Saka M, Ates Y, et al. Enteral nutrition via percutaneous endoscopic gastrostomy and nutritional status of patients: five year prospective study. *J Gastroenterol Hepatol*. 2005;20:1002–1007.

5. Mincheff T. Metastatic spread to a percutaneous gastrostomy site from head and neck cancer: case report and literature review. *JSLS*. 2005;9:466–471.

6. Lin HS, Ibrahim HZ, Kheng JW, Fee WE, Terris DJ. Percutaneous endoscopic gastrostomy: Strategies for prevention and management of complications. *Laryngoscope*. 2001;111:1847–1852.

7. Park R, Allison M, Lang J, et al. Randomised comparison of percutaneous endoscopic gastrostomy and nasogastric tube feeding in patients with persisting neurological dysphagia. *BMJ*. 1992;304:1406–1409.

8. Loser C, Wolters S, Folsch U. Enteral long-term nutrition via percutaneous endoscopic gastrostomy in 210 patients: a four year prospective study. *Dig Dis Sci*. 1998;43:2549–2557.

9. Suzuki Y, Urashima M, Ishibashi Y. Covering the percutaneous endoscopic gastrostomy (PEG) tube prevents peristomal infection. *World J Surg*. 2006;30:1450–1458.

10. Sharma V, Howden C. Meta-analysis of randomized controlled trials of antibiotic prophylaxis before percutaneous endoscopic gastrostomy. *Am J Gastroenterol*. 2000;95(11):3133–3136.

11. Schrag S, Sharma R, Jaik N, et al. Complications related to percutaneous endoscopic gastrostomy (PEG) tubes. A comprehensive clinical review. *J Gastrointestin Liver Dis*. 2007;16:407–418.

12. Foutch P, Talbert G, Waring J, Sanowski RA. Percutaneous endoscopic gastrostomy in patients with prior abdominal surgery: virtues of the safe tract. *Am J Gastroenterol*. 1988;83:147–150.

13. Russell T, Brotman M, Norris F. Percutaneous gastrostomy: a new simplified and cost-effective technique. *Am J Surg*. 1984;148:132–137.

14. Sabnis A, Liu R, Chand B, Ponsky J. SLiC Technique: a novel approach to percutaneous gastrostomy. *Surg Endosc*. 2006;20:256–262.

15. Choudhry U, Barde C, Markert R, Gopalswamy N. Percutaneous endoscopic gastrostomy: a randomized prospective comparison of early and delayed feeding. *Gastrointest Endosc*. 1996;44:164–167.

16. Stein J, Schulte-Bockholt A, Sabin M, Keymling M. A randomized prospective trial of immediate vs. next day feeding after percutaneous endoscopic gastrostomy in intensive care patients. *Intensive Care Med*. 2002;28:1656–1660.

17. Kozarek R, Ball T, Ryan J Jr. When push comes to shove: a comparison between two methods of percutaneous endoscopic gastrostomy. *Am J Gastroenterol*. 1986;81:642–646.

18. Alley J, Corneille M, Stewart R, Dent D. Pneumoperitoneum after percutaneous endoscopic gastrostomy in patients in the intensive care unit. *Am Surg*. 2007;73:765–768.

19. Wiesen A, Sideridis K, Fernandes A, et al. True incidence and clinical significance of pneumoperitoneum after PEG placement: a prospective study. *Gastrointest Endosc*. 2006;64:886–889.

15

Chest Drainage

Gabriel T. Bosslet and Praveen N. Mathur

■ INTRODUCTION

Physicians charged with the task of caring for the critically ill will inevitably encounter patients who require drainage of the pleural cavity, e.g., those with pneumonia, central lines, and mechanical ventilation. Practitioners caring for these individuals should be comfortable with placement and management of chest tubes.

■ HISTORY

Hippocrates was the first to describe surgical drainage of the pleural cavity using metal tubes and cautery in the fourth century BCE.[1] The next detailed accounts of the procedure were published in the late nineteenth century, when Playfair described the successful aspiration of an empyema[2] and Hewett detailed the technique of closed chest drainage.[3] Empyemata associated with the great influenza epidemic of 1918 drove further

P.N. Mathur (✉)
Departments of Pulmonary and Critical Care Medicine, Indiana University,
550 N University Blvd, Suite 4903, Indianapolis, IN 46202, USA
e-mail: pmathur@iupui.edu

H.L. Frankel and B.P. deBoisblanc (eds.), *Bedside Procedures for the Intensivist*,
DOI 10.1007/978-0-387-79830-1_15,
© Springer Science+Business Media, LLC 2010

study. The recommendation of routine drainage of empyemata by Evarts Graham led to dramatic reductions in associated mortality;[4] however, use of pleural drainage for management of traumatic injuries did not become standard until World War II.[5]

■ THE PLEURAL SPACE

The parietal pleura is a serous membrane that lines the inner portion of the chest wall and diaphragm. The visceral pleura meets the parietal pleura at the lung hila, and covers the lung parenchyma. The potential space between these two serous layers is the pleural space which normally contains a very thin layer of pleural fluid that acts as a lubricant between the two pleural surfaces during respiration. The outward elastic recoil of the chest wall coupled with the constant inward recoil of the lung makes the pressure in the pleural space negative during all phases of quiet breathing.

■ INDICATIONS FOR PLEURAL DRAINAGE

When the buildup of fluid or air in the pleural space becomes clinically relevant, drainage becomes necessary. Indications for pleural drainage include:

- Hemothorax
- Empyema
- Complicated parapneumonic effusion
- Pneumothorax–tension, large, or symptomatic
- Bronchopleural fistula
- Postthoracotomy
- Pleural effusions: large or symptomatic
- Pleurodesis

Elimination of pleural accumulations can take place either medically (e.g., with treatment of congestive heart failure) or surgically (e.g., aspiration of air in the case of a pneumothorax). The surgical drainage of pleural collections will be discussed here.

Pneumothorax

Pneumothorax, the presence of air in the pleural space, can occur via perforation of the visceral pleura and introduction of air into the pleural space via the lung parenchyma (as in barotrauma related to high airway pressures) or through perforation of the parietal pleura (via trauma or iatrogenic- associated with central line placement or thoracentesis). The incidence of iatrogenic pneumothorax in one large ICU cohort was found to be 1.4% at 5 days, and 3.0% at 30 days.[6]

Pneumothoraces can be classified as either spontaneous or traumatic. Spontaneous pneumothoraces may be either primary (without associated intrinsic lung disease) or secondary. While always pathologic, air in the pleural space will resolve on its own, as long as the initial air leak is resolved. The rate at which pleural air resorbs has been found to be approximately 1.25% of the volume of the hemithorax per day.[7] At this rate, a 40% pneumothorax would take approximately 50 days to resolve. Because of the slow rate of resolution, larger stable pneumothoraces are usually aspirated.

A tension pneumothorax occurs when the air that enters the pleural space disrupts the mediastinal structures, causing cardiovascular compromise. This entity requires urgent drainage, or death can occur. Although spontaneous tension pneumothoraces have been described, they are rare.[8,9]

Fluid in the Pleural Space

There are multiple causes of pleural fluid collections in the intensive care unit. One prospective study found pleural effusions in 62% of ICU patients, 92% of which were quantified as small.[10] Small pleural effusions usually do not require drainage. They can be observed for progression, and if there is concern for infection or if the cause is not clinically apparent, they should be sampled. In addition, transudative effusions are generally only drained when maximal medical therapy is not adequate for control of symptoms. Although not all pleural fluid collections require drainage, hemothoraces, empyemas, complicated parapneumonic effusions, and large effusions that cause respiratory compromise should be drained.

■ CONTRAINDICATIONS

Most contraindications to tube thoracostomy are relative to the clinical situation. Pleural effusions that recur in a hemithorax that has undergone pleurodesis or pleurectomy are best managed with close surgical consultation, as adhesions can complicate the procedure. Placement of a chest tube through infected skin or cancerous lesions can spread infection or tumor to the pleural space and should be avoided. As with any procedure, care should be taken to correct any coagulopathies prior to instrumentation.

■ ANATOMY

A tour of the body from the skin to the pleural space traverses several layers. Skin covers subcutaneous and adipose tissue. A deeper fascial layer then overlies the three layers of intercostal muscles, which, in turn, lie over and between the ribs. The parietal pleura that covers the inner cavity of the chest is the final tissue layer before the pleural space.

The intercostal neurovascular bundle that runs along the inferior aspect of each rib can be avoided by entering the pleural space just *superior to* a rib. Likewise, operators should take care to avoid the internal mammary arteries and veins that run parallel to the sternum, approximately 2 cm lateral to each border.

Bedside tube thoracostomy is generally performed in one of two anatomical locations (Fig. 15-1). The anterior second intercostal space is preferred for emergent decompression of tension pneumothoraces and for aspiration of small pneumothoraces. Because the intercostal space is smallest anteriorly, only smaller tubes are accommodated here (generally less than 18 French). This space is located by first finding the sternomanubrial junction. The second rib inserts at the sternomanubrial junction. The chest tube should be placed in the second intercostal space just superior to the third rib in the mid-clavicular line.

The lateral location is preferred for draining pleural effusions and larger pneumothoraces. Here, the intercostal space is at its widest, and as such there is capacity for a larger tube. This insertion site is located in the mid- or anterior-axillary line at the fifth or sixth intercostal space.

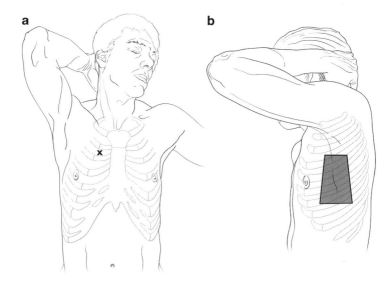

Figure 15-1. The preferred anterior site of entry (**a**) is the second intercostal space in the mid-clavicular line. Laterally (**b**), the shaded area demonstrates the area of entry, usually the fifth or sixth intercostal space in the mid-axillary line.

■ EQUIPMENT

Cook (Bloomington, IN), Argyle [Sherwood Medical (Tullamore, Ireland)], and Arrow International (Reading, PA) are the manufacturers of the three most commonly used commercial chest tube kits in the United States. Each manufacturer makes a variety of tube types and sizes for pleural drainage. In addition, many hospitals prepare their own packaged chest tube kits that contain most, if not all, of these materials for chest tube insertion:

- Chlorhexidine antiseptic solution
- Sterile gauze pads
- Sterile towels and drapes
- 1 or 2% lidocaine ± epinephrine, 10–20 cc
- 10-cc syringes
- 22- and 25-gauge needles
- Scalpel
- Kelly forceps
- Chest tube
- Silk suture, size 2–0
- Needle driver
- Scissors
- Drain dressings
- Petrolatum gauze
- Silk tape
- Drainage system or Heimlich valve

The preferred type of chest tube for pleural evacuation depends largely upon the indication. Tension pneumothoraces can urgently be evacuated using any catheter device. Pneumothorax kits containing 12 French pigtail drainage catheters are convenient for this indication. However, a 2-in. large-bore IV catheter or a spinal needle attached to IV tubing and placed into a container of sterile water or saline can be used if no kit is available and the clinical scenario necessitates urgent decompression. Small caliber chest tubes, less than 24 French, can also be used to drain less viscous fluid collections. These tubes have the advantage of multiple insertion techniques which can decrease pain and require smaller entry sites. They may also have the advantage of a lower complication rate.[11] In addition, they may be required for individuals with a smaller intercostal distance. Smaller chest tubes are often placed under ultrasound guidance into loculated pleural fluid collections.

Larger caliber chest tubes, 24 French and greater, are usually used in adults with persistent air leaks. These are purchased with or without a trocar for ease of placement. Accordingly, patients with large bronchopleural fistulas requiring mechanical ventilation may require a larger-bore tube in order to adequately vent the pleural space; larger fistulas may even require two tubes in order to keep the lung expanded.

For purulent empyemata, blood, or more viscous fluids, a larger-bore 28- to 32-French tube is appropriate, to decrease the likelihood of luminal obstruction. According to Poiseuille's law, flow in a tube is proportional to the diameter of the tube to the fourth power and inversely proportional to the length of the tube.[12] Therefore, a small increase in the diameter of the chest tube can greatly increase evacuation capability.

■ SETUP, PREPARATION, AND POSITIONING

Once informed consent is obtained, equipment (as outlined above) should be gathered and organized on a bedside table. As with any procedure, operator preparation and patient sedation, analgesia, and positioning are of utmost importance.

The patient should be positioned so that there is maximal exposure of the surgical field with minimal obstruction from tubes, lines, and wires. The bed and table should be raised to an optimal height for operator comfort. For anterior tube placement, the patient is placed in the supine position and the head of the bed is raised to about 20° both for patient comfort and to allow air in the pleural space to gather just below the area of tube insertion. For the lateral insertion site, a towel should be rolled and placed beneath the patient so that the surgical site is at approximately 20° (Fig. 15-2a).

Care should be taken to adhere to strict sterile technique. The area of interest should be clipped of hair but not shaved and sterilized with chlorhexidine solution. Sterile drapes can then be used to outline the field. Often it is helpful to use a sterile skin marker to outline the rib margins in the area of interest in order to facilitate placement.

■ ANESTHESIA

The parietal pleura is heavily innervated and proper anesthesia and analgesia is essential to successful chest tube placement. While chest tube insertion can be performed without the use of sedation, most operators prefer to use small doses of benzodiazepines and/or narcotics to lessen patient discomfort. Generally, 20–30 cc of 1–2% lidocaine is sufficient to completely anesthetize the area of interest.

First, a small 0.5-in, 25-gauge needle is used to raise a small intradermal wheal at the planned incision site. Next, a larger needle is used to anesthetize the deeper structures in a wide subcutaneous area so as to minimize patient discomfort. Care should be taken to fully anesthetize the nearby periosteum of the rib above and below the insertion site. Once this is complete, the needle should be passed just superior to the rib below while the operator aspirates pleural fluid or air, signaling passage through the parietal pleura. Withdrawing the needle while continuing aspiration on the plunger until air or fluid no longer returns identifies when the tip

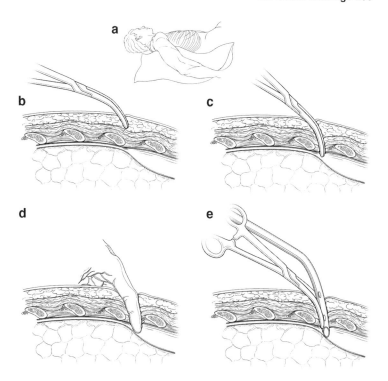

Figure 15-2. Blunt dissection for chest tube insertion. The lateral decubitus position (**a**) is preferred for placement of a lateral chest tube. After local anesthesia and incision, the forceps are used to bluntly dissect just superior to the rib to the level of the pleura (**b**). The forceps are then advanced through the parietal pleura (**c**), usually resulting in return of air or fluid. A finger can be placed into the pleural space to inspect and ensure the absence of significant adhesions that may preclude tube placement (**d**). The distal end of the chest tube is grasped with the forceps and placed in the pleural space (**e**).

of the needle is at the parietal pleura. Generous amounts (5–10 cc) of anesthetic should be injected into this area of the parietal pleura to minimize the pain of tube insertion.

■ TECHNIQUES

There are several different insertion techniques, depending on the type of tube being used. These insertion techniques are discussed separately below.

Blunt Dissection

Insertion of a larger-bore chest tube requires this technique, as it creates a larger entrance site for insertion (Fig. 15-2b–e). Blunt dissection also allows for digital palpation of the pleural space, which makes it the preferred insertion technique for complex fluid collections. This technique can be used at either the anterior or lateral insertion sites, although it is more commonly employed laterally, since the intercostal distance is larger there than in the anterior position. The steps are as follows:

1. Setup, sterilize, drape, and anesthetize as described above.
2. Using a scalpel, make an incision through the skin parallel to the rib that lies immediately below the intercostal space of interest.
3. With a Kelly forceps, bluntly dissect through the subcutaneous tissues by inserting the closed forceps and then opening them after advancing within the tissue. Once the dermal fascia has been opened it is often easy to use one's index finger to help with further dissection to the level of the rib.
4. Using the Kelly forceps, locate the lower rib of interest. Walk the forceps over the superior margin of the lower rib, and penetrate the intercostal muscles and pleura with the forceps closed. Usually penetration is confirmed by a rush of air or fluid. Open the forceps within the pleural space to ensure an adequately large tract.
5. Use an index finger to probe into the pleural space and palpate the thoracic structures. The lung should freely move away from the parietal pleura with palpation. Digitally palpate the parietal pleura 360° around the insertion site to ensure that there are no pleural adhesions that would impede tube insertion.
6. Tube insertion can be done in one of two ways, depending on the presence or absence of a trocar:
   (a) When not using a trocar, clamp the end of the tube that is to be inserted with the Kelly forceps, and use the forceps to direct the tube into the pleural space. The Kelly can be inserted several centimeters into the chest to ensure proper placement. Unclamp the chest tube and push it into the pleural cavity. When pleural fluid is anticipated, it is often helpful to have a second hemostat or Kelly forceps clamped to the distal end of the tube, so that fluid does not rush onto the floor or bed.
   (b) When using a trocar, the technique is similar. Load the tube onto the trocar and insert both as a unit into the pleural space. The trocar can be used to direct the tube several centimeters in the pleural space to help with tube positioning. Be careful not to advance the trocar into the chest cavity too far, as its sharp point can damage vital structures. Advance the tube as the trocar is removed to the desired position. It is often helpful to have an assistant ready with a hemostat to clamp the tube if a rush of fluid is anticipated.
7. For a pneumothorax, the tube should be directed anteriorly and apically. For a pleural effusion, the postero-basal position is favored.

8. The depth of insertion depends upon individual patient anatomy, but generally 12–14 cm is adequate. If the most proximal hole is within the subcutaneous tissue rather than the pleural space, subcutaneous emphysema can develop. If this fenestration lies outside the body, a false air leak or pneumothorax can develop.

9. Connect the tube to a pleural drainage device (see instructions below) making sure that connections are secure. Disconnect any clamps on the tube in order to begin draining any pleural fluid.

10. Secure the tube with oversized suture, dressings, and tape (see below).

11. Confirm placement of the tube with a radiograph. The most proximal side hole of the chest tube can be seen on plain film as a break in the radiopaque line that runs the length of the tube. This break should always be located within the chest cavity. If the proximal fenestration is outside the chest cavity, the tube should be pulled and a new one placed if drainage is still required. Advancement of the tube into the pleural space is not acceptable unless the sterile field has not been broken, as this risks contaminating the pleural space.

Seldinger Technique

In 1953, Dr. Sven Ivar Seldinger introduced the technique for vascular access that bears his name.[13] This technique (Fig. 15-3) has been employed for access to a variety of hollow organs, including the pleural space. Several companies manufacture Seldinger-based pleural access kits. These tubes come in either the straight or pigtail variety. While this technique is generally reserved for insertion of smaller chest tubes (<20 French), Seldinger kits are available in sizes that range up to 36 French. The Seldinger technique has the advantage of being less traumatic than blunt dissection. However, there is no opportunity for palpation of the pleural space by the operator, and the ability to direct the orientation of the chest tube in the pleural cavity is limited. For this reason, this technique is not generally indicated for loculated fluid collections.

The Seldinger insertion technique is as follows (reading the manufacturer's instructions prior to insertion is recommended, as each manufacturer may utilize slightly different equipment):

1. Setup, sterilize, drape, and anesthetize as described above.

2. Using a scalpel, make an incision at the superior aspect of the rib lying just below the intercostal space of interest. This incision should be just greater than the diameter of the tube to be inserted, and should pierce the skin and immediate subcutaneous tissue.

3. Using the percutaneous entry needle attached to a syringe, advance the needle until the superior aspect of the previously anesthetized rib is encountered. Slowly walk the needle over the superior margin of the rib. Aspiration of fluid or air (depending on the indication of insertion) denotes entry into the pleural space.

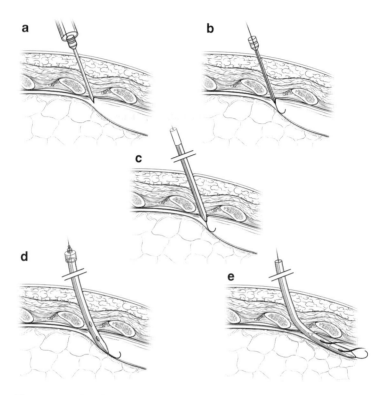

Figure 15-3. The Seldinger technique for chest tube insertion. After local anesthesia, the introducer needle is advanced into the pleural space just superior to the rib (**a**). When a rush of air or fluid is returned, the syringe is removed and the wire is fed through the introducer needle into the pleural space (**b**). The introducer needle is then removed. After a small incision is made in the skin around the wire, a dilator is used to create a tract for the chest tube (**c**). The tube is then placed into the pleural space over the wire (**d**) and the wire is removed (**e**).

4. Carefully remove the syringe from the needle and insert the wire through the introducer needle and into the pleural space. The wire should easily advance 4–6 cm into the chest to ensure its secure position in the pleural space. Advancing the wire too deeply increases the possibility of compromise of deeper thoracic structures.
5. Remove the introducer needle from the wire, taking care to leave the wire within the pleural space.
6. For larger sized tubes, there may be one or several serially sized dilators included. Place the smallest dilator over the wire, and

advance through the chest wall and into the pleural space. Insertion of dilators can be facilitated by rotating the dilator as it is advanced. Be careful to control the wire at all times during dilation. The ability to easily oscillate the guidewire within the dilator insures that the guidewire has not folded up in the subcutaneous space. Use each dilator in succession until the tract is able to accommodate the chest tube.

7. Seldinger chest tubes are sometimes packaged with an insertion device (see manufacturer's instructions). Insert the chest tube and insertion device (if included) over the wire. In general, insertion of the tube to the hub of the catheter is preferable, unless specific patient anatomy warrants a more shallow insertion.

8. Remove the insertion device and wire, taking care to leave the chest tube in position.

9. Connect the tube to a pleural drainage device (see instructions below).

10. Secure the tube with a single stitch of oversized suture at the hub of the catheter and place a sterile dressing over the catheter hub.

11. Confirm placement of the tube with a chest radiograph.

Catheter-Over-Needle

The catheter-over-needle technique is the quickest and easiest way to access the pleural space. These catheters are small, generally 8 or 8½ French. They are best used for aspiration of simple pneumothoraces, and can be used as a temporizing measure for tension pneumothorax until a more suitable catheter can be inserted. Because of the smaller size and the tendency toward luminal obstruction, they are not typically used for drainage of fluid collections in the ICU.

Generally these catheters are used to access the pleural space via the anterior mid-clavicular line. Insertion is quick, easy, and can be done by even minimally experienced operators in emergent situations. There are several commercially available pneumothorax kits that come prepackaged with all needed supplies, including a Heimlich valve (see description below) and tubing.

Insertion steps are as follows (in the rare situation of life-threatening tension pneumothorax, these steps may be truncated):

1. Setup, sterilize, drape, and anesthetize as described above.

2. Attach a syringe to the needle-catheter. Advance the needle through the skin and subcutaneous tissues until the superior portion of the rib is felt.

3. Walk the catheter over the rib while aspirating the plunger. Entry into the pleural space is signified by the return of air into the syringe.

4. Advance the needle approximately 0.5 cm further. Carefully push the catheter into the pleural space over the needle without further

advancing the needle. Generally, when placing these tubes in the anterior position for a pneumothorax, directing the catheter toward the apex of the lung is advised.

5. Once the catheter is in place to the hub, remove the needle. Attach the tubing and a Heimlich valve or a pleural drainage device.
6. Secure the tube with a simple suture at the hub of the catheter. Place a sterile dressing over the catheter hub.
7. Ensure placement of the tube with a chest radiograph.

Suture Technique

It is imperative that the tube be securely fashioned so that it is not inadvertently pulled out. Smaller tubes, such as the catheter-over-needle and smaller (<20 French) Seldinger kits are easily secured at the hub with a suture and sterile dressing. Larger tubes that are placed via blunt dissection are not as easy to secure, as there is no specific hub to suture to the patient, and the point of insertion is larger than the tube itself.

The general method for securing the tube involves placing sutures through the incision on both sides of the tube. These sutures are tied securely to close the lateral margins of the incision and used as anchors to which the chest tube is tied with several knots. The suture material should be nonabsorbable and of significant tensile strength, such as 0 or 1–0 silk. Two suture techniques can be employed to secure the tube. Regardless of the suture technique employed, care must be taken to avoid skin necrosis at the tube entry site.

The first technique places two purse string sutures around the tube through the incision, oriented 180° to each other (Fig. 15-4). Both sutures are tied with a surgeon's knot to the skin, leaving ample excess suture to tie to the tube. The excess suture is then used to place several firm knots around the tube, securing it to the body. The purse string sutures serve both to anchor the chest tube and to close the incision around the tube.

The second technique employs vertical mattress sutures on either side of the chest tube. The vertical mattress technique allows for firm closure of both superficial and deeper tissues. Again, a surgeon's knot is used to approximate the incision on each lateral border of the tube, with plenty of suture remaining to firmly tie the tube to the skin. Both sutures are wrapped around the tube several times and secured tightly to the tube with several knots.

■ DRESSING THE CHEST TUBE

Clean and well-placed dressings can be as important as sutures in keeping the tube in place. First, petrolatum gauze should be wrapped around the tube at the insertion site to help prevent air leaks. Then place a drain sponge, which contains a slit for placing around the tube, over the insertion

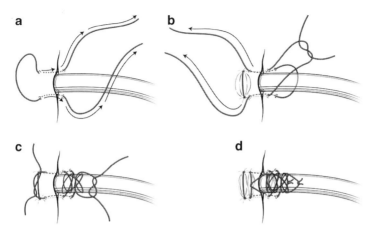

Figure 15-4. Pursestring suture technique for securing a chest tube placed by blunt dissection.

site and the petrolatum gauze. Silk tape can then be used to cover the site, using ample tape to ensure a secure dressing.

Just distal to the insertion site, it is advisable to secure the portion of the tube lying outside the chest cavity to the thorax using omental tags of tape (Fig. 15-5). To do this, place the tube in the center of a long (approximately 25 cm) piece of silk tape. The tape is wrapped around the tube so that the adhesive portions are approximated, except for the last 5–6 cm of each side. This portion is used to adhere to the patient's thorax. Two or three omental tags of tape can serve to further anchor the tube to the patient, but allow for enough tube movement to prevent kinking.

■ DRAINAGE DEVICE

A drainage device is attached to the chest tube both to drain any fluids from the pleural space and to form a seal that prevents air from entering the pleural space from the chest tube. The "three-chamber system" of pleural drainage is the preferred method of pleural drainage. This setup consists of three chambers connected in series to the chest tube, each with a separate and specific function (Fig. 15-6). The first chamber collects pleural fluid. This is connected to the water seal chamber, which prevents air from entering the chest from the system and allows for visualization of any air leaks. The third chamber is the suction regulator, which allows for adjustment of negative pressure in the system when suction is applied. There are several available brands of commercial drainage devices that provide a three-chamber system in one sterile, disposable unit.

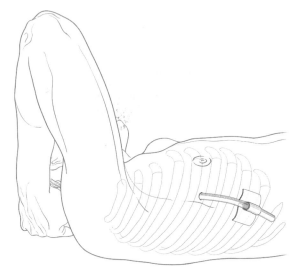

Figure 15-5. An omental tag allows for some movement of the chest tube without inadvertent removal.

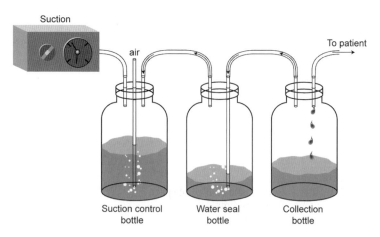

Figure 15-6. The three-bottle system for pleural drainage.

The chest tube is attached via a connector piece to the tubing provided with the drainage system. It is important that the tube connections be secure as disruption of the integrity of the drainage system increases the risk of air leak in the system and/or introduction of infection into the pleural space. A thin strip of tape spiraled around the connections ensures integrity of the tube connections.

It is customary to place the chest tube to suction (-20 cm H_2O) for assistance in drainage of pleural fluid collections; however, this practice is not supported by data.

In the setting of a pneumothorax there is no consensus on whether or not the application of suction is indicated. Powner demonstrated in 1985 that suction applied to a chest tube in a patient with a bronchopleural fistula may either increase or decrease the flow through the fistula, depending on the specific patient.[14] Since then, multiple studies have demonstrated equivocal results between management of pneumothorax with suction vs. water seal.[15,16] Unless a large air leak is suspected, it is reasonable to place the chest tube to water seal when placed for pneumothorax. If the chest radiograph does not demonstrate resolution or significant decrease in the size of the pneumothorax, then -20 cm H_2O can be applied in an effort to help with re-expansion of the lung.

In the case of a simple iatrogenic or spontaneous pneumothorax, in which only a small air leak is anticipated, a Heimlich valve can be used in lieu of a larger drainage device. The Heimlich valve is a device that allows air to escape the system, but does not allow air to enter. It is imperative that the Heimlich valve be oriented in the correct direction when attached to the chest tube, as a backward connection will result in the tube being unable to vent the pleural space and can lead to a tension pneumothorax. Most Heimlich valves are labeled with an arrow indicating the direction of flow; this arrow should be oriented away from the patient to allow for proper venting. Heimlich valves should not be used when draining fluid collections because the fluid can clog the valve and cause it to malfunction.

■ COMPLICATIONS

As with any procedure, there are inherent risks related to the placement and management of chest tubes:

- Insertion site bleeding
- Pain
- Infection – insertion site or pleural space
- Subcutaneous emphysema
- Intercostal neuralgia
- Hemothorax
- Re-expansion pulmonary edema
- Thoracic organ laceration/puncture

The most common complications of chest tube placement are pain, infection, and bleeding. Pain can be controlled with the liberal use of analgesic medication and careful attention to local anesthesia during placement.

Infectious risks can be minimized with strict sterile technique upon insertion and by keeping the insertion site clean and covered.

Bleeding is a specific concern. As discussed above, the neurovascular bundle can be avoided by inserting the tube just superior to the lower rib of an interspace. Anatomic irregularities exist which can lead to inadvertent laceration of these vessels and significant bleeding. Correction of any existing coagulopathy is the first step. Local pressure to the bleeding vessel can be applied by inserting a Foley catheter through the chest tube incision into the pleural space, inflating the balloon on the catheter with saline, and then placing traction on the inflated balloon to pull it against the inner portion of the chest wall.[17] These steps should be taken while a surgical consultation is initiated as bleeding refractory to these steps may require surgical correction.

Kinks in the chest tube or obstructions of the drainage system can impede flow from the chest cavity and can be a serious complication leading to tension pneumothorax in the setting of a large air leak.

Subcutaneous emphysema can occur when the proximal hole of the chest tube lies in the subcutaneous tissues. This complication, although sometimes distressing in cosmetic appearance, is usually self-limited with correction of the chest tube placement. Intercostal nerve impingement can lead to neuralgia.

Drainage of large pleural effusions that are associated with compressive atelectasis can lead to re-expansion pulmonary edema. This complication usually occurs several minutes to hours after drainage and is often heralded by the development of dyspnea and hypoxia. The radiograph demonstrates alveolar infiltrates in the distribution of the expanded lobe. Supportive care is usually adequate, although mortality rates as high as 20% have been reported.[18] To decrease the incidence of this complication, the British Thoracic Society recommends limiting drainage of large effusions to 1.5 L at a time.[19]

It is rare that major organ damage occurs. The heart, esophagus, major vessels, lung, diaphragm, liver, or spleen can be injured by misplacement of a chest tube. While rare, these complications can require surgical intervention and can be life-threatening.

■ ASSESSMENT OF FUNCTION AND TROUBLESHOOTING

Daily assessment of tube output and function is an important part of management of chest tubes. Tube placement should be evaluated with a daily chest radiograph. In addition, tube function can be assessed by respiratory tidal motion either in the tubing or in the water seal chamber. In a spontaneously breathing patient, the column in the water seal chamber should move up with inspiration and down with expiration. This tidal pattern may be reversed in patients on positive pressure ventilation. Temporarily discontinuing wall suction from the drainage device can be helpful if tidal motion is difficult to visualize with the suction applied. If no tidal motion is noticed, sitting the patient upright and asking him to cough forcefully can increase the force transmitted to the tubing and should move the column if the tube is functioning. Absence of tidal motion with respiration or cough indicates that the tube is misplaced, kinked, or occluded.

If the tube has been placed for a pneumothorax, an assessment for an air leak should be performed frequently. Bubbling in the water seal chamber indicates that air is entering the system. If an air leak is present, regular chest radiographs should be obtained to search for a pneumothorax. Persistent bubbling indicates that there is either a bronchopleural fistula or an air leak. If a leak in the tubing is suspected, first check all tubing connections. If these appear to be satisfactory, then temporarily clamp the chest tube near the entrance site at the chest. Continued bubbling implies an air leak in the tubing, while cessation of bubbling implies either that the proximal hole of the tube is outside of the chest or that an active air leak still exists in the lung.

Evaluation of fluid output is important when the tube has been placed for an effusion. Care should be taken by nursing staff to record the output of the chest tube at least every shift, and marks should be placed on the collection chamber with a date and time so that accurate recordings are kept.

In the setting of a suspected occluded chest tube, the tube can be disconnected under sterile conditions and attempts can be made at flushing it with sterile saline. Successful expulsion of clogged material is heralded by the easy flow of saline through the tube. A tube that cannot be cleared by flushing with sterile saline should be removed and replaced if the situation requires further pleural drainage. Replacement should take place in a new site, as placement of a new tube through a previous insertion site increases infectious risk.

■ REMOVAL

Timing of tube removal depends upon the indication for tube placement. In the case of a pneumothorax, it is usually wise to wait until the patient is off positive pressure ventilation before pulling out the chest tube, although there are situations where this may not be possible. First confirm that there is no air leak in the water seal chamber with respirations or coughing and that the chest radiograph demonstrates re-expansion of the lung. At this point, it may be appropriate to clamp the chest tube for several hours and to repeat the chest radiograph to provide reassurance that it is safe to pull out the tube. A small, stable pneumothorax can be tolerated as long as the chest radiograph is stable after several hours of tube clamping and the patient remains asymptomatic.

Timing of chest tube removal for pleural effusions is more variable. The mechanism by which the effusion was created should be remedied before discontinuation of the tube which should result in a significant decrease in chest tube output. Although there are no strict guidelines for the amount of chest tube output required for removal, less than 200 mL/day in the setting of an improving clinical picture is usually adequate.

The removal process is as follows:

1. Sterile gloves should be worn and the area should be cleaned with chlorhexidine solution prior to removal.
2. Place occlusive petrolatum gauze dressing on a stack of 4×4 gauze. This will serve to form an airtight seal over the incision site.
3. Remove any sutures.
4. In the spontaneously breathing patient, the tube should be pulled during active exhalation, so that the pleural pressure is greater than atmospheric pressure. This helps to reduce the chance of air entering the chest tube site as the tube is pulled. The easiest way to ensure that this is the case is to have the patient hum while pulling the tube. A patient receiving mechanical ventilation should have his tube pulled during a positive pressure breath, when the pleural pressure is most likely to be positive.
5. Immediately upon withdrawal of the tube, place the occlusive dressing over the incision site.
6. Secure the gauze dressing to the skin securely with tape.
7. Obtain a chest radiograph to ensure absence of pneumothorax.

■ SUMMARY

Pleural disease is a common problem in the critically ill patient. The safe placement and management of pleural drainage devices requires both a thorough knowledge of indications, anatomy, techniques, and complications as well as procedural experience.

■ REFERENCES

1. Hippocrates. *Genuine Works.* Vol 2. New York: William Wood and Company.
2. Playfair G. Case of empyema treated by aspiration and subsequently by drainage: recovery. *BMJ.* 1875;1:45.
3. Hewett C. Drainage for empyema. *BMJ.* 1876;1:317.
4. Graham E, Bell R. Open pneumothorax: its relation to treatment of empyema. *Am J Med Sci.* 1918;156:839–871.
5. Brewer L. Wounds of the chest in war and peace, 1943–1968. *Ann Thorac Surg.* 1969;7:387–408.
6. de Lassence A, Timsit JF, Tafflet M, et al. Pneumothorax in the intensive care unit: incidence, risk factors, and outcome. *Anesthesiology.* 2006;104(1):5–13.

7. Takahashi S, Yokoyama T, Ninomiya N, Yokota H, Yamamoto Y. A case of simultaneous bilateral spontaneous pneumothorax developed into tension pneumothorax. *J Nippon Med Sch.* 2006;73(1):29–32.

8. Holloway VJ, Harris JK. Spontaneous pneumothorax: is it under tension? *J Accid Emerg Med.* 2000;17(3):222–223.

9. Kircher LT Jr, Swartzel RL. Spontaneous pneumothorax and its treatment. *J Am Med Assoc.* 1954;155(1):24–29.

10. Mattison LE, Coppage L, Alderman DF, Herlong JO, Sahn SA. Pleural effusions in the medical ICU: prevalence, causes, and clinical implications. *Chest.* 1997;111(4):1018–1023.

11. Whitaker S. *Introduction to fluid mechanics.* Englewood Cliffs, NJ: Prentice-Hall; 1968.

12. Beamis J, Mathur P, eds. *Interventional Pulmonology.* New York: McGraw-Hill; 1999.

13. Seldinger SI. Catheter replacement of the needle in percutaneous arteriography; a new technique. *Acta radiol.* 1953;39(5):368–376.

14. Powner DJ, Cline CD, Rodman GH Jr. Effect of chest-tube suction on gas flow through a bronchopleural fistula. *Crit Care Med.* 1985;13(2):99–101.

15. So SY, Yu DY. Catheter drainage of spontaneous pneumothorax: suction or no suction, early or late removal? *Thorax.* 1982;37(1):46–48.

16. Reed MF, Lyons JM, Luchette FA, Neu JA, Howington JA. Preliminary report of a prospective, randomized trial of underwater seal for spontaneous and iatrogenic pneumothorax. *J Am Coll Surg.* 2007;204(1):84–90.

17. Urschel JD. Balloon tamponade for hemorrhage secondary to chest tube insertion. *Respir Med.* 1994;88(7):549–550.

18. Mahfood S, Hix WR, Aaron BL, Blaes P, Watson DC. Reexpansion pulmonary edema. *Ann Thorac Surg.* 1988;45(3):340–345.

19. Laws D, Neville E, Duffy J. BTS guidelines for the insertion of a chest drain. *Thorax.* 2003;58(Suppl 2):ii53–ii59.

16

Intracranial Monitoring

R. Morgan Stuart, Christopher Madden,
Albert Lee, and Stephan A. Mayer

■ INTRODUCTION

The critical care management of patients who have suffered catastrophic neurological injuries such as intracerebral hemorrhage, traumatic brain injury, ischemic stroke and subarachnoid hemorrhage has undergone significant advances in the last few decades. The intensivist caring for these patients now has a full armamentarium of invasive and noninvasive monitoring techniques for gathering real-time information regarding the physiology and metabolism of the injured brain in patients who are comatose, rendering the neurological examination unreliable or incomplete. The monitoring techniques available today in the ICU allow for measurement of intracranial pressure (ICP), cerebral perfusion pressure (CPP), cerebral blood flow (CBF), oxygenation, temperature, cerebral cellular metabolism, and, most recently, intracortical electroencephalography.

S.A. Mayer (✉)
Neurological Intensive Care Unit, Department of Neurology, Columbia New York Presbyterian Hospital, 710 West 168th Street Box 39,
New York, NY 10032, USA
e-mail: sam14@columbia.edu

H.L. Frankel and B.P. deBoisblanc (eds.), *Bedside Procedures for the Intensivist*,
DOI 10.1007/978-0-387-79830-1_16,
© Springer Science+Business Media, LLC 2010

The data yielded from intracranial monitoring in this subset of critically ill patients provides information down to the cellular level, helping to guide management and improve outcomes.[1,2]

■ INDICATIONS AND CONTRAINDICATIONS

In the case of catastrophic neurological brain injury, the patient is often comatose and unresponsive, requiring mechanical ventilation. In this situation, the physical exam and the neurological exam may fail to yield important information regarding the patient's neurological status. Furthermore, in many cases of devastating brain injury, management of increased ICP requires that a patient remain deeply sedated and further confounding the neurological exam. This subset of neurologically critically ill patients can represent a "black box" to the intensivist, as he or she is left with limited methods both to assess the status of the injured brain and to guide therapy. It is for these patients that intracranial monitoring is essential. The injuries for which intracranial monitoring may be indicated include traumatic brain injury, ischemic stroke, subarachnoid hemorrhage, intracerebral hemorrhage, intraventricular hemorrhage, or status epilepticus.

The type of monitoring employed depends on the disease process, its severity, and the relative stability of the patient. Typically, for a stable, large intracerebral hemorrhage where increased ICP is the main concern, an ICP monitor alone can suffice, while for poor-grade aneurysmal subarachnoid hemorrhage, where hydrocephalus, rebleeding, vasospasm, and seizures are all potential serious adverse consequences, multimodal monitoring of ICP, CBF, oxygenation, metabolism, as well as electroencephalography can all provide clinically relevant data to guide management. Some monitoring devices, such as the extraventricular drain (EVD) can also be used to treat elevated ICP.

As understanding of the utility of this information has evolved and as technological advances have allowed various monitoring devices to be "bundled" together at the bedside, practice standards have migrated toward the use of multimodality monitoring in most patients for which intracranial monitoring is of potential benefit.

Before placement of any invasive cerebral monitoring device, a patient's coagulation status must be assessed. Recommended coagulation values prior to beginning the procedure are:

- Platelets >100,000
- INR <1.5
- PTT within normal range
- No history of aspirin or clopidogrel use within 7 days

Any coagulopathies must be corrected prior to insertion, owing to the potentially devastating consequences of intracerebral hemorrhage.

Patients with head or brain injuries frequently have abnormal coagulation parameters; however, no best practice guidelines exist for acceptable coagulation values for placement of invasive intracranial monitors. Fresh frozen plasma infusions are commonly used for correction of elevated prothrombin and partial thromboplastin times, but excessive transfusions can delay time to monitor placement and treatment of increased ICP, as well as expose patients to potential transfusion reactions.[3]

The practice management guidelines from the National Institutes of Health and the College of American Pathologists for fresh frozen plasma (FFP) transfusion recognize that abnormal bleeding does not generally occur until clotting factor activity is below 20–30% and includes recommendations for correction of microvascular bleeding only if the PT or PTT are > 1.5 times normal or the INR is >1.6 (approximately 40–50% of factor activity).[3-5] These represent commonly accepted values for placing an intracranial monitoring device or external ventricular drain among neurosurgeons. Davis et al[3] also found that the use of FFP to correct an INR below 1.6 for placement of an ICP monitor is of no benefit in preventing hemorrhagic complications. If a patient is taking aspirin, platelets are generally infused during the procedure. For platelet-aggregation inhibitors such as clopidogrel and ticlopidine that cannot be reversed by transfusion, the increased risk of monitor placement must be carefully weighed by the clinician on an individual case basis against the potential for emergent therapeutic benefit.

Injection of desmopressin (DDAVP) 0.3 μg/kg IV and platelet transfusion are also reasonable alternatives for patients with clinically suspected platelet dysfunction, such as those with renal failure or alcohol abuse. Recombinant activated factor VIIa (rFVIIa, NovoSeven, Novo Nordis A/S, Bagsvaerd, Denmark) given as a 40 vg/kg or 2.4 mg IV injection can immediately correct coagulapathy due to warfarin use, and has been reported to safely expedite the emergency placement of intracranial monitors when it is considered a life-saving procedure. Pretreatment with rFVIIa has also been reported to be useful for the placement of intracranial monitors in coagulopathic patients with fulminant hepatic failure and cerebral edema.

In cases of large intracerebral hemorrhage where the etiology has not been elucidated and an underlying mass lesion has not been excluded, great care must be taken not to place the device within the hemorrhagic nidus, due to the potential to disturb or rupture an underlying tumor, aneurysm, or arteriovenous malformation. Placement of monitors within clot or infracted tissue can also result in spurious values that are of no clinical value. The risk of infection secondary to intracranial monitor placement is very low. For intracranial monitors confined to the parenchymal space (as opposed to external ventricular drains which are placed within the ventricular system) antibiotic prophylaxis has not shown to be of benefit and is not routinely practiced.[6]

■ MONITORING DEVICES

Integra Neurosciences (Plainsboro, NJ) and Codman (Codman/Johnson & Johnson, Raynham, MA) are the manufacturers of the most commonly used commercial ICP-monitoring devices in the United States. Each manufacturer provides proprietary probes, insertion devices, connection cables, and bedside monitors. The probes can be inserted through a bolt device which screws into a prefashioned burr hole in the skull, or tunneled under the skin and inserted directly into a burr hole.

The LICOX (Integra, Plansboro, NJ) is a combined brain oxygen and temperature monitoring system available in three different configurations. The IP2.P features a dual-lumen introducer, a combined oxygen and temperature probe, and a bolt to fix the device to the skull. The IT2 model also features a combined temperature and oxygen probe, but the introducer is designed to be tunneled underneath the skin rather than fixed to a bolt device. Finally the IM3 features a triple lumen introducer, bolt, and separate oxygen and temperature probes. Each model is designed to provide an extra lumen that can be used to place another compatible monitoring device, such as an ICP monitor, or a microdialysis catheter.

CMA/Microdialysis (North Chelmsford, MA) manufactures the microdialysis system used in the USA. The microdialysis catheter contains a miniature dialysis tube that functions essentially as an artificial blood capillary. The catheter is infused via a small portable battery-powered pump with a sterile perfusion fluid that approximates the composition of CSF. When inserted into the brain, the perfusate diffuses passively and equilibrates with interstitial fluid outside the probe (De Georgia, Ungerstedt). The subsequent concentration gradient drives chemicals across the membrane, where they are collected in small vials attached to the proximal end of the catheter. The samples are then deposited in a special analyzer that uses enzymatic reagents and colorimetric measurements to report the concentrations of various small molecules (<20 kD) within the CSF. The catheter is available either as a tunneled catheter, or as a bolt catheter, though CMA does not manufacture a proprietary bolt. The MD 70 bolt-fitting catheter is compatible with the LICOX multi-lumen introducers.

The Hemedex Bowman Perfusion Monitor (Hemedex, Cambridge, MA) monitors continuous, real-time capillary blood flow and is the only commercially available bedside device that measures cerebral blood flow. The probe for this device is tunneled under the skin to a small burr hole, where it is inserted directly into the brain parenchyma. The method by which the probe measures CBF is known as thermal diffusion. The probe consists of two small thermistors that measure the tissue's ability to dissipate heat; the greater the blood flow, the greater the dissipation of heat.[7,8] The Bowman Perfusion Monitor may be placed into the brain parenchyma using either a tunneling or a bolt-fixed technique, both of which are described below. In order to auto-callibrate, the Hemedex probe must be placed at least 2 cm into brain tissue parenchyma.

■ SETUP, PREPARATION, AND POSITIONING

After informed consent is obtained the equipment specified should be placed on a bedside table in an ordered fashion. A Cranial Access Kit™ (Codman, Raynham, MA) contains most, if not all, of the following materials:

- Razor or electric shaver
- Chlorhexidine prep tray
- Hat, mask, eye protection
- Sterile gown and gloves
- Sterile clear plastic drape and burn sheet or other large drape
- Four pack of sterile towels
- Sterile ruler and marking pen
- Sterile drill kit and appropriate bit (± guard)
- Toothed forceps, hemostat, and needle driver
- Skin knife with #11 and #15 blades, ± scissors, ± small retractor
- 3–0 nylon suture
- 10-cc syringe with 24- and 18-gauge needles
- 1% lidocaine with epinephrine
- 30 cc of sterile preservative-free saline
- 4" breathable transparent medical dressing

One of the challenges in performing bedside intracranial procedures is negotiating the setup of monitors, IV drips, and mechanical ventilator in the patient's room, that are typically positioned behind the patient's head, precisely where the procedure is to be performed. Newer ICUs are equipped with rotary arms for monitors and IV drips, so that they may be swung aside to make room if an intracranial procedure needs to be performed. Some dedicated NICUs position the feet first in the room for ease of access to the head. A careful examination and rearrangement of the bedside equipment can greatly improve the ease with which placement of an intracranial monitoring device is achieved.

Positioning of the patient is key to the success of any procedure. The patient's head should be elevated to a 30–45° level to allow the best exposure and insertion trajectory, as well as to prevent any transient elevations in ICP that may result in laying the patient flat for the procedure. The hair is shaved, preferably with clippers and the skin meticulously prepped. The choice of side of placement is the subject of some debate. The "at-risk penumbra" is the area of relatively uninjured brain tissue immediately adjacent to the area of hemorrhage or infarct. The penumbra is commonly considered to be the ideal placement for the LICOX/microdialysis catheters because this area of the cortex is most susceptible to further injury from ischemia or hemorrhagic extension. However, technical difficulties may preclude penumbra placement. In cases of aneurysmal subarachnoid hemorrhage, in which the aneurysm has been secured via surgical clipping, a craniotomy site may be present over the otherwise preferred site of monitoring access. Drilling through a bone flap is not advised. The treating clinician may wish to preserve the dominant hemisphere so the side of hemispheric dominance may also dictate placement. Ultimately, the placement of each intracranial monitoring device will be dependent on a host of patient-specific factors that are at the discretion of the intensivist or neurosurgeon responsible for the patient's care. Preparation issues are:

- ABC's – secure the airway, monitor vital signs, and pulse oximetry
- Restraints – especially in an awake patient
- Head of bed elevated to 30–45°
- Head in neutral position and apex slightly off the top of the bed
- Shave half of the head across midline and back to coronal suture, and down to zygomatic arch
- Point of entry is Kocher's point: 1–2 cm anterior to the coronal suture in mid-pupillary line or 11 cm posterior from the glabella and 3 cm lateral from midline (Fig. 16-1).
- Right (nondominant) frontal lobe is preferred unless:
  - Scalp lacerations/abrasions.
  - Previous craniotomy or complicated fracture with absent bone.
  - Large hemorrhage on right (catheter will have an tendency to clot).
  - Proposed future surgery on right.
- Tract may go through AVM or mass.

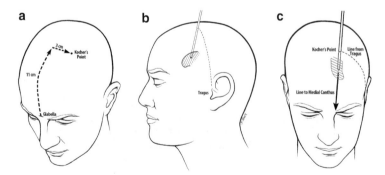

Figure 16-1. Depiction of ideal ventriculostomy placement at Kocher's point: (1–2 cm anterior to the coronal suture in mid-pupillary line or 11 cm posterior from the glabella and 3 cm lateral from midline). The ideal trajectory is toward the ipsilateral medial canthus with the catheter maintained in the same coronal plane as the tragus.

■ ANESTHESIA

The patient must be adequately sedated so involuntary movement does not occur during skin incision or drilling of the burr hole. Typically, the patient is deeply comatose and local anesthetic can suffice, as the most painful part of the procedure is the skin incision. Occasionally, a small bolus of propofol 50–100 mg or midazolam 2–4 mg is required. A generous wheal should be raised in the area where the small 2–3 cm linear skin incision is to be made. Care should be taken to inject local anesthetic all the way to the periosteum. If a tunneling procedure is planned, the local infiltration should extend to the site (typically a few centimeters lateral to the incision) to which the device will be tunneled. Satisfactory local anesthesia can usually be achieved with <10 cc of 1–2% lidocaine.

■ INSERTION TECHNIQUES

Whether placing a single ICP-monitoring bolt or a LICOX with microdialysis catheter, the initial opening technique is similar:

1. Setup, sterilize, drape, and anesthetize as described above.
2. Mark a 2–3 cm linear incision in the sagittal plane approximately 2–3 cm off midline and at least 2 cm anterior to the coronal suture. Kocher's point is commonly used for placement of external ventricular drains and can be employed similarly for placement of neuromonitoring devices. Because placement of a transcutaneous monitoring catheter within the ventricular system does not require high precision in location of the skin incision, erring slightly anterior and lateral to Kocher's point is usually advised in order to avoid the motor strip and any large draining veins to the sagittal sinus, respectively.
3. Using the 15-blade scalpel to make the skin incision. Be sure to incise all the way down to, and through, the periosteum.
4. Carefully sweep the periosteum away on each side to expose the calvarium. The self-retaining retractor may be inserted at this point to maximize exposure and keep the periosteum retracted away. The retractor is also useful in stopping any superficial scalp bleeding which occurs.
5. Attach the drill bit *that is included with the monitoring device to be placed.* This is an important point because the Cranial Access Kit comes with two additional drill bits that *cannot be used* for insertion of a bolt-secured monitoring device (such as LICOX). These drill bits will create a burr hole that is either *too large* or *too small* for the bolt to screw into. It is therefore a good idea to dispose of these extra drill bits prior to beginning the procedure. A small Allen wrench is included with the device-specific drill bit to adjust the drill bit guard.
6. A nurse or assistant may be employed to stabilize the patient's head from beneath the surgical drapes while the burr hole is fashioned.

Hold the drill in the gun position. Care must be taken to orient the drill perpendicular to the skull to prevent skiving of the drill. The proper drilling technique involves using high revolutions with minimal downward force, to avoid plunging the drill through the dura inadvertently. After the outer cortical bone layer is passed and the thinner, cancellous bone is encountered, the drilling becomes easier. When the inner cortical bone layer is reached, the drilling becomes more difficult again, signaling the inner surface is near. At this point the drilling should be more cautious and deliberate to ensure the drill just penetrates no further than up to the dura.

7. At the inner cortex, the drill will catch. Remove the drill by rotating the handle in the opposite direction and pulling back away from the brain. Occasionally the drill bit will dislodge from the drill, requiring manual removal with a hemostat.

8. Remove bone debris from the hole using forceps, gauze, and saline irrigation.

9. The small Allen wrench used to adjust the drill bit guard may be used to delicately feel inside the burr hole to make sure the bone is completely gone. With experience the characteristic feel of the dura can be appreciated, indicating the drill work is adequate. Importantly, the wrench can be used to feel circumferentially around the extent of the burr hole, to make sure the opening is even and concentric. Since the bolt will occupy the entirety of the burr hole, any uneven bony edge or fragment will prevent the probes from inserting. Occasionally the drill must be reinserted and carefully spun to complete the burr hole opening.

10. The method used for dural opening varies. At our institution we routinely use the 18-gauge needle. A very small dural puncture is made, which is expanded bluntly using the Allen wrench. Extreme care must be taken not to puncture the pia beneath the dura, as this may cause pial or cortical hemorrhage that is almost impossible to control through such a small bony opening. Care must also be taken, however, to ensure the dural opening is large enough to accommodate the monitoring probes.

11. At this point the desired monitoring device may be placed.

Once dural access has been obtained insertion of the monitoring device should follow manufacturer guidelines. Techniques for several common devices are summarized below.

Ventriculostomy

Additional equipment needed:

- Minimum of four sutures, preferably 3–0 nylon (× 3) and 2–0 or 0 silk (× 1)

- Camino tray with bolt, drill bit, and fiber-optic cable.
- Ventriculostomy catheter and appropriate stylet, adapter/connectors, and trochar
- Buretrol™ burrette system (Baxter, Deerfield, IL)
- Pressure transducer
- Additional 50–250 cc of preservative-free sterile saline
- 50 cc syringe
- Additional 18-gauge needle
    1. Set up a sterile field, and prepare the ventriculostomy catheter. The ICU nurse can setup the burrette system as the catheter is placed. The dura is entered as described above.
    2. After puncturing the dura with the needle, grab the ventriculos- tomy catheter and its stylet with the right hand at the tip. The left hand should have index and thumb at 6 cm to prevent passing it too far (Fig. 16-2). The trajectory is defined by the ipsilateral medial canthus and ipsilateral tragus.
    3. If a "pop" is felt at approximately 5 cm and CSF is seen, remove the stylet carefully and soft pass the catheter to 7 cm at the skin, tunnel the device out of a subgaleal tract approximately 3–4 cm away from the incision along the anesthetized tract. Use a non-

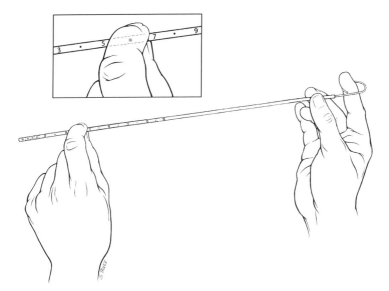

Figure 16-2. Depiction of proper hand positioning for ventriculostomy place- ment. One hand should hold the catheter at approximately the 6-cm mark to pre- vent passing it too deep.

toothed device to hold the catheter at the bone and prevent movement while tunneling.

4. If there is no spontaneous flow, remove the stylet and drop the distal end of the catheter to check for CSF.

5. Before reattempting another pass, clean out all the brain/blood material. Three passes is generally considered the limit when trying to place a Camino™ or Codman™ device.

6. When CSF is obtained, connect the plastic connector and cap the distal end to prevent further loss of CSF.

7. Close the incision at Kocher's point using a running 3–0 nylon suture.

8. While taking care to avoid occluding the catheter, suture it in place using a standard drain stitch. Create 1–2 loops of catheter and suture them down to create slack in case of an accidental tug.

9. Use a nylon or silk tie to secure the plastic connector to the catheter then connect the Buretrol system and zero the transducer.

ICP Bolt (CAMINO™, VENTRIX™)

Additional equipment needed:

- One suture, preferably 3–0 nylon
- Camino box with cables. (manufacturer published drift 0 ± 2 mm Hg for first 24 h, then ± 1 mmHg/day, http://www.integra.com)
    1. Place the Camino box within easy reach. Only use the drill bit included in the tray.
    2. Prep, anesthetize, and mark landmarks appropriately. Placing this device slightly anterior to Kocher's point, leaves the option for placing a ventriculostomy behind it without major risk for increasing hemorrhage or venous infarctions.
    3. Make a 0.5 cm or 1 cm incision in the skin down to through the pericranium. Use the toothed end of the forceps to clear the periosteum.
    4. Setup the guard at 1.5–2 cm again if desired. Line the drill up perpendicular, and begin to drill.
    5. After penetrating the inner cortex remove the bone debris, and perforate the dura with an 18-gauge needle.
    6. Screw in the bolt to finger tight. There are different depths for the bolt to enter into the skull, and a spacer can be used to offset the Camino.
        (a) Neonatal 2–3 mm
        (b) Pediatric 3–5 mm
        (c) Adults 0.5—1 cm
    7. Lightly confirm with the stylet that the dura has been entered. If resistance is felt perforate again with the 18 gauge needle.

8. Place the stylet back in the Camino bolt before zeroing the Camino.
9. The probe must be precalibrated and zeroed to ambient air pressure prior to insertion.
10. Pass the fiber-optic probe through the bolt prior to insertion in order to measure the depth to which the probe is to be inserted. Markings on the extracranial portion of the probe can be referenced to determine depth. For adults we usually place the Camino at 6.25 cm from the top of the cap and then pull back to about 6 cm.
11. Place the bolt into the hole, perpendicular to the skull, securing by turning clockwise.
12. Insert the stylet to ensure the dura is open.
13. Rotate the compression cap to secure it loosely. Fully tightening the compression cap at this time will prevent removal of the stylet.
14. Remove the sylet.
15. Delicately place the probe into the bolt, securing it at the desired depth.
16. Tighten the compression cap until a snug fit is achieved. Pull back gently on the fiber-optic cable to make sure it does not slide
17. Secure the skin edges around the bolt using a U-stitch, and re-approximate any remaining portion of the skin incision using simple interrupted 3–0 nylon suture.
18. Wrap the base of the bolt in a strip of petroleum gauze.
19. If desired, a redundant loop of the probe may be secured to the scalp with an additional 3–0 silk suture to prevent inadvertent probe dislodgement.

LICOX

The following instructions pertain to the LICOX IM3.ST that features a triple lumen introducer and bolt. Though manufactured for insertion of a temperature probe, an oxygen probe, and an ICP probe through each of the three lumens, respectively, other probes, such as the CMA 70 Bolt-Fixed Microdialysis catheter, may be used. The particular array of monitoring probes selected is at the discretion of the intensivist.

Additional equipment needed:

- One suture—preferably 3–0 nylon
- Camino tray without the bolt or drill bit. This is the only one that will properly fit into the Licox combination device.
- Licox tray with bolt, drill bit, and the Licox introducer (should have 3 ports on the distal side)
- 6–8 Tegaderms (4" size)
- Two packs of sterile gauze
- Chlorhexidine prep

- Licox box and cable (cables look different from the Camino cables)
- Camino box and cable
  1. Remove the Licox probe protector and protecting tube from the probe.
  2. Insert probe into introducer as far as possible
  3. Hold the Luer-lock and rotate clockwise to secure
  4. Prepare, prep, drape, and drill through the skull as described above.
  5. When opening up the Licox portion of the kit, hand off the calibration card to the nurse. If this card is lost or damaged, the device will not calibrate properly. Have the nurse turn on and place the card in the Licox box to make sure the box and the card are functioning properly. If there is a problem use another box and cable.
  6. Zero the Camino to air.
  7. Place the bolt device as described above and perforate the dura with the 18-gauge needle.
  8. Now use the included attachment device with the three ports. Port #1 (labeled "Temp") is the port where the temperature probe is to be placed (or alternatively a microdialysis catheter if desired), port #2 (labeled "ICP") is where the Camino is to be placed, and port #3 (labeled P02) is where the Licox PB02 monitor is to be placed.
  9. Place the Licox device(s) first and then the Camino.
  10. When attaching the Licox introducer keep the stylets in place. If there is any resistance when trying to mate the Licox Introducer to the bolt, stop, and reperforate the dura. Do not use the stylet to open the dura.
  11. Once through the dura, take the stylet out and replace it with the appropriate cap. Then lightly screw on the Licox introducer's butterfly nut to the bolt (also know as the Luer-type fitting), half turn.
  12. Now place the Licox PB02 and temperature probes. Simply place the devices in their respective ports and twist down the connectors to secure them in place. If a microdialysis catheter is to be placed instead of either the temperature or PB02 probe, it is recommended to place the microdialysis catheter first, as this catheter is relatively delicate and can be difficult to pass if other probes are already in place. For the PB02 and temperature probes, do not connect the distal cabling yet.
  13. Now connect the Camino. Use the previous steps with the following changes:
     (a) The Camino goes into port #2 labeled "ICP."
     (b) Push the Camino until the white plastic sleeve touches the compression cap of the Camino Make sure the Licox introducer butterfly nut is well set into the bolt.
     (c) Pull back until you can visualize the black ring. The tip of the Camino catheter will extend beyond the bolt by approxi-

mately 1.5 cm when the plastic sleeve is touching the compression cap. Tighten the compression cap of the Camino.

(d) If the Camino is not needed, place the "ICP obturator device" to prevent CSF from leaking at port #2.

14. Screw down the Licox introducer butterfly nut until it is hand-tight. The goal distance between the two butterflies should be approximately 2 mm. Check for leakage of CSF. The nurse may now calibrate the LICOX probes, as well as connect the portable pump to the MD catheter, if used.

Codman ICP Monitor

This is an ideal device for placing on the side where a decompressive craniotomy has been performed. The device must be "zeroed" underwater and must be tunneled before inserting into the brain.

Additional equipment needed:

- Four sutures 3–0 nylon
- Codman tray, Codman box with cables, and ICP wire
- Tunneling device
- 1–2 Tegaderms (4" size)
- Small piece of paper tape or sticker to record the calibration number.

1. Position, shave, prep, mark, and drill in the same manner as the ventriculostomy.
2. Drill as described above at Kocher's point.
3. Tunnel before piercing the dura. Start at an appropriate site away from Kocher's point in the sterile field. Aim for the incision at Kocher's point. Extend the incision if needed to help with tunneling.
4. Remove the metal stylet and leave the metal sheath.
5. Use the metal sheath to place the catheter from the tunneling insertion site to the incision.
6. Remove the metal sheath pulling a little bit extra through the skin is acceptable to help with zeroing.
7. Calibrate the Codman by handing the distal portion to the bedside nurse to connect to the cable of the Codman box. Maintain sterility of the wire on the operative field. Place the transducer under sterile saline. Turn on the box and go to the calibrate screen. Record the calibration number and tape it to the box.
8. If an error during calibration occurs, it usually means that the box cannot read the transducer, which could be caused by the following:

(a) The Codman box needs to be reset: Turn off the box and make sure all connection are snug and turn it back on.

(b) The Codman box or cable does not work: change the box and/or the cable.

    (c) A defect or kink in the wire, either at the transducer or a kink from the transducer to the cable: Retunnel another wire.

9. Now pierce the dura with an 18-gauge needle. Bend the Codman wire by hand at approximately 2–2.5 cm. Insert the Codman into the parenchyma to approximately 1.5 cm.

10. An ICP number should appear on the box.

11. Pull back any slack, and visualize that the bend in the wire is at the bone edge, and the wire is not pulled out. Make certain there is no tension on the wire.

12. Place the "drain stitch" to secure the wire, before closing the wound. This allows inspection of the wire at the bone edge before closing the wound.

13. Suture and loop the wire, and close the wounds. Clean up and place a Tegaderm, and tape down the cable to the shoulder.

Tunneling Insertion Technique

Occasionally, it is desirable to tunnel an intracranial monitoring probe under the skin, rather than place it through a bolt device. A tunneled probe may be used in cases where a low profile set-up is advantageous, such as in either the uncooperative or agitated adult or the small child. In these situations the exposed hardware of the bolt is susceptible to damage or inadvertent removal. Tunneled probes are often placed in the operating room at the time of a craniotomy. Virtually every probe for every monitoring modality is available in tunneled and bolt-affixed versions, and the use of one versus the other is at the discretion of the intensivist. The insertion of a tunneled probe involves the use of a trocar to which is attached a small piece of plastic tubing, both of which are included with most tunneled probes.

    General principles for inserting a tunneled probe are:

1. The skin incision and the burr hole are fashioned in the same manner described above. However, when using a tunneled probe, the exact drill bit used is less critical, as there is no specific bolt device to which the size of the burr hole must be matched. Any size burr hole that accommodates the probe is acceptable, though smaller is better.

2. Make a second stab incision (just large enough to accommodate the tunneling trocar) a few centimeters away from the first incision. This second incision should not extend through the periosteum.

3. Bend the tunneling trocar into a "C" shape and attach the plastic tube.

4. Insert the trocar into the stab incision and push until the tip emerges from the first incision. Pull the trocar out through the incision.

5. Using scissors cut the plastic tubing from the trocar, leaving an open tube which extends from the stab incision to the incision which overlies the burr hole.
6. Carefully thread the probe (ICP monitor, MD catheter, etc.) through the plastic tube.
7. Pull the tube out from the initial incision, leaving the probe, which can then be inserted into the burr hole to the desired depth.
8. Close the initial incision in standard fashion. Place a U-stitch around the probe where it exits the skin.
9. To further secure the probe against inadvertent dislodgement, create a gentle, redundant loop that can then be anchored to the skin with a few 3–0 silk sutures.

■ COMPLICATIONS

At computed tomography (CT) scan should be obtained immediately following insertion to verify placement as well as to make sure no large hemorrhage has occurred. The catheter and probe tips are readily visible on CT. If a small cortical hemorrhage is found along the insertion tract, serial CT scans should be performed to verify that the bleeding is stable. Any residual coagulopathy should be aggressively reversed. If there is evidence of large or expanding hemorrhage the device should be removed immediately. Routine antibiotic prophylaxis with cephalosporins or vancomycin (for those with a penicillin allergy) should be performed at the time of EVD placement and continued while the EVD is inserted. Infection related to intraparenchymal ICP monitors is rare and antibiotic prophylaxis is not indicated.[6] However, the use of antibiotic prophylaxis with multimodality monitors such as the LICOX is generally advised.

■ REMOVAL

Prior to the removal of any intracranial monitoring device, the same criteria for acceptable coagulation values used for insertion should be met. The area where the device enters the skin should be prepped and sterilized. If the device is sutured to the skin, all sutures should be carefully removed. Remove all intracranial probes in a stepwise fashion before unscrewing the bolt attachment. Each probe should be backed out of its lumen in a slow, deliberate fashion to prevent disruption of cortical or pial vessels during removal. When the last probe is removed, the bolt may be unscrewed from the skull. At this point, the skin incision should be closed in an expedient fashion to prevent air from entering through the dural opening. Typically a 3–0 absorbable chromic or a 3–0 nylon suture is used. A CT scan is generally not necessary if the removal was uneventful.

If there is suspicion of infection (particularly with EVD catheters), the tip may be sent for routine culture and sensitivities.

■ CONCLUSIONS

The care of the critically brain-injured patient has undergone significant advances in recent years, as significant advancements in brain monitoring technologies allow the intensivist to continuously monitor a host of neurophysiological parameters. Advanced invasive neuromonitoring attempts to detect neurological deterioration at a time when intervening may prevent permanent brain injury. As the utility and applicability of these monitoring technologies continues to grow, the intensivist must remain familiar with the technical aspects of device placement. If performed correctly, the insertion of advanced intracranial monitoring devices can be done safely and efficiently at the bedside in the ICU and should be considered in any patient suffering from catastrophic brain injury, in whom the neurological exam is limited or unreliable.

■ REFERENCES

1. Spain D, McIlvoy L, Fix S, et al. Effect of clinical pathway for severe traumatic brain injury on resource utilization. *J Trauma*. 1998;45(1):101–105.
2. Simons R, Eliopoulos V, Laflamme D, Brown D. Impact on process of trauma care delivery 1 year after introduction of trauma program in a provincial trauma center. *J Trauma*. 1999;46(5):811–816.
3. Davis JW, Davis IC, Bennink LD, et al. Placement of Intracranial Pressure Monitors: Are "Normal" Coagulation Parameters Necessary? *J Trauma*. 2004;57(6):1173–1177.
4. American Society of Anesthesiologists Task Force on Blood Component Therapy. Practice guidelines for blood component therapy. *Anesthesiology*. 1996;84:732–747.
5. Office of Medical Applications of Research, National Institutes of Health. Fresh frozen plasma: indications and risks. *JAMA*. 1985;253:551–553.
6. College of American Pathologists. Practice parameters for the use of fresh-frozen plasma, cryoprecipitate and platelets. *JAMA*. 1994;271:777–781.
7. Stoikes NF, Magnotti LJ, Hodges TM, et al. Impact of intracranial pressure monitor prophylaxis on central nervous system infections and bacterial multi-drug resistance. *Surg Infect*. 2008;9(5):503–508.
8. Carter LP, Weinand ME, Oommen KJ. Cerebral blood flow (CBF) in intensive care by thermal diffusion. *Acta Neurochir Suppl (Wien)*. 1993; 59:43–46.
9. De Georgia MA, Deoaonkar A. Multimodal monitoring in the neurological intensive care unit. *Neurologist*. 2005;11(1):45–52.

17

Billing for Bedside Procedures

Marc J. Shapiro and Mark M. Melendez

■ INTRODUCTION

In the USA, in the year 2000, critical care medicine accounted for 14.4% of inpatient days and 0.56%, or $55.5 billion, of the gross domestic product.[1] The act of billing for these services has become an art with all the rules and regulations that must be adhered to in order to get compensated for the work that one does. To have a clear understanding of the billing process, this chapter begins with an introduction into the US billing and reimbursement program and then progresses to the process of cognitive and procedural reimbursement.

M.J. Shapiro (✉)
Department of Surgery, SUNY – Stony Brook University Medical Center,
HSC T-18-040, Stony Brook, NY, 11794-8191, USA
e-mail: mjshapiro@notes.cc.sunysb.edu

H.L. Frankel and B.P. deBoisblanc (eds.), *Bedside Procedures for the Intensivist*,
DOI 10.1007/978-0-387-79830-1_17,
© Springer Science+Business Media, LLC 2010

■ PATIENT CARE CODES

In 1966, the first Current Procedural Terminology (CPT) manual was published by the American Medical Association (AMA). CPT's intent is to standardize terminology used for billing for procedures and direct patient care. The direct patient care codes are known as evaluation and management, or E/M codes. For each code listed in the manual, which comes out yearly, there is a complete description as well as a designated five-digit code. In addition to administrating the CPT process, the AMA also administrates the Relative Update Commission (RUC), a diverse group that maintains a Resource-Based Relative Value System (RBRVS), which establishes the relative value units (RVUs) that CPT codes represent and determines the payment that the health care provider receives. The total RVU value is made of three parts:

- The work RVU, which represents 55% of the total
- The malpractice RVU, which represents about 3%
- The practice expense RVU, which represents about 42% of the total RVU

There is also a controversial conversion factor (the sustainable growth rate) and a geographic Practice Cost Index, which factors into this payment. This system is used by the Centers for Medicare and Medicaid Services (CMS) and most major health insurance providers.[2]

■ CRITICAL CARE CODES

Critical care is "the direct delivery by a physician(s) of medical care for a critically ill or critically injured patient."[3] This critical condition is defined by a preeminent or life-threatening condition that occurs to one or more organ systems, impairing the health of that individual by potentially or actually placing them in a life-threatening situation. Although accounting for 30% of all inpatient health care expenditures, critical care medicine involves taking care of the "sickest of the sick," using the most advanced state-of-the-art technology for diagnosis and treatment. "Critical care involves high complexity decision-making to assess, manipulate, and support vital system function(s) to treat single or multiple vital organ system failure and/or to prevent further life-threatening deterioration of the patient's condition."[3] The intense acuity and the high level of competence involved in complex and intricate decision making make this aspect not only one of the most fiscally rewarded cognitive areas but also the most challenging for the clinician. Billing for critical care is a time-based code that applies not only to treating complex severe disease and organ dysfunctional states but also includes the time and manipulation to prevent patients from approaching these critical states. The various vital systems included in evaluation and treatment include, but are not limited to the central nervous system, shock due to neurological, traumatic, circulatory or septic etiologies, circulatory failure, renal failure, hepatic failure, metabolic or toxic failure, and/or respiratory failure. As long as the patient's condition requires this intricate, detailed and constant vigilance, critical care – when documented – can be provided over multiple days, weeks, or months, even if the life-threatening event has improved or is being aggressively treated to prevent progression.

Critical care is most commonly given in an intensive care unit (ICU) such as medical (MICU), surgical (SICU), pediatric (PICU), coronary care unit (CCU), emergency department, respiratory care unit, or any other acute care setting. Critical care is given when the patient exhibits a life-threatening or potentially life-threatening condition. Care of a non-critical nature, even if provided in an ICU setting, is reported with other noncritical care E/M codes.

The two primary critical care codes (Table 17-1) are time based. The E/M code 99291 is for the evaluation and management of the critically ill or injured patient for the first 30–74 min in a 24-h period. It can only be used once per given date. If the time is less than 30 min, another code (e.g., 94002 or 94003 for ventilatory management) should be used. The code 99292 is listed separately, added once for each additional 30 min. Thus, 120 min of critical care would be coded 99291 + 99292 × 2. Included within this code and as part of the time are interpretations and performance of:

- Cardiac output measurements (93561, 93562)
- Chest radiographs (71010, 71015, 71020)
- Pulse oximetry (94760, 94761, 94762)
- Blood gases
- Patient information:
  - EKGs
  - Labs
  - Vital signs
  - Extensive interpretation of multiple databases
- Gastric intubation (43752, 91105)
- Temporary transcutaneous pacing (92953)
- Ventilatory management (94002–94004, 94660, 94662)
- Certain vascular access procedures (36000, 36410, 36415, 36540, 36600).

Table 17-1. 99291 and 99292 critical care E/M codes.

Code	Total duration of critical care
Appropriate E/M codes	Less than 30 min (less than 30 min)
99291 × 1	30–74 min (30 min to 1 h 14 min)
99291 × 1 and 99292 × 1	75–104 min (1 h 15 min to 1 h 44 min)
99291 × 1 and 99292 × 2	105–134 min (1 h 45 min to 2 h 14 min)
99291 × 1 and 99292 × 3	135–164 min (2 h 15 min to 2 h 44 min)
99291 × 1 and 99292 × 4	165–194 min (2 h 45 min to 3 h 14 min)
99291 and 99292 as appropriate (see illustrated reporting examples above)	195 min or longer (3 h 15 min, etc.)

99291. Critical care: evaluation and management of the critically ill or critically injured patient; first 30–74 min
99292. Each additional 30 min (list separately in addition to code for primary service)

Any services that are necessary and not included above can be billed separately with the appropriate modifier.

Critical care codes 99291 and 99292 are the total time spent in providing critical care in a calendar clock 24-h period of time, even if that time is not continuous. Only one physician may bill for a given hour of critical care, even if more than one physician is providing care to the patient. However, during the time reported the physician must devote their full attention to only that patient. This time may also include time reviewing imaging studies and/or test results as well as discussing care with other medical and nursing staff, posting progress notes, discovering clinical findings, writing orders in the medical record, discussing with family members or surrogate decision makers for purposes of obtaining a medical history, reviewing the patient's condition or prognosis, or discussing treatment or limitation(s) of treatment when unable to discuss this with the patient due to incompetence or the patient being clinically unable. Conversation time directly bearing on the management of that patient may also be included. Time spent in teaching sessions with residents may not be counted as critical care time whether conducted on rounds or in other venues. Time spent teaching or by the resident in the absence of the teaching physician is not billable, whereas time spent together directly involved in that particular patient's care may be counted.

To include time in the critical care codes, the clinician must be immediately available to the patient. Thus, telephone calls outside the ICU proximity and time which does not directly impact or contribute to the treatment of the patient cannot be counted as critical care. However, time spent during the transport of a critical patient over 24 months of age from a facility or hospital may be included. For pediatric patients under 24 months of age, codes 99293–99296 should be used.[3–6]

Documentation is crucial to coding. The adage that if it is not written then it did not occur is particularly true with critical care coding. Notes should document that the critical care provided was time based and be legible and detailed (Fig. 17-1). Proper documentation will support the coding, prevent time-consuming resubmissions, avoid denials, and avoid claims of fraud and abuse.[7]

■ MODIFIERS

Modifiers are added to the CPT code when there is unusual or additional evaluation, management, and procedures performed on the same patient during various times of their hospital stay. The modifiers most often used with critical care codes[2, 3] are:

- 25: Significant, separate identifiable evaluation and management service by the same physician on the same day of the procedure or other service.

a

* S U 2 C 0 2 0 *

Smart Medicine
STONY BROOK
UNIVERSITY HOSPITAL
Expert Care

INTENSIVE CARE NOTE
TRAUMA AND SURGICAL CRITICAL CARE
DAILY PROGRESS NOTE

RESIDENT DOCUMENTATION

Date: ____________ Time: ________ Hospital/Post op day: ____/_____

Brief history:

Major events overnight:

VS: TMax: ________ TCurrent ________ BP ________ HR ________ RR ___

Ventilator/O2 Settings: ____________

ABG: PH ________ Pco2 ______ Pao2 _____ Sat ________ BE ________

PA Readings: PA ____ RA/CVP ____ Co ____ CI ____ PCWP ____ SVRI _____

Central Line day: ____________ Arterial Line day: ________

IV Fluids ________ at ________ mL/h. Total Fluids: ________ mL/hr.

Tube Feedings ____________ at ________ mL/hr. Residuals ______ mL

1/0 ______ / ______ NGT ________ Drains ________ Chest tube ______

DVT prophylaxis: ☐ Chemical ☐ Mechanical ☐ Filter

GI Prophvlaxis: ☐ Yes ☐ No

Labs:

Cultures:

Chest X-ray:

RESIDENT EXAMINATION:

HEENT: ____________

Neck: ____________

Lungs: ____________

Lymph nodes: ____________

Skin: ____________

CV: ____________

ABD/GI: ____________

GU: ____________

Extremities: ____________

Neuro/psych: ____________

Breast: ____________

Other: ____________

Medications:

Infusions:

Antibiotics (day#):

Attending History & Physical Exam/assessment: I have Examined the patient & reviewed the history, physical, & care plan with the Resident & revise/confirm as follows

SIDE 1 OF 2

SU2C020 (3/05)

Figure 17-1. Example of a SICU note used to document critical care. Used with permission.

– Used when, on the same day that a procedure or service is provided (e.g., 99291), the patient's condition requires a significant and separately identifiable E/M service or procedure above and

b

Smart Medicine		
STONY BROOK		
UNIVERSITY HOSPITAL		
Expert Care		

INTENSIVE CARE NOTE
TRAUMA AND SURGICAL CRITICAL CARE
DAILY PROGRESS NOTE

Attending circle Diagnosis related	Resident Assessment/Plan	Attending Physician History & Physical Exam/Assessment: I have examined the patient and reviewed the interdisciplinary care plan with the resident and revise/confirm as follows:
To encounter: Acidosis Anemia Blood Loss ARDS Aspiration Atelectasis Cardiac Contusion Cardiac Failure Coagulopathy Concussion DVT Electrolyte Imbalance Empyema Fever Hemothorax Hypoxemia Hypertension Hypoxemia Liver Failure Liver Insufficiency Malnutrition Muscle Weakness Pain Pancreatitis Pleural Effusion Pneumonia Pneumothorax Pulm Contusion Pulm Edema Pulm Embolus Renal Failure Renal Insufficiency Resp. Failure Resp Insufficiency Rib Fracture Sepsis Tachycardia Thrombocytopenia Hypotension Cerebral vasospasm	CV: Pulmonary: GI/Nutrition: ID: Renal: Neuro: _____ Resident Signature ID# Date Time I personally examined the patient, reviewed the History, Physical exam and decision making as done by the Resident/Fellow: _____ Attending/Teaching Physician Signature ID# Date Time Time in Critical Care _____minutes	

SIDE 2 OF 2   SU2C020 (3/05)

Figure 17-1. (continued)

beyond the other service provided or beyond the usual pre and postoperative care associated with the procedure (Table 17-2).
– If any procedure is done that is not already bundled into the critical care codes and cognitive critical care is being provided, the modifier should be used.

Table 17-2. Critical care procedure codes for commonly performed procedures.[2, 3]

CPT code	Procedure
36620	Insertion arterial line
36556	Insertion nontunneled central line over 5 years old
93503	Placement PA catheter
33210	Insertion temporary transvenous pacemaker
37620	IVC interruption
31500	Intubation – emergency, endotracheal
31622	Bronchoscopy
31645	Bronchoscopy with therapeutic aspiration
31624	Bronchoscopy with bronchial-alveolar lavage
31600	Tracheostomy
31502	Tracheotomy tube change prior to established tract
32421	Thoracentesis
32551	Tube thoraocostomy
49080	Puncture peritoneal cavity
92950	Cardiopulmonary resuscitation
43752	Placement naso- or oro-gastric tube
43246	PEG

- Failure to use the modifier may lead to payment denial.
- Example:
  - (a) Providing 70 min of critical care
  - (b) Placing a central line for hypotension
  - (c) Coding would be 99291 plus 36556–25
- Any procedure that is not included in the 99291/99292 coding must not have its time included in the time-based code.
- 51: Multiple procedures.
  - Use when multiple procedures are performed outside of the E/M service at the same session as the first procedure
  - Append this modifier to the other procedures.
- 59: Distinct procedural service.
  - Use to indicate that a procedure or service was distinct or independent from other services performed on the same day.
  - This will prevent these procedures from bundling into each other such as putting in bilateral chest tubes, where each is reimbursed separately.
  - When another modifier is appropriate, it should be used in preference to modifier 59.
- 76: Repeat procedure by the same physician.
  - Use for a repeat procedure or service performed subsequent to the original procedure such as performing therapeutic bronchoscopy three times on the same day.
  - Add 76 to the third bronchoscopy (34645, 31646, 31646–76).
- 77: Repeat procedure by another physician.
  - Use for a repeat procedure by another physician such as repeating a therapeutic bronchoscopy on the same patient later in the day.
  - Add 77 to the second physician's bronchoscopy code.

■ MEDICAID AND MEDICARE

Many practice plans negotiate rates with private carriers including rates for critical care. Medicaid is a program established in 1965 and, although funded by state and federal governments jointly, is administered by the state and pays for medical assistance for certain individuals and families with low incomes and resources. The more global federal Medicare program is the single largest provider of healthcare insurance in the USA, accounting for approximately 30% of annual payments to hospitals in 2002. In addition to being the primary program to provide healthcare insurance to the elderly, Medicare also covers disabled individuals and those with end-stage renal disease. In 2003, Medicare covered more than 35 million elders and more than 6 million disabled Americans. Previously administered by the federal Health Care Financing Administration (HCFA), in 2001 it was renamed the Centers for Medicaid and Medicare Services (CMS).[8]

The two principle parts of Medicare include:

- Part A, which pays hospitalization to institutions and healthcare facilities and helps subsidize training programs in the USA.
- Part B is voluntary and supplemental, covering inpatient and out-patient physician services, outpatient hospital services, ambulatory services and certain medical supplies, and other services for eligible participants. It has been estimated that Medicare pays for more than 50% of all ICU days.

Interestingly, without proper documentation for ICU care, the denial rate for claims tends to be high when compared to other physicians, being 15.7% for the 12-month period ending June 30, 2003. The most common reasons for denials, in addition to absence or deficiency of documentation of critical care delivery, are failure to document time, failure to subtract procedure time, and failure to use modifiers after E/M codes.[6, 8] Point of care billing using portable or electronic methods will hopefully improve accuracy and facilitate timely bill submissions, but does not substitute for adequate and timely documentation.[9] Such programs as "Pay for Performance" recognize excellence and quality healthcare and lead to premium reimbursement. In contrast, CMS and insurance carriers will soon begin denying payment for certain in-hospital complications, such as pulmonary embolism or surgical wound infections, with a secondary goal of driving up quality care and perhaps competition.[10]

■ REFERENCES

1. Halpern NA, Pastores SM, Thaler HT, Greenstein RJ. Critical care medicine use and cost among medicare beneficiaries 1995–2000: major discrepancies between two United States federal Medicare databases. *Crit Care Med.* 2007;35(3):692–699.

2. Dorman T, Loeb L, Sample G. Evaluation and management codes: from current procedural terminology through relative update commission to Center for Medicare and Medicaid Services. *Crit Care Med.* 2006;34(suppl 3):S71–S77.

3. American Medical Association (AMA). *CPT 2009*. Chicago, IL: American Medical Association; 2009:17–18.

4. Mabry C. The global surgical package – let's get the facts straight. *J Trauma.* 2008;64(2):385–387.

5. Department of Health and Human Services. *Medicare Reimbursement for Critical Care Services.* Washington, DC: Office of Inspector General, Department of Health and Human Services; 2001, OEI:05:00:00420.

6. Marinelli AM. *Optimizing Critical Care Coding.* ATS; 2007. http://www.thoracic.org.

7. Fakhry SM. Billing, coding, and documentation in the critical care environment. *Surg Clin N Am.* 2000;80(3):1067–1083.

8. Gerber DR, Bekes CE, Parrillo JE. Economics of critical care: medicare part A versus part B payments. *Crit Care Med.* 2006;34(suppl 3):S82–S87.

9. Fahy BG. Implementation of a handheld electronic point of care billing system improves efficiency in the critical care unit. *J Intensive Care Med.* 2007;22(6):374–380.

10. Reed RL, Luchette FA, Esposito TJ, Pyrz K, Gamelli R. Medicare's global terrorism: where is the pay for performance? *J Truama.* 2008; 64(2):374–389.

Index

Printed in the United States of America